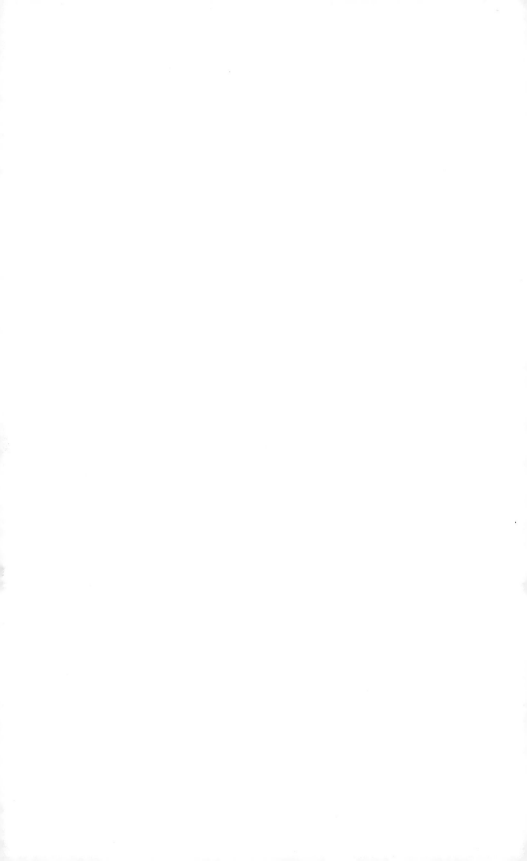

Public Health and Aging

Steven M. Albert, PhD, MSPH, is Professor of Behavioral and Community Health Sciences at the Graduate School of Public Health at the University of Pittsburgh. He is trained in anthropology (PhD, University of Chicago) and epidemiology (MS, Columbia University) and completed postdoctoral fellowships in aging and health policy (Rutgers University) and aging and cognition (Columbia University). Dr. Albert has 20 years of research in aging and public health, with completed projects investigating disability transitions in old age, mental health at the end of life, cross-cultural variation in health and chronic disease, home health care, family caregiving, and medication adherence. He conducted fieldwork in Papua New Guinea as a Fulbright Scholar. Current projects include studies of medication review in senior housing, dynamic computational modeling of health behavior, worksite health promotion for chronic disease management, and assessment of home care technologies. He cofounded the Aging and Public Health MPH Program at Columbia University and teaches courses in aging and public health and research methods in aging research. Dr. Albert is the author or editor of 3 books and over 100 peer-reviewed articles. He has served as an officer in the Behavioral and Social Sciences section of the Gerontological Society of America and the Gerontological Health Section of the American Public Health Association.

Vicki A. Freedman, PhD, MA, is a Research Professor at the Survey Research Center of the Institute for Social Research at the University of Michigan. Dr. Freedman has published extensively on topics related to population aging, disability, and long-term care. Her recent research focuses on the causes and consequences of late-life disability trends; measuring disability, time use, and well-being among older couples; evaluating the population-level effects of interventions to maximize functioning; and neighborhoods and late-life health and functioning. She has served on over a dozen national advisory panels for federal agencies, including the Institute of Medicine's Committee on the Future of Disability in America, and currently serves as Co-Principal Investigator for the National Health and Aging Trends Study and the Panel Study of Income Dynamics. She earned her doctorate in Epidemiology from Yale University and master's in Demography from Georgetown University.

Public Health and Aging

Maximizing Function and Well-Being

Second Edition

STEVEN M. ALBERT, PhD, MSPH
VICKI A. FREEDMAN, PhD, MA

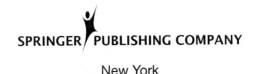

SPRINGER / PUBLISHING COMPANY

New York

Springer Publishing Company, LLC
11 West 42nd Street
New York, NY 10036
www.springerpub.com

Acquisitions Editor: Sheri W. Sussman
Project Manager: Mark Frazier
Cover Design: TG Design
Composition: Apex CoVantage, LLC

E-book ISBN: 978-0-8261-2152-3

12 / 5 4 3 2

The author and the publisher of this Work have made every effort to use sources believed to be reliable to provide information that is accurate and compatible with the standards generally accepted at the time of publication. The author and publisher shall not be liable for any special, consequential, or exemplary damages resulting, in whole or in part, from the readers' use of, or reliance on, the information contained in this book. The publisher has no responsibility for the persistence or accuracy of URLs for external or third-party Internet Web sites referred to in this publication and does not guarantee that any content on such Web sites is, or will remain, accurate or appropriate.

Library of Congress Cataloging-in-Publication Data

Albert, Steven M. (Steven Mark), 1956-
  Public health and aging : maximizing function and well-being /
Steven M. Albert and Vicki A. Freedman. — 2nd ed.
      p. ; cm.
  Includes bibliographical references and index.
  ISBN 978-0-8261-2151-6 (alk. paper)
  1. Community health services for older people.   2. Preventive
health services for older people.   3. Older people—Medical care.
4. Public health.   I. Freedman, Vicki A.   II. Title.
  [DNLM: 1. Health Services for the Aged.   2. Aging—psychology.
3. Public Health. WT 31 A333p 2009]
  RA564.8.A438   2009
  362.198'97   dc22   2009032284

Printed in the United States of America by Hamilton Printing.

*To our cherished teachers: our mentors,
students, and beloved older members
of our families and communities.*

Contents

Preface

Cultural conceptions of the aging experience are many and often recognize a long arc of development followed by decline in later life. Consider Shakespeare's "seven ages of man" (*As You Like It,* II, 7). "One man in his time plays many parts, his acts being seven ages." The seven stages include infancy, "whining schoolboy . . . creeping unwillingly to school," lover, soldier ("seeking the bubble reputation even in the cannon's mouth"), judge or administrator, retirement based on frailty ("his big manly voice, turning again towards childish treble"), and finally "second childishness and mere oblivion . . . sans teeth, sans eyes, sans taste, sans everything."

Religious traditions also provide guidance on approaches to old age. Through a series of anecdotes, for example, the Talmud (i.e., Jewish law) teaches the obligation of honoring elderly parents. Stories feature parents who are physically frail and in some cases senile. Honoring parents involves what is now recognized as help with activities of daily living: offering food, helping with dressing, and assistance in getting around (*Bavli, Kiddushin* 31b). This obligation is traced back to an unusual source: the treatment of the first tablets of commandments, which were broken by Moses in anger upon seeing the Golden Calf. The fragments of the broken tablets were not discarded but rather kept alongside the new tablets that replaced them. Both were carried by the Israelites as they wandered through the desert (*Berakhot* 8b). The old shattered tablets were considered valuable by the community, not only in their own right, but also because they were linked to the newer tablets.

When the first edition of this book appeared in 2004, it noted that age is a dominating factor in health, as it is in so many social, psychological, and economic spheres. To see the centrality of age, consider these comments from our university alumni magazine (Cornell University, Spring, 2002). The 1995 graduate (age 30 or so) exhorts his classmates in this way: "May all your weddings be perfect, babies brilliant, exams easy, jobs fun, and friends true." The 1945 graduate (age 77 or so) makes this report: "Nothing to do and not enough time to do it." The 1938 graduate (age 84 or so) reports, "Angina in April, pacemaker in July, angioplasty in August. Otherwise, fine." And the 1934 graduate reports this: "My theme song now at 94 is 'Don't get around much any more!'" The same issue reports on the oldest living graduate of the college, a man from the class of 1916, aged 108. This long-time gardening columnist resides in an assisted living facility. Four generations of descendents attended his birthday party, which he remarked was "just a lot of fuss over me." This man's age puts him near the oldest-oldest old; the 2000 U.S. Census reported just 1,400 people over age 110 (of some 285,000,000).

Today aging poses a number of challenges for both individuals and the societies in which they live. The biomedical challenge is to develop ways to delay, prevent, or remediate much of the frailty and dementia that we observe in late life. The epidemiologic challenge is to identify risk factors that affect the incidence and progression of the chronic conditions that characterize old age, and that accordingly increase the prevalence of disability. The sociological challenge is to understand why different segments of populations experience old age and aging so differently, with groups defined by socioeconomic status or race already entering old age with very different resources, including cognitive and physical resiliency and social capital. The ethical challenge is to understand when to shift the goals of medical treatment from maximizing care to minimizing suffering.

These challenges have taken on a new urgency in the face of the imminent demographic change facing the United States and countries around the world. Over the next few decades older adults will reach numbers—and proportions—never before seen in human history. As we discuss in Chapter 5, longer life does not necessarily mean worse health and functioning. But the shift toward older ages is not simply a temporary phenomenon, but likely a permanent structural change with which public health must grapple.

Indeed, these different approaches to the challenges of aging come together in the public health approach to aging, the focus of this book. Unlike in Shakespearean or Biblical times, today, public health and aging must address a much more heterogeneous aging experience. Rather than only focusing on the prevention of disease and its debilitating effects, we argue in this volume that a broader lens is needed to address the many faces of aging, whether robust, physically frail, living with dementia, approaching death, or compensating and adapting to changes in capacity.

The public health challenge is to promote the development and maintenance of optimal physical, mental, and social function, irrespective of acquired disease and with due recognition of the senescent changes that accompany late life. In the case of public health and aging we argue that "health promotion and disease prevention," the mantra of public health, needs to be broadened to stress *maximizing function and well-being*. Hence, the subtitle of this book.

We also call for greater appreciation of the earlier-life origins of many features of health in old age. What happens in the first 50 years of life matters a great deal for the second 50 years. For this reason we prefer "public health and aging" over "public health gerontology" to describe the field.

In the first edition of this book, we sought to define the field of public health and aging and to identify the research tools and designs most fruitful in this area. We noted that public health and aging was still a developing field that lacked a unified treatment or overarching framework. The first edition of the book applied such a framework to a series of large questions that are still with us: How can we ensure a healthy old age? Why are some segments of society able to enter old age with greater physical and cognitive resources than others? To what extent can physical and cognitive disability be prevented? To what extent can they be remediated? Does it make sense to speak of the prevention of frailty or other forms of primary prevention in late life? These issues have become more pressing with population aging. By 2050, we can expect to see 15–20% of the world's population over age 65, in both more and less developed economies, and in some countries (such as Japan) as many as a third.

But in the half decade or so that separates the two editions of this book, the field of public health and aging has also changed. The Administration on Aging (AoA), state health departments, the CDC, the Centers for Medicare and Medicaid Services (CMS), as well as managed care organizations, corporate employers, and advocacy organizations, have all started, in their own ways, to *practice* public health and aging. For example, in collaboration with CDC and AoA, state health departments are developing community-wide health promotion and disease prevention efforts in the areas of chronic disease self-management, care management, physical activity, nutrition, environmental modification, and falls prevention. CMS has added a preventive health care visit and additional screening to Medicare's basic package of services. Many state governments now have integrated blueprints for healthy aging, and communities increasingly seek "elder-friendly" impact assessments for planning and development.

These developments, we would argue, make this new edition even more valuable. It is still unclear how best to link current public health efforts for seniors to the many other services they may require, such as medical care, pharmacy management, long-term and end-of-life care, allied health services, and supportive aging services. Too narrow a focus on promoting health may miss opportunities for promoting function. As we argue in Chapter 1, in the real world of imperfect screening tests, invasive diagnostic technologies, and difficult decisions about treatment in the context of declining health and the approach of death, promoting health and promoting function may not always correspond. In public health and aging, supportive care and services are often as important as medical treatment once we recognize that function and disability, rather than diagnosis, should guide population-focused policies. For this insight, we thank M. Powell Lawton, who came to this realization in the 1960s, long before either of us considered research on aging as a possible career.

The second edition of this book expands the first considerably, with fully a third more pages. We have added new chapters on the aging services network and public health (Chapter 3), chronic disease (Chapter 4), long-term care (Chapter 9), and ethical issues in public health and aging (Chapter 11). Other chapters have been substantially revised to reflect advances in thinking about population aging (Chapter 2), physical functioning and disability (Chapter 5), and cognitive disability (Chapter 6). We have updated the remaining chapters to reflect the explosion of knowledge and interest in the years between the editions and provide updates on demographic and epidemiologic perspectives (Chapter 2), affective and social function (Chapter 7), quality of life (Chapter 8), and mortality (Chapter 10). Our overall perspective begins with the "compensating, adaptive elder," who alters daily tasks, relies on spared abilities to compensate for deficits, and selectively invests physical, cognitive, and affective effort to maximize the likelihood of social participation and activity despite health-limiting conditions (Chapter 1).

The current volume reflects our understanding of public health and aging as a field today. Inevitably, important topics have been omitted, and, in places, classic references have been retained in place of newer studies. These choices reflect our desire to present a balance of breadth and depth.

We crafted this new edition with reviews of the first edition in mind. These reviews were favorable, but suggested that our focus on the tools of public health and aging should include, as well, discussion of how public health efforts are actually delivered to older people. We have tried to address this earlier gap in several chapters, which now examine development of "healthy aging networks" (Chapter 3), the growing preventive services emphasis of Medicare (Chapter 4), national efforts to reduce falls and make communities elder-friendly (Chapter 5), interventions to support family caregivers (Chapter 6), evidence-based depression management programs (Chapter 7), and efforts enhancing long-term care (Chapter 9).

We have designed this book to serve as the main text for an undergraduate or graduate class in aging as it relates to the core fields of public health: epidemiology, population studies, health systems and policy, and health behaviors. It may also be used as a supplementary text in gerontology and geriatrics, population studies, the allied health sciences, and sociology. An accompanying teaching guide is available for use of the book in the classroom. (Qualified instructors may e-mail textbook@ springerpub.com to request a copy.) Beyond the classroom, this book represents an integrated treatment of one of the greatest challenges of our time, how to maximize functioning in later life, which we hope will be of interest to researchers across the clinical, behavioral, and population sciences.

We thank Sheri W. Sussman of Springer Publishing for her encouragement and patience, as well as the many colleagues who have helped us think through these issues. To our families, young and old, we add special thanks, for this revised edition would not have been possible without their support.

Steven M. Albert, PhD, MSPH
Vicki A. Freedman, PhD, MA
June 2009

1 Introducing Public Health and Aging

What is public health and aging? Although we understand each component reasonably well, this burgeoning interdisciplinary field is clearly more than the sum of its parts. Thus, the field of public health *and* aging has not been well defined. It draws on the more well-known population sciences of epidemiology and demography but often focuses on subpopulations, such as frail elders, healthy elders at risk for disability, or elders whose health is surprisingly robust. It requires an understanding of health behaviors and prevention, health systems and policy, research methods and statistical analysis, and social and environmental risk factors, but favors no single disciplinary approach. It not only draws on geriatric medicine to promote health outside the clinic and beyond the clinician-patient encounter, but also shares an affinity with gerontology more generally as a multidisciplinary study of aging. Nevertheless, it is distinct from these disciplines in its focus on populations rather than patients and its proactive recognition that health and functioning in later life are rooted in much earlier experiences.

To better demarcate the domains of this emerging field, we first provide an overview of what constitutes public health. We then provide a primer on aging, highlighting the most common archetypes of later life. Next, we introduce the life course perspective, providing examples particularly germane to public health and aging. We end the chapter with a discussion of healthy aging as a key goal and the corresponding domains of public health and aging.

ESSENTIAL SERVICES OF PUBLIC HEALTH

Open any introductory textbook on public health and you will inevitably find lists of what public health does, how public health serves, and what tools public health uses. In the mid-1990s, the Public Health Service, the U.S. agency responsible for public health at a national level, developed a consensus document in collaboration with other major public health organizations that outlined what constitutes public health practice. The lists have been adopted as a framework for identifying the responsibilities of local public health systems and evaluating public health efforts.

As shown in Box 1.1 public health has responsibilities in six distinct areas, summarized broadly as health promotion and disease prevention. What you will not see on this list is explicit mention of older adults, aging, or aging communities. In part, this reflects the tradition in public health of being concerned with communities at large without respect to age. Although any of these functions could easily be extended to an older population (e.g., from preventing epidemics and the spread of disease among older adults to assuring the quality and accessibility of health services for seniors), no explicit aim in this list of what public health does speaks directly to aging.

Box 1.1

WHAT PUBLIC HEALTH DOES

1. Prevents epidemics and the spread of disease
2. Protects against environmental hazards
3. Prevents injuries
4. Promotes and encourages healthy behaviors and mental health
5. Responds to disasters and assists communities in recovery
6. Ensures the quality and accessibility of health services

Source: http://www.health.gov/phfunctions/public.htm

A second common "to do" list explicitly addresses how public health serves communities. These 10 bullets constitute the essential services of public health (Box 1.2). The list includes critical tasks such as monitoring and investigating health, educating and mobilizing communities, developing policies and plans, evaluating services and programs, ensuring safety, linking people to services, assuring a competent workforce, and conducting research to solve public health problems. Together these essential services support public health's overarching goal: "assuring conditions in which people can be healthy" (Institute of Medicine [IOM], 1998).

Box 1.2

THE 10 ESSENTIAL SERVICES OF PUBLIC HEALTH

1. Monitor health status to identify and solve community health problems.
2. Diagnose and investigate health problems and health hazards in the community.
3. Inform, educate, and empower people about health issues.
4. Mobilize community partnerships and action to identify and solve health problems.
5. Develop policies and plans that support individual and community health efforts.
6. Enforce laws and regulations that protect health and ensure safety.
7. Link people to needed personal health services and ensure the provision of health care when otherwise unavailable.
8. Ensure a competent public and personal health care workforce.
9. Evaluate effectiveness, accessibility, and quality of personal and population-based health services.
10. Research for new insights and innovative solutions to health problems.

Source: http://www.health.gov/phfunctions/public.htm

Again, although there is no explicit mention of aging, certainly each of these services can be readily applied to an older population. For example, "monitor the health status *of older adults*" would clearly fall within the first essential service and "inform, educate, and empower *older* people about health issues" fits squarely within the third function. But public health and aging is clearly more than the application of these essential services to older people.

The distinctive yet varied tools of public health stem from the core areas of study found within schools of public health. The names and scope of these core areas may vary slightly across teaching institutions, but each offers methods and materials for investigating populations, prevention, and policy.

- *Population sciences* provide demographic and epidemiologic tools to study population dynamics and the health of populations. These tools help describe population-level phenomena and identify risk factors for disease and disability.
- *Behavioral sciences* (also health education and community health programs) emphasize methods to design and implement programs to influence health and health behaviors. Essential tools from this subspecialty include evidence-based health behavior modification programs and community participatory research.
- *Environmental health sciences* are concerned with measuring and manipulating factors in the environment to influence health. Understanding the environment is critical to disease prevention, but it is also key for tertiary prevention of disability. That is, people with physical or cognitive deficits may remain above the threshold of disability in supportive environments. Environment is thus a malleable component of disability.
- *Health systems and policy* draws on policy analysis and economics to understand and improve health service delivery, including health planning, organization, and policy formulation. This subspecialty recognizes that public health programs do not operate in isolation but require linkage to existing systems and policies if they are to be sustained.
- *Biostatistics* draws on statistical tools and research methodology to characterize or investigate health problems and programs.
- *Public health genomics, infectious disease microbiology, global health, public health informatics, public health law, and emergency preparedness* represent emerging areas of public health

that will likely grow in importance as the field matures and adopts methods from adjacent fields.

As we will discuss in this chapter, researchers and practitioners in public health and aging bring to bear these varied and powerful toolkits to promote what we will call "healthy aging." *The aim of public health and aging is healthy aging: to balance prevention of disease and injury with promotion of behaviors and environments in a way that maximizes functioning and well-being across the life span.* The emphasis is decidedly population based rather than patient focused and recognizes that early and midlife status have implications for health in later life. Just how are the tools of public health implemented to achieve these ends? To answer this question requires a deeper understanding of the phenomenon that we call aging and a basic understanding of changes that individuals encounter as they age.

WHAT IS AGING?

All individuals, whether young or old, are aging. Annual birthday celebrations mark the passage of chronological age. But aging also occurs at the cellular level according to a biological clock. Changes that occur because of cellular aging are often difficult to discern from those caused by disease processes. Here, we discuss the distinctions between chronological and biological aging and between senescence and disease.

Chronological vs. Biological Aging

Aging is the maturation and senescence of biological systems. "Maturation" and "senescence" imply time-dependent changes: with time, our minds and bodies change in a variety of ways, and these changes are what we mean by "aging." With each additional decade of life, adults will see a decrease in reaction time, psychomotor speed, and verbal memory; declines in strength and walking speed; a decreased rate of urine flow; loss of skeletal muscle; and greater mortality, among many other changes. They will also see declines in addictive behaviors and crime, reduction in severe psychiatric disorders, and stability in psychological well-being; continuing increases in vocabulary; greater selectivity in friendship and increased contact with close family; less need for novel stimuli; and increases in leisure time and altruistic behaviors, among many other changes. The popular understanding of aging mostly stresses the first set, the negative changes; but a more complete and accurate understanding would more profitably stress both kinds of change, because both are relevant to a public health perspective on aging.

These changes, positive and negative, occur with the longer life or greater age of the organism. It would be useful to distinguish the two meanings of "aging." The first is simply the number of years an organism has survived, that is, chronological aging. Chronological age is marked solely by the passage of time since birth. Hence, two persons born on the same day, by definition, are the same chronological age, although one may live to an older age. The second definition involves the ticking of some kind of mechanism that governs the "maturation and senescence" of biological systems, and may vary from person to person. One 84-year-old may be biologically vigorous, whereas another born on the same day may lack vitality; hence, despite identical chronological ages, their biological aging, the rate of maturation of their biological systems, may be quite different.

Declines in health may be more prevalent in later life because they are, in fact, expressions of senescence and maturation. Or these declines may be more prevalent simply because of the greater length of time older people have lived, and hence the greater opportunity they have had to experience the risks or exposures that produce these effects. This is a key distinction. It is more than likely that some combination of true senescence and greater exposure to risk factors is likely to be responsible for the changes we consider "aging." For example, the highest audible pitch people can hear declines with greater age, suggesting that this change is a senescent feature of the auditory system. But it is also likely that long years of occupational exposure to noise, untreated ear infections during childhood, neurological conditions, and an accumulation of minor injuries might also contribute to loss of hearing in old age. Senescent changes, long periods of exposure to disease risk factors, and the interaction between the two are confounded in the lay understanding of aging, but a successful public health approach to aging must distinguish between them.

Senescence vs. Disease

Senescence is the progressive, cumulative deterioration in function or loss of physiological capacity associated with greater chronological age. Current thinking suggests that senescence is a biological feature of many physiological systems and that it is best measured as decreased reserve and reduced resistance to stressors. It is evident in a "diminished availability of redundant systems necessary for physical and social well-being" (Crews, 1990). For example, research suggests that sarcopenia, loss of skeletal muscle and lean body mass (and greater infiltration of fat cells in muscle), is a universal, involuntary change that is distinct from pathological wasting syndromes (such as those common in cancer) and cachexia (seen in patients with rheumatoid arthritis, congestive heart failure, or end-stage renal disease). Nonetheless, these senescent changes put older people at risk for pathological changes and, in this sense, can be considered "the backdrop against which the drama of disease is played out" (Roubenoff & Castaneda, 2001). A senescent change, such as sarcopenia, puts the body at risk for disease and poor recovery from disease; for example, "a body already depleted of protein because of aging is less able to withstand the protein catabolism that comes with acute illness or inadequate protein intake" (Roubenoff & Castaneda, 2001).

Hence, senescence and disease are related but distinct. We only see senescence in organisms that have lived a long time, but a longer time alive also means a greater opportunity to develop disease or suffer health insults that are actually distinct from these senescent changes.

Consider cancer. It is often said to be a disease of aging. This presumption is probably based on the higher death rate from malignant neoplasms evident among older adults. Indeed, the mortality rate from cancer among adults aged 85 and older in 2005 was 1,637.7 per 100,000, much higher than the rates of 118.6 among people aged 45–54 and 326.9 among people aged 55–64 (Arias, 2007, Table 38). Of the 512,894 deaths due to cancer in the United States in 2005, 388,322, or 69.4%, involved older adults (Arias, 2007, Appendix Table 32). But the larger number of cancer deaths in older adults does not mean that cancer is a feature of aging. In fact, cause-specific mortality from cancer is actually higher in the 45–64 age group; 32.6% of deaths in this group were due to cancer, compared with 21.7% of deaths in the older age group. Cancer incidence is also lower in the 7th and 8th decade of life, compared with the 5th and 6th decades (Hadley, 1992). Here again, we see confounding between old age as a time for longer exposure to disease agents that may lead to cancer, and old age as an expression of senescent changes that may lead to cancer directly (i.e., dysregulation of cellular processes, such as apoptosis), or that put one at risk for cancer (such as slower bowel motility, development of polyps, and onset of colorectal cancer).

This combination of disease- and senescence-determined factors complicates public health efforts for older adults. In the setting of late-life declines in physiological reserve, what is "normal" senescence and what is disease? Put another way, what is an age-determined relationship (senescence) and what are age-related phenomena (disease)? Wallace (1997) describes some of the different ways disease and senescence may be related. First, the pathogenesis of some diseases is likely to be altered with age. Declines in immune response, for example, a feature of aging, may turn a viral infection into pneumonia rather than a less complicated respiratory tract infection. Second, an age-determined change in one physiological system (which may not cause overt disease in that system) may increase susceptibility to disease in another system. An example mentioned by Wallace is an increase in stroke related to age-determined hypotension. Third, age-determined changes can make older people more susceptible to disease when exposed to environmental challenges. Older adults develop reductions in glucose tolerance, for example, that may lead to frank diabetes under certain conditions. Wallace also points out that some age-determined changes may actually retard development of disease. Lactose intolerance, an age-determined change to the extent that it increases with age, may lead to less fat intake and reduced risk of atherogenesis.

Why make the distinction between age-determined and age-related phenomena? Whether age-determined or age-associated, if changes in later life lead to loss of reserve and put one at risk for disease, are they not appropriate targets for intervention? They may be, but distinguishing changes that are due to senescence from those that are due to external risk factors may help sharpen the appropriate intervention strategy. Moreover, science has made great strides in understanding the risk factors for many of the common diseases of later life, but has yet to identify the specific biological mechanisms responsible for senescence.

Aging and "Social Age"

When people think of old age, they first think of years or some other indicator of the passage of time (for example, in societies where people do not use year-based calendars, these indicators might include the number of harvests completed, the number of ritual cycles conducted, or the number of relocations of dwellings). But even in contemporary American culture, "old age" is not simply a matter of chronological age or the biological expression of senescence. Fry (1980) used a technique drawn from cognitive anthropology to show that cultural dimensions, such as productivity, vulnerability, and reproductive potential, underlie judgments of "young," "middle-aged," and "old." In her pile-sort study, respondents were asked to group hypothetical age-linked social statuses according to similarity. Multidimensional scaling analyses revealed a clear chronological age dimension, but also second- and third-order dimensions, showing, for example, that respondents also grouped older people and children together as opposed to people of middle age. This finding is consistent with research on the "infantilization" of older people (Albert & Brody, 1996; Ryan, Bourhis, & Knops, 1991). "Baby talk" is often applied to older people with cognitive impairment or other disabilities, and terms typically reserved for children are often applied to older people. For example, older people are often spoken of as "cute" and elicit a protective urge seen with infants, such as a desire to hug or comfort.

The reverse is also true. Younger adults who are not active, not interested in new experiences or travel, not willing to switch careers, or who are slow, deliberate, or narrow-minded, are often called "old." They are said to be "old before their time." These negative features of aging— negative, at any rate, when applied to younger people—are meant to criticize or embarrass young people. This use of language also suggests a social component in our understanding of aging. People are old not only because of their age, but also because of their behavior, their health, their attitudes, their choices, and even their politics.

More generally, evidence from cross-cultural studies suggests that the defining characteristics of old age include chronological age, as well as many other criteria, such as achieved social status, having grandchildren, holding political office, oratorical skill, and physical changes. In societies with high mortality and short life expectancy, having children reach adulthood is associated with a change in status to "elder" and associated honorific terms (Albert & Cattell, 1994). Again, the other side to social age needs to be mentioned. In American society, adults can refuse to "grow up," and people can insist on "not acting their age." This can take a variety of forms: not leaving a parent's home, not marrying at an appropriate age, refusing to establish clear career goals, marrying someone much younger than you are, and even buying consumer products associated with a different age stratum.

Thus, old age has a social dimension. For public health efforts, this social component is most relevant in its bearing on expectations for health and function in later life. Even this brief discussion of the use of age criteria to label behaviors suggests that attitudes toward aging and old age are mostly negative. Old age is seen as a time of decline, withdrawal, and vulnerability. In this view, aging is not welcome, and little should be expected of older people; instead, we are expected to ease their decline, provide care, and protect them from exploitation or danger related to their increased vulnerability. These are the elements of "ageism" (Butler, 1969; Palmore, 1999): assumptions of disability, lack of ability, or vulnerability (and, hence, need for protection) based on age, rather than on actual competencies.

The pervasiveness of ageism should not be underestimated. Older persons who miss a word because of a hearing problem are considered too old for conversation and patronized with simplified language. Words may be put in their mouths and their opinions ignored. Older people who forget a name are called "senile," dissatisfaction with illness-related activity restrictions is called "crankiness," and expressions of sexual interest make one a "dirty old man or woman." Even medical personnel are not above recourse to ageist stereotypes.

This sort of ageist thinking has consequences for public health. If missing a word is considered a feature of "getting old," families (and older people themselves) may not take advantage of tertiary treatments available to manage hearing loss, such as hearing aids. Losing track of names may indicate mild cognitive impairment, not just aging; and people with mild cognitive impairment may benefit from cognitive prostheses, environmental modification, antidementia drugs, or increased supervision by family members. "Crankiness" may be depression, or genuine dissatisfaction with unpalatable symptoms, a complaint against undesirable housing, or simply a bad mood, any of which would otherwise be understood as features of daily life for people of any age. From a public health perspective, these expressions of ageism are doubly damaging. They falsely label potentially treatable medical conditions (such as memory or hearing loss) as "aging," and also turn everyday complaints, dissatisfactions, interests, and behaviors into pseudomedical aging syndromes ("crankiness," "childishness," "the dirty old man").

Ageist thinking is revealed for what it is when one compares preconceptions about older people with the facts at hand. For example, younger people mostly imagine old age as a time of sickness, disability, and loss of autonomy. In fact, nearly 80% of people aged 65 and older have no disability of any sort and less than 5% reside in nursing homes. For all our fears of cognitive decline and Alzheimer's disease as invariant features of aging, it is mainly a disease of the very old; most surveys find an Alzheimer's disease prevalence of 6% for people aged 75–84 and 20% for people aged 85 and older (Brookmeyer, Gray, & Kawas, 1998; GAO, 1998). A recent prevalence survey for a nationally representative sample of Americans aged 71+ puts the prevalence of Alzheimer's disease at 9.7% and any dementia at 13.9% (Plassman et al., 2007). Evidence also suggests that the prevalence and incidence of both physical and cognitive limitations in later life may be declining (Schoeni, Freedman, & Martin, 2008). Clinical depression is also not more common in older people (see Chapter 9); it is often a comorbid feature of physical illness and bereavement and, for this reason, seems more common among older people.

Myths About Aging

Many of these ageist attitudes have been elicited by use of questionnaires, such as "What Is Your Aging IQ?" (Special Committee on Aging, 1991). The questions present typical preconceptions about aging and in this way highlight ageist thinking. One version of the questions is shown here, with suggested correct answers:

True or False?

1. Baby boomers are the fastest growing segment of the population. *False.*
2. Families don't bother with their older relatives. *False.*
3. Everyone becomes confused or forgetful if they live long enough. *False.*
4. You can be too old to exercise. *False.*
5. Heart disease is a much bigger problem for older men than for older women. *False.*
6. The older you get, the less you sleep. *False.*
7. People should watch their weight as they age. *True.*
8. Most older people are depressed. Why shouldn't they be? *False.*
9. There's no point in screening older people for cancer because they can't be treated. *False.*
10. Older people take more medications than younger people. *True.*
11. People begin to lose interest in sex around age 55. *False.*
12. If your parents had Alzheimer's disease, you will inevitably get it. *False.*

13. Diet and exercise reduce the risk of osteoporosis. *True.*
14. As your body changes with age, so does your personality. *False.*
15. Older people might as well accept urinary accidents as a fact of life. *False.*
16. Suicide is mainly a problem for teenagers. *False.*
17. Falls and injuries "just happen" to older people. *False.*
18. Everybody gets cataracts. *False.*
19. Extremes of heat and cold can be especially dangerous for older people. *True.*
20. You can't teach an old dog new tricks. *False.*

These questions elicit ageist stereotypes well. They reflect unrealistic fatalism and therapeutic nihilism ("everybody gets cataracts," "falls and injuries just happen to older people," "there's no reason to treat older persons with cancer," and "most older people are depressed"), false assumptions about the aging process ("you can't teach an old dog new tricks," "people begin to lose interest in sex after age 55," and "the older you get, the less you sleep"), overestimates of the heritability of late-life disease ("If your parents had Alzheimer's disease, you will inevitably get it"), sociological naïveté ("American families have by and large abandoned their older members"), and underrecognition of the truly negative aspects of aging, such as the increased risk of suicide among older White men and the greater use of prescribed medicines. Sometimes the problem is a misplaced recognition of a problem, such as the claim of less sleep with greater age. It is true that older people sleep for shorter durations, and this is related to poorer quality of sleep. However, older people also nap more during the day, resulting, in fact, in greater amounts of sleep overall than younger people have.

Together, these prejudices suggest that aging is mostly misunderstood. Overall, the negative features are exaggerated and the positive features ignored. This social or cultural component of aging should be recognized as a potential obstacle to successful public health interventions for older people.

When Does Old Age Begin?

So far, we have examined aging and older persons without specifying when someone is old. From what we have said already, we see that the question is unreasonable. There is no single age at which we can say that people cross the threshold into "old age." People age at different rates; hence, for any given age, there will be great variation in all proposed biomarkers of aging or phenotypes of healthy aging. "Old age" does not have a biological definition, only a social one. For example, in the United States, establishment of the Social Security system linked old age to age 65. This definition of old age was more a product of social perceptions and economic necessity than anything else.

But people do have an idea of when people become old. A number of surveys have asked at what age someone is old. The start of "old age" can be assigned to a wide range of chronological ages. This assigned age may reflect attitudes toward aging and older persons. For example, assigning the start of old age to increasingly older ages means that many aspects of aging, once considered hallmarks of old age, now fall short of making someone old. It also stands to reason that many of the characteristics of the respondents, such as age and social status, are likely to be related to judgments regarding the start of old age. One may imagine that minority groups with a shorter life expectancy might date the onset of old age to earlier ages than other more advantaged groups.

Someone who reports that old age begins at age 55 clearly has a different attitude toward aging than someone who asserts that it begins at age 75. In the one case, a larger portion of the life span is considered the period of "old age," with the physical and psychological changes of the 5th and 6th decade already considered signs of senescence. In the other, only changes typical of the 7th decade and beyond qualify as "old age," and senescence is pushed ahead to a point closer to death and the maximum biological life span. Respondent choices of an age for "old age" tell us the decade when people are expected to slow down, retire, and focus on self-maintenance rather than new careers or goals.

Figure 1.1 shows the age at which respondents consider women to be old. These data are drawn from the National Council on Aging *Myths and Realities of Aging* survey, conducted in 2000 in a national probability sample of the United States. The data are weighted to reflect the sampling scheme and overrepresentation of older people and minorities. The figure plots the mean age that "the average woman" is said to be old by respondent's age and sex.

Note the strong relationship between a respondent's age and his or her report of when women are old. Young people clearly consider the start of old age to be much earlier than older people do. For people at about age 20, women are old at age 45. By the time people reach the

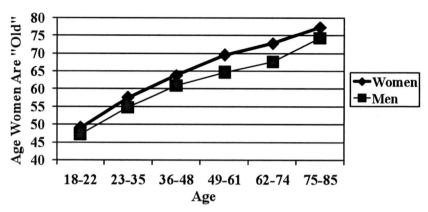

Figure 1.1 Age at which women are "old," by respondent age and sex (United States).

Source: From National Council on Aging (NCOA), 2001; weighted data.

6th and 7th decade, old age is pushed back to the late sixties and early seventies. Note too that women date the start of old age to a later age than men do, whatever the respondent's age. Women consider old age to begin 2–4 years later than men do. They push old age further back than men do, not only for themselves, but also in their reports of the start of old age for men (Albert, O'Neil, Muller, & Butler, 2002d). Moreover, the age at which old age is said to begin now seems to be far more correlated with one's own age than in earlier surveys.

FIVE FACES OF AGING

The experience of late life is varied and complex. To better understand the aims of public health and aging, it is useful to delve into some of the most common experiences of aging. Gillick (1994), a clinical geriatrician, has provided an excellent account of the most common faces of aging. As a geriatrician with a primary care focus, one of the few physicians who still make home visits, her experience offers important guidance on what it is like to be old, ill, and in need of medical care. She begins her account with an overriding principle: "Only if we start with a deep understanding of what being sick is like can we hope to reach a consensus on what kind of health policy is appropriate for the elderly" (Gillick, 1994, p. 10). In her account, Gillick identifies four types of elder and has provided clinical vignettes of the particular challenges and opportunities specific to each type.

The Robust Elder

The robust older persons are "physically vigorous, mentally acute, a fount of wisdom and experience for their families, [and] busy accomplishing all the things they never previously had the time to undertake." However, as Gillick reminds us, they typically have accumulated at least some chronic conditions in their 70 or 80 years of life, such as arthritis, hypertension, diabetes, hearing loss, glaucoma or macular degeneration, essential tremor, and other treatable but only minimally impairing conditions. Hence, "their date books are sprinkled with doctor's appointments; they carry a packet of their medicines in their pockets; their night tables are lined with containers for hearing-aids, glasses, and dentures." A defining feature of this type of elder is increases in health care use, but lack of disability.

An example of a robust elder described by Gillick was Mrs. Landsman (a pseudonym), who at age 96 was quite active until she developed anemia, which led to detection of an advanced colorectal cancer. As a competent adult, she had to choose between surgery (and a risk of immediate death) and symptomatic treatment, where the progression of the cancer would ultimately lead to increasing morbidity and disability and later death. Gillick (1994, pp. 55–56) describes Mrs. Landsman's response in this way:

> Mrs. Landsman thought long and hard about the various options. She had no illusions about her own mortality, and in fact was quite ready to depart from this world. But there was one thing she was quite clear about: she did not wish to be a burden to others, nor did she wish to be dependent on others, which she regarded as equivalent. The prospect of repeated visits to the hospital for transfusions or treatment for chest pain or fractures was dismal. The prospect of fading away over an extended period of time, becoming increasingly dependent, was even more unappealing.
>
> Mrs. Landsman opted for surgery. Ironically, an operation that would probably prove to be curative was performed because it provided the best palliation available. The simplest, most humane, and cheapest way to provide comfort for this very elderly woman was to perform major surgery.

Studies suggest that the robust senior is not an uncommon experience. Indeed, 20%–33% of older adults are robust without any chronic disease (Strawbridge, Wallhagan, & Cohen, 2002). An even greater proportion of older adults—perhaps as much as 40%—experience minimal interruption of usual activities and maintain social participation in the face of disease. Seventy-five to 80% of Americans over age 65 report no disability in personal self-maintenance activities, such as bathing or dressing.

The Frail Elder

Gillick (1994, p. 105) describes frail older people as "hav[ing] no one overriding health problem. Instead they suffer from impairments in multiple domains . . . that collectively render them vulnerable to the slightest perturbation."

She describes Mr. Schaeffer, age 83, who had diabetes, hypertension, congestive heart failure, psoriasis, and emphysema. Fatigue and weakness led him to live an increasingly less active life. He was unable to babysit for his grandchild on his own, could not go out unless he had a ride from someone, could not read the newspaper through without falling asleep, and employed a homemaker to do grocery shopping, cooking, laundry, and cleaning. He then developed repeated bouts of pneumonia, which led to repeated hospitalizations. At the hospital he was diagnosed with aortic stenosis, which was treated with a valvuloplasty, but he subsequently developed delirium, lost weight, acquired a nosocomial infection, and became increasingly less mobile. His family then recognized that he could not safely live independently and would not be able to return to his apartment. He became a candidate for the nursing home. He had a cardiac arrest, however, while still in the hospital, which led to the last of his three intubations. This time, however, he could not be revived and died.

These are the prosaic but important details of medical care for the frail elder. They are not glamorous. As Gillick writes, "autobiographical and fictional accounts of aging focus on the drama, but seldom on the prosaic details that make all the difference to the frail older person. I have yet to read a story in which the elderly protagonist describes his intense embarrassment upon suddenly developing incontinence, only to be rescued by a geriatric consultant who determines that his problem has been caused by the new blood pressure medicine he has been taking" (1994, p. 106).

Efforts to establish frailty as a phenotype have resulted in an explosion of research on this topic in recent years. One proposed operationalization consists of the following components: shrinking (unintentional loss of 10 lbs or more), weakness (scores in the lowest 20% of the distribution of grip-strength values), poor endurance (reports of exhaustion when performing daily activities), slowness (scores in the lowest 20% of the distribution of timed gait speeds), and low activity (scores in the lowest 20% of activity profiles, as determined by estimated expenditure of calories). Older adults with three or more of these characteristics are considered to be frail (Fried et al., 2001). This concept overlaps with, but is distinct from the notion of disability, more generally defined as a gap between an individual's capacity and the challenges of his or her environment. Estimates of frailty in clinically based samples have ranged from about 12% to 16% (Rockwood, Andrew, & Mitnitski, 2007).

The Elder With Dementia

Dementing disease is one of the central challenges of public health and aging. Although many diseases cause the global, progressive, irreversible impairment in cognitive function that we call "dementia," the most prevalent sources are vascular disease and Alzheimer's disease. These diseases of later life, for the most part, pose extreme challenges to caregiving families and medical providers. As Gillick remarks,

> The dilemma of when to stop treating, or when to provide less than maximally intensive care, is never more poignant than with the elderly person who has Alzheimer's disease or one of several types of dementia. Dementia, the gradual loss of multiple facets of the mind such as memory, language, and judgment, robs people of their ability to understand what is happening to them when they get sick. Illness becomes as incomprehensible to these patients as its treatment. Moreover, the future they are vouchsafed if they are successfully cured of pneumonia or appendicitis is one of relentless decline. If they live long enough, they will likely pass from a state of mild forgetfulness to apathy and incontinence, and ultimately to a bed-bound existence. (1994, p. 17)

Older adults with dementia have varied symptoms, which may include memory loss, difficulty understanding or using words, inability to carry out motor activities (despite physical ability to do so), and failure to identify or recognize objects. Dementia is often accompanied by behavioral disturbances (e.g., wandering, pacing, and repetitive questions). Although approximately 10% of adults aged 71 and older have frank dementia, as many as 22.2% in addition may have cognitive impairment short of dementia (Plassman et al., 2008; see Chapter 8). Most seniors who meet criteria for dementia are cared for in the home by relatives or paid caregivers and the remainder live in residential care settings (e.g., nursing homes, assisted living facilities).

The Dying Elder

"Late life," as the term implies, is the period of life closest to death. Although it is not always clear when the dying process starts (and, as a result, when medical care goals should shift further toward palliation), care of the dying elder is a key component of geriatric care and an important consideration in public health and aging.

One challenge in meeting the needs of the dying elder is the lack of realistic appraisal of the risk of dying by patients and their families, which, in some cases, unfortunately is encouraged by clinicians. These unrealistic appraisals may lead to poor choices in medical care, such as recourse to invasive procedures that have little or no chance of success. Clinicians may be as uncomfortable with end-of-life choices as patients, but with proper communication of risk, this situation can change. As Gillick (1994, p. 80) writes, "if instead of being told that they had a 10% or 20% chance of survival with ICU care, patients were told they had an 80% to 90% chance of dying with ICU treatment, and a 99% chance of dying without it . . . how many in fact would choose the ICU?" This is an interesting question worth a study in itself (see Chapter 10).

A second challenge for this type of elder is the issue of control and autonomy at the end of life, which may be complicated further by mental health issues. Gillick describes Mrs. Renan, who is dying of cancer. Mrs. Renan sought physician-assisted suicide and would not accept reasonable medical management of her condition, which included blood transfusions and easily available palliative treatments. "She accused me of abandoning her because I said I would not and could not give her a lethal injection." Gillick distinguishes reasonable medical care goals, such as strategies to reduce disability and relieve symptoms, and inappropriate goals, such as elimination of existential suffering.

Was I a failure as a doctor if I could not cure . . . her overwhelming sadness and rage over aging? My role was supportive. I could try to make Claire as functional as possible during her final months or years. This entailed such things as blood transfusions to improve her strength and prescribing a wheelchair to help her maintain some degree of mobility. I could try to make her as comfortable as possible by treating her arthritic pain with medication and trying to regulate her bowels with a judiciously selected combination of stool softeners and cathartics. I could provide relief by simply being there, by acknowledging her misery and promising not to abandon her. But [I do not] think that physicians must at all costs obliterate suffering, if necessary by causing death. (Gillick, 1994, p. 90)

Nearly 2 million older adults die each year. So, liberally, 5%–7% of the older population faces end-of-life issues in a given year. Trajectories to death also vary widely. Lynn and Adamson (2003) describe three prototypical descents experienced by Medicare beneficiaries: a short period of decline, typical of many cancers; a longer period of limitations with multiple exacerbations and sudden death, typical of organ system failure; and a slow, prolonged decline typical of dementia, disabling stroke, and frailty. Lunney, Lynn, and Hogan (2002) have found that about one fifth of deaths in a given year occur in a manner consistent with the first trajectory, another one fifth follow the second profile, and as many as two fifths follow the prolonged trajectory.

Trajectories of dying are an active area of research. Could the type of trajectory influence the kind of dying one faces (such as death at home or in the hospital, or perhaps the likelihood of transitions between health care settings)? Or could the type of trajectory influence expectations for dying and decision making at the end of life? Both questions fall within a growing subdomain of public health and aging, namely, the public health impact of the end of life (Anderson & Smith, 2005; GAO, 1998).

The Compensating, Adaptive Elder

Cutting across these archetypes of aging is the reality of being old, the need to maintain function and accomplish daily goals in the face of declining abilities, often pressing symptoms of chronic disease, and awareness in some cases of impending death. As in people with disabilities or younger people facing life-limiting illness, older people alter daily tasks, rely on spared abilities to compensate for deficits, and selectively invest physical, cognitive, and affective effort to maximize the likelihood of social participation and activity. The psychological analog to such modification of daily life in the face of declining abilities is "selective optimization with compensation" (Baltes & Baltes, 1990).

Research in compensation is still in its infancy. Baltes and colleagues have shown for psychological processes that even quite frail older people are active in the management of dependency. They may accept personal self-maintenance care to allow them the physical strength or energy to accomplish more valued activities, such as social activity or leisure pursuits. Unable to go outside or even ambulate indoors, the elder with mobility limitation may seek a strategic position in a home, perhaps a chair with a commanding view. This too can be considered a selective investment of resources to compensate for a deficit and in this way optimize experience in the face of disability. Recourse to personal assistance equipment is a similar accommodation. The essence of selective optimization with compensation is development of strategies that allow older adults to retain control or accomplish some goal in the setting of declining ability.

Researchers are just beginning to generalize this paradigm to physical function (Agree & Freedman, 2000; Verbrugge & Sevak, 2002; Weiss, Hoenig, & Fried, 2007). For example, it stands to reason that the elder with lower extremity disability may rely more heavily on preserved upper body function to accomplish daily tasks. The elder able to do so will likely report less disability and perhaps better mental health, signs of effective adaptation. At the microscopic ergonomic level, people make such accommodations all the time, changing the way in which they reach or grasp in the face of arthritic pain, making lists or using elaborate mnemonics in the case of memory impairment, or avoiding hills or simply slowing down in the case of dyspnea. Compensatory processes may also cross physiological domains. In our experience, elders with severe physical deficits but preserved cognition manage to figure out ways to complete physical activities.

Studying compensation would probably be valuable, because it may be possible to teach such optimization strategies. In fact, Clark and colleagues have completed a series of occupational therapy interventions designed to do just this and have shown benefit in mental health, self-efficacy, quality of life, and range of activities accomplished. They have taken the research further to examine the physical and neuroendocrine effects (Clark et al., 1997) of such compensatory efforts.

Table 1.1 summarizes these types of aging experience and goals of medical care and public health. We will return to these issues in later chapters.

Table 1.1

TYPES OF AGING EXPERIENCE AND GOALS
OF MEDICAL CARE AND PUBLIC HEALTH

TYPE OF ELDER	GOAL OF MEDICAL CARE	GOAL OF PUBLIC HEALTH
Robust	Life prolongation, cure	Prevention of frailty and disability
Demented	Maximization of function, palliation	Prevention of excess morbidity; excellent custodial care
Dying	Palliation ("upstreamed")	Reduction of isolation, maximization of choice
Frail	Upper bound: maximum medically tolerable intervention Lower bound: medical care based on best interest of patient	Environmental modification to reduce task demand; rehabilitation to increase capacity by developing spared abilities
Compensating	Occupational, physical, speech therapy; rehabilitation; cognitive remediation	Provision of appropriate aging services; promotion of maximally integrated setting

HEALTHY VS. SUCCESSFUL VS. OPTIMAL AGING

It is salutary to try and explain the functions of public health and aging to the audience for our efforts, the people who have experienced old age and who confront the risk of frailty and chronic disease. One case will speak for many. Hannah is a 92-year-old Israeli. She has lived on a kibbutz, a collective settlement, for over 50 years, a hard but supportive environment for older persons that has been shown to confer important health advantages (Walter-Ginzburg, Blumstein, & Guralnik, 2004). At age 92, she was quite frail and required 24-hour personal care assistance, which was provided by the kibbutz. She used a walker for indoor mobility, left her small home to go outside only rarely, and required help with dressing, toileting, and meal preparation. She had given up housework, shopping, and travel. In contrast, she took medications and used the telephone independently, kept track of her affairs quite efficiently, and, despite pain from osteoporosis and some dyspnea from a heart condition, appeared to be active within her home.

She asked one of us (SA) what public health could do for her and whether she was an example of healthy aging. Put on the spot, I first asked her about her health. She explained that she suffered from many chronic conditions: heart disease, hypertension, osteoporosis, osteoarthritis, kyphoscoliosis, diabetes, and hearing and vision loss. She needed to take 10 different medicines daily, from digoxin to diuretics. What could I do for her, she wanted to know, and what could she do to promote healthy aging? I then asked if she found her days more or less satisfying and interesting. "Oh yes," she said, "I am always reading, I hear from my daughter and grandchildren on the telephone everyday, I make sure I check off medicines and meals on my chart throughout the day, and people come and visit all the time. I enjoy some of the shows on television, especially basketball, and make sure I watch the news everyday."

"You mean you find each day satisfying despite your poor health?"

"Of course."

"Well, then," I said, "I would say you are a very good example of healthy aging. Public health could learn from you. How is it that your days are so full and satisfying despite all the illness and pills?"

"My mind is clear, I have the help I need, and I still can appreciate books, friends and neighbors, and my children and grandchildren. But are you sure there is nothing else I should be doing?"

I demurred. Aside from checking for adverse effects from polypharmacy and perhaps some minor environmental modifications of the home, this 92-year-old serves as an excellent illustration of one kind of healthy aging: high risk of poor health and disability typical of very old age, but also engagement in daily projects, expert in self-care and disease management, maximally supported to promote independence in the face of frailty, well-connected to family and community, funny and feisty.

Indeed it is useful to contrast the notion of "healthy aging" with the perhaps more popularized notion of "successful aging." Rowe and Kahn (1987) define the latter as consisting of three elements: absence of disease and the risk factors for disease, maintenance of physical and cognitive abilities, and engagement in productive activities. They viewed the three elements as roughly hierarchical: absence of disease allows maintenance of physical and cognitive skill, and preservation of these skills in turn allows engagement in productive activity. Their key insight was recognition of variation in aging, which allows us to raise the bar for goals and expectations about health in old age. If successful aging is possible, then we can aim higher than "usual aging." They stress that aging is more than disease and disability, and that there is more to successful aging than avoiding disease and disability. In their view, successful aging includes avoiding disease and disability, which may involve interventions that enhance cognitive and physical function. This may also require that we develop a society that provides individuals opportunities of continuing engagement in life.

Rowe and Kahn (1987) did not specify what proportion of older people met this definition of successful aging, or, more critically, what proportion, given any particular age stratum, would be a reasonable goal for public health. Nor did they try to operationalize the three criteria. Attempts to use existing measures to partition the older population in this way (and relaxing criteria to stress minimal rather than absence of disease or disability) show that only 20%–33% of community-resident older Americans meet the criteria for successful aging (Strawbridge et al., 2002).

Other working definitions of successful aging have been proposed that are closer to the notion of healthy aging. An alternative approach stresses minimal interruption of usual activities and maintenance of social participation in the face of disease. By this criterion a majority of older adults, including the 92-year-old described earlier, could be considered successful agers. As we have seen, one mechanism for this preservation of activity and social participation is "selective optimization with compensation," that is, doing well with remaining strengths by recruiting preserved abilities to compensate, when possible, for areas of weakness (Baltes & Carstenson, 1996).

Most recently, researchers have recognized that neither "successful aging" nor "healthy aging" are the right terms. Elders who reach old age with chronic conditions or who develop disabilities would be considered examples of "failed" aging by using the first term. Likewise, because most seniors have some declines in function and chronic disease (or ultimately will develop them), the focus on "healthy aging" narrowly construed misses the point of maintenance of function and well-being despite these common features of old age. Perhaps the better term is "optimal aging," defined as a range of values for clinical indicators that we would expect more in people of younger ages. Thus, a 90-year-old with a gait speed typical of a 75-year-old can be said to have met the optimal aging criterion in this one key phenotype.

The focus on optimal aging is superior to prior approaches because it is norm-driven and uses chronological age as a criterion. It also allows an individual to age optimally in one area but perhaps not in another (although in practice these will be highly correlated). An elder at age 85 can have memory performance 1.5 *SD* above the norm for her age and education, making her equivalent in this domain to a 75-year-old. This is optimal aging in a cognitive domain. The same may be true for grip strength, light-touch pressure sensation, visual contrast sensitivity, insulin or glucose chemistries, bone mineral density, systolic blood pressure, or wound healing. We prefer this approach because it opens the door to more reasonable endpoints in clinical trials and better characterization of the health of older populations.

Such notions of optimal or healthy aging are important to keep in mind in articulating the boundaries of public health and aging. Assuring conditions for health promotion in late life must be considered along with conditions to foster successful adaptation to states of ill health. Both are reasonable goals for public health promotion, and the mix of emphasis on the two may change with age. That is, while assurance of the conditions for health should be the goal at all ages, with very old age the more critical goal may be assuring conditions to promote successful compensation in the face of disease and disability. Our 92-year-old *kibbutznik* failed all three of the Kahn and Rowe criteria but had successfully optimized her remaining abilities to live well.

HOW THE FIRST 50 YEARS MATTER FOR HEALTH RISKS IN THE SECOND 50 YEARS: THREE ILLUSTRATIONS

Gillick's portraits provide rich and varied snapshots of later life. Yet, as we explained earlier in this chapter, aging begins at birth and continues throughout the life course. How these earlier life experiences influence outcomes in later life is a growing area of interest. Hayward and Gorman (2004), for example, have referred to this phenomenon as the "long arm of childhood" in their study demonstrating important childhood influences on male mortality in later life.

It is challenging to study the ways in which health and risk behaviors in the first half of life may affect health in the second 50 years and even more difficult to generalize public health applications from such studies. Imagine the definitive cohort study that follows prospectively an entire birth cohort until each and every member dies or reaches very old age. Such a study would lend itself to precise measurement of risk factors in early life and allow researchers to relate them to outcomes in later life. Despite decades of gerontological research, we still do not have a prospective cohort study that has observed people from birth to death. Even if we did have such a cohort, what we could learn from studying such a cohort that would apply to today's public health system is unclear, because the members of the cohort would have been born over 100 years ago.

In practice, most gerontological research cohorts usually begin at age 65, or perhaps at preretirement, at age 50 or 55. Therefore, we often do not have direct evidence of health at earlier ages. As a result, we are forced to use proxy measures, or sometimes retrospective measures, to summarize health and risk experience in the first half of life. These proxy measures typically include such factors as:

- Occupation, to assess environmental exposures during work years
- Education and literacy, to assess cognitive engagement over the life span
- Parent occupation and education, to assess perinatal and childhood conditions
- Recollections of childhood health and experiences
- Household income, to assess access to health services over the life span
- Birthplace, to assess environment and access to health care in migrating populations
- Birth weight and stature, to assess pre- and postnatal nutritional status
- Race and ethnicity, to assess the effects of culture and potentially restricted access to health services

Recent progress in molecular genetics, environmental health, and imaging technologies now allows derivation of biological indicators, in some cases, for these lifelong factors. For example, some genes, such as APOE, are more common in particular racial or ethnic groups. If a sociocultural group is more at risk of a disease associated with this gene, such as a cardiovascular condition or Alzheimer's disease, we can now begin to separate sociocultural and genetic factors. Likewise, long-term environmental exposures leave a DNA signature, just as long-term cognitive engagement, evident in educational attainment and literacy, may be visible in functional magnetic resonance images.

We turn now to case studies that illustrate well the different legacies from the first 50 years that affect the health resources older adults have when they enter later life. These examples also show some of the difficulties involved in public health research, where biological and clinical factors are often confounded with socioeconomic status. The first two focus on relationships over the life course at the individual level, and the second brings a population-level perspective.

Entry Into Late Life With Lower Cognitive Reserve

African Americans face a higher risk of Alzheimer's disease (AD) than White Americans. This difference remains when we stratify samples by *APOE* e4 status, a well validated risk factor for Alzheimer's disease. Figure 1.2 compares the incidence of AD in Whites, African Americans, and Hispanic Americans living in northern Manhattan, New York City. Only people with the e3/e3 variant of *APOE* (the so-called wild type) are included, thus removing the effect of this genetic risk factor. The cumulative incidence curves in the figure plot the risk by age in the three race-ethnicity groups. As in all incidence studies, people included in the analysis were free of the disease initially, and all were followed up at regular intervals with a common cognitive assessment battery to identify the age at which people first met criteria for AD.

As the figure shows, minorities were significantly more likely to meet criteria for AD. By age 75, 2% of the Whites and 9% of the minorities developed the disease. By age 80, approximately 9% of the Whites and 21% of the minorities met AD criteria. These large differences in incidence persisted even with statistical control for differences between the race-ethnicity groups in a great variety of risk factors for AD, such as years of school, family history of AD, number of comorbid chronic disease conditions, and behaviors such as smoking and head injury. Tang and colleagues (1998) also recalculated incidence by use of a stricter definition of dementia to identify only clear and obvious cases of AD. This strategy eliminated more mild forms of AD as "cases" and, as a result, also should have helped to eliminate subtle diagnostic biases, either from clinicians interpreting cognitive tests or from the tests themselves, and in this way to reduce any differential misclassification. Even with this conservative approach to diagnosis, differences between the race-ethnicity groups persisted.

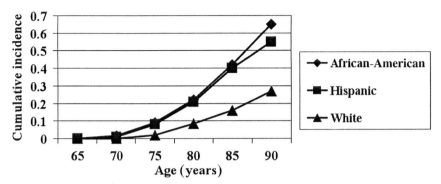

Figure 1.2 Cumulative risk of AD, by race-ethnicity, limited to APOE e3/3.

Source: From "The APOE-Epsilon4 Allele and the Risk of Alzheimer Disease Among African Americans, Whites, and Hispanics," by M. X. Tang et al., 1998, *Journal of the American Medical Association, 279*, Table 1. Copyright © (1998) American Medical Association. All rights reserved.

These differences in the risk of AD raise important questions. Do we overdiagnose minorities (and if so, why?), or do we underdiagnose Whites (and again, if so, why?). Graphically, is the cumulative incidence curve for the minorities too high, or is the cumulative incidence curve for Whites too low? Why should minorities be at greater risk for developing AD? Is it because they enter later life with previously poorer abilities, so that they start follow-up at age 65 or 70 closer to the threshold of the low cognitive ability used to define AD? Or do they enter late life with abilities similar to Whites, but decline at a faster rate in old age? The first factor suggests an effect in the first 50 years of life; the second implies an effect in the second half of life.

We investigated this issue in a related sample of 871 older adults drawn from the same community and assessed with the same clinical battery and diagnostic paradigm. We selected all people who had at least three cognitive assessments, where the AD diagnosis, if made for a respondent, was made at the last of the series of assessments. Of the 871 people, 138 met criteria for AD at their last assessment, whereas the remainder never met criteria for AD.

To assess whether the race-ethnicity groups entered old age with different cognitive resources, we examined scores on the Selective Reminding Test, a test of memory, at baseline, that is, when no one had yet met criteria for dementia. The test asks respondents to repeat a list of 12 words over six trials, for a maximum score of 72 and minimum of 0. Mean scores at baseline were significantly lower among minorities. If we divide the distribution into tertiles (upper third, middle third, lower third), the lower third included scores with a range from 8 to 34. Of Whites 16.3% scored in the lowest tertile, but 32.4% of African Americans and 44.4% of Hispanics scored in this range. This difference strongly supports the claim of earlier life events as a predictor of a key later life outcome. Minority elders enter later life with poorer memory scores and, hence, less cognitive reserve.

By contrast, the slope of memory score change over the serial assessments, that is, the mean rate of decline, was not significantly different across the three race-ethnicity groups. Age, education, and initial memory score were all independently associated with rate of decline in memory performance, but in a regression model that included these factors, race-ethnicity was not significantly associated with rate of decline. Thus, cognitive performance in minorities did not decline at a faster rate. Baseline differences, differences that predate old age, seem to be responsible for the higher risk of AD among minorities. Of course, poorer memory performance at baseline very likely reflects an early stage of disease progression, prodromal AD. But this too is consistent with earlier life experience as the source of greater risk of AD in later life.

Entry Into Late Life With Differences in Physical Reserve

Rantanen and colleagues (1999) examined a cohort of men aged 45–68 and found that grip strength at this age was a strong predictor of disability 25 years later. These men, all from the Honolulu Heart Program—Asia Aging Study, were first assessed in 1965–1968 and were reassessed between 1991 and 1993, when participants were 71–93 years old. Grip strength is correlated with strength in other muscle groups and for this reason is considered a good indicator of overall strength. Grip strength performance was assessed with a handheld dynamometer, and hand strength at midlife was categorized into low (<37 kg), middle (37–42 kg), and high (>42 kg) performance tertiles.

Men with low performance in midlife were significantly more likely to report disability in late life. These men reported nearly twice as much disability as men in the upper tertile in doing heavy household work (25% vs. 14%), walking (26% vs. 15%), bathing (8% vs. 3%), as well as a variety of other indicators of disability and functional limitation (i.e., walking speed, ability to rise from a chair). Men in the middle tertile fell between these two groups in risk of disability in late life. The increased risk of disability in old age associated with low grip strength in midlife persisted in regression models that controlled for age, height, weight, education, occupation, smoking, physical activity, and chronic conditions at the examination in which disability status was established.

This finding is extremely important. "Muscle strength is found to track over the life span: those who had higher grip strength during midlife remained stronger than others in old age" (Rantanen et al., 1999). For this reason, these men entered late life with a greater reserve in strength, and this reserve helped forestall onset of disability. Rantanen and colleagues mention a number of alternative hypotheses for this finding, which are also of note: (1) grip strength may be a marker of physical activity, which may itself prevent disability; (2) low grip strength may reflect early disease processes that later progress and cause disability; and (3) grip strength may be related to motivation to stay fit and through this mechanism lower the risk of disability in late life. Each of these hypotheses merits investigation, but all suggest the critical role of health factors in midlife as predictors of late-life outcomes.

It turns out, as well, that grip strength in midlife is related to birth weight. In the UK Medical Research Council National Survey of Health and Development, 2,815 men and 2,547 women born in 1946 were observed through 1999, when they were 53 years old (Kuh et al., 2002). Men and women in the highest fifth of the distribution of birth weight had 10% greater grip strength at age 53, compared with people in the lowest birth weight group. A 1-kg increase in birth weight was associated with a 1.9-kg increase in grip strength for men and a 1.2-kg increase for women 53 years later. This relationship persisted even with control for weight and height and "suggest[s] the importance of prenatal influences on muscle development that have persisting consequences through to later adulthood."

Thus, grip strength in middle age is related, at least in part, to prenatal environment. And grip strength in midlife is related to disability in late life. These investigations represent a rare case in which a single important risk factor or health indicator has been investigated across the whole life span and related to outcomes at different points in the life span. They suggest the unity of the life span, where a risk factor acquired at the earliest ages is expressed in different ways across the life span. More research of this type will be required if we are to understand health outcomes in late life.

Early and Midlife Influences on Late-Life Disability Trends

The prevalence of activity limitations in later life has declined in the United States over the past 25 years. Efforts to understand why this is so have been hampered until recently by the inability to sort out factors that occur in the early, intermediate, and late phases of the life course (Schoeni, Freedman, & Martin, 2008). A study analyzing survey data from the 1995–2004 Health and Retirement Study (HRS) sheds light on this question by sorting out the influence of early and midlife factors on recent late-life activity limitation trends (Freedman, Grafova, Schoeni, & Rogowski, 2008).

The HRS is a national study designed to provide both snapshots of the experience of adults aged 50 and older in the United States and dynamic assessments of changes as individuals age. Respondents are selected in such a way (with a known probability of selection) that responses can be weighted to reflect national experience. More than 20,000 individuals aged 50 and older are observed over time, with individuals newly turning 50–55 years of age added every 6 years.

In this analysis, the samples were limited to between 4,500 and 4,700 persons aged 75 and older in 1995, 1998, 2000, 2002, and 2004. Measures of activity limitations included both difficulty with activities of daily living (ADLs, e.g., bathing, dressing, grooming, using toilet) and with instrumental activities of daily living (IADLs, e.g., managing money, using the telephone, light cleaning, managing medications). Early-life measures included self-reported race-ethnicity; recollections of region of birth, mother's education, childhood socioeconomic status, and childhood self-rated health; and an estimate of having lower than average peak stature, obtained by adjusting initial reports of current height. In addition, three indicators of midlife were included: completed education; whether the respondent was a veteran; and lifetime occupation.

Between 1995 and 2004, the profile of the older population changed in many ways. Reports of difficulty with ADLs declined significantly from 30.2% in 1995 to 26.0% in 2004. There were also fewer reports of smoking, increases in reports of many common chronic conditions, including obesity and hearing problems, and improvements in self-rated vision. In addition, more older adults were classified in the highest levels of income and wealth.

The profile of early and midlife factors among those very old adults also shifted during this period. For example, older adults in 2004 reported more years of school completed for themselves and their mothers and better health in childhood. In 2004 they were also more likely to have worked in a white-collar or pink-collar occupation, and to be a veteran. The question is whether these shifts in early and midlife factors can account for the changes observed in the prevalence of activity limitations in late life.

With use of multinomial logistic regression techniques our study demonstrated that early-life factors were independent predictors of late-life disability. For example, respondents who rated their childhood health as fair or poor had an increased odds (1.3 times) of reporting limitations in ADLs in later life compared with those who reported excellent childhood health. And respondents who had service sector and secretarial occupations had an increased odds of IADL limitations compared with those in white collar professional and managerial positions. These findings persisted even after controlling for other early-life, midlife, and contemporaneous factors.

Moreover, shifts in the older population with respect to education, mothers' education, health during childhood, and lifetime occupation all contributed to the declines in the prevalence of ADL limitations. Improvements in late-life vision and increases in wealth also appeared to contribute to the declines, but reports of increased chronic conditions in late-life offset these gains. Analysis of changes in ADL onset and recovery over the time period suggested that early and midlife factors contributed, along with late-life factors, to U.S. late-life disability trends, mainly through their influence on the onset of, rather than recovery from, limitation.

As with any study, this analysis had limitations worth reviewing because they highlight the difficulty in conducting research on ways in which the first 50 years of life influence the latter 50 years. Although rich in details about current health and economic status, some of the earlier life measures used were less than ideal. For example, lifetime occupation (based on work histories) could not be ascertained for a significant portion of the sample, and measures of childhood socioeconomic status and health relied on long-term memory. Measures of midlife health were also not available. And because the HRS began in the 1990s, only a decade's worth of trends could be assessed (at least thus far).

What are the public health implications of such findings? One certainly cannot go back and intervene in the early-life circumstances of today's oldest members of society. Rather, the findings are instructive in what they suggest about the persistence of early and midlife effects on late-life activity limitations. The health and economic circumstances of today's children and adults can have a profound influence on the health and functioning of the nation's future elders. In other words, the target of public health and aging efforts is not just the older adults of today but the children and adults who are the future elders.

THE DOMAINS OF PUBLIC HEALTH AND HEALTHY AGING

We are now ready to address the domains of public health and aging. As mentioned earlier, the majority—although certainly not all—of older adults have already developed chronic disease and many have developed disability, frailty, and cognitive impairment. Hence, the aims of public health in an aging society arguably go well beyond creating circumstances that support health and prevent disease and injury. Instead, the overarching aim of public health and aging is to promote the development and maintenance of optimal physical, mental, and social well-being and function, irrespective of acquired disease. Examples of what public health does to promote healthy aging are provided in Box 1.3.

The true test of this approach to public health and aging is whether it is broad enough to meet the needs of each of the illustrative faces of aging described earlier (see Table 1.1). Recall the robust elder with chronic disease. For those meeting the criteria of robust aging, health promotion and disease prevention may be ample, but those with chronic disease need additional attention to disease management and prevention of disability. For the frail elder, the public health goal is not solely to slow progression of disease but to maximize function and well-being. This typically takes two forms: environmental modification programs to reduce task demands and rehabilitation to increase capacity and adapt spared abilities. For the elder with dementia, the public health goals include excellent supportive care that addresses both quality of care and quality of life, support of informal caregivers, and, when possible, physical and cognitive remediation. For the subset of the population who are dying, public health goals may depend on the nature and course of the trajectory (Lynn & Adamson, 2003), but, in all cases, maximizing well-being and providing the opportunity for patient and family to experience a "good death" are of interest. For all groups, support for compensatory strategies is appropriate. These draw on the allied health and rehabilitation fields (occupational, physical, and speech therapy; physical medicine), nursing, social work care management, and new specialties such as certified driving rehabilitation specialists, doula support for dying, and cognitive remediation for patients with Parkinson's and stroke.

Box 1.3

EXAMPLES OF WHAT PUBLIC HEALTH DOES TO PROMOTE HEALTHY AGING

1. Prevent epidemics and the spread of disease
   - Influenza immunization
   - Screening for chronic disease
2. Protect against environmental hazards
   - Recognition and reduction of environmental health risks in the homes of older adults
   - Development of aging-friendly communities that promote physical activity in later life
3. Prevent injuries
   - Fall prevention programs
   - Wander prevention programs for dementia care
   - Interventions to reduce motor vehicle crashes among older adults
4. Promote and encourage healthy behaviors and mental health
   - Promotion of later life engagement (senior centers, life-long learning, volunteerism)
   - Enhancement of self-management of chronic disease
5. Respond to disasters and assist communities in recovery
   - Development and implementation response strategies that address unique concerns of older adults
6. Ensure the quality and accessibility of health services
   - Development of quality indicators for aging experiences (home care, assisted living, end-of-life care, nursing home care, etc.)
   - Training of medical professionals about aging experiences.

How does all this differ from current approaches? How does the field of public health and aging, as we envision it, differ from clinical geriatrics and gerontology? These differences should now be clear. Clinical geriatrics stresses medical management of chronic disease and rehabilitation in the face of disabilities related to these conditions (and now, increasingly, "prehabilitation" to delay the onset of disability due to disease and frailty) (Gill et al., 2002). Wallace and Gutierrez (2005) explain that, unlike clinical geriatrics, public health and aging places emphasis on prevention, proactive measures to preserve and promote health, rather than on the reactive treatment of disease. Moreover, public health focuses on the population rather than on the individual, and its programs and policies therefore address the community as a whole.

Public health and aging also overlaps with social and clinical gerontology. Like public health and aging, gerontology is concerned with the study of human aging, and involves attention not just to health, but also to the social and policy context of aging. Like geriatrics, gerontology mostly focuses on individuals rather than the experience of populations. Moreover, public health and aging is explicit in its use of population-based public health tools to address primary and secondary prevention of frailty, disease, and disability in later life. For these reasons, public health and aging represents an emerging field with a distinct focus, along with developing tools and study designs that we describe in later chapters.

POPULATION AGING AND THE GOALS OF PUBLIC HEALTH: BEYOND DISEASE PREVENTION AND HEALTH PROMOTION

As we have discussed, the goal of public health is to create circumstances under which a population is likely to achieve health. More commonly, this aim is referred to as "health promotion and disease prevention." Here, we review this goal and take up a question that is implicit in our approach to public health and aging. In an aging society, where an increasing proportion of the population survives into older ages, is the goal of health promotion and disease prevention sufficient? We argue that the focus in some cases should be broader to encompass *promotion of function*. Promoting health and promoting function may not always correspond in the real world of imperfect screening tests, invasive diagnostic technologies (whose harm is often underappreciated), otherwise successful treatments that may yet put patients at risk for new medical challenges (such as methicillin-resistant *Staphylococcus aureus* [MRSA] or *Clostridium difficile* infection in the hospital setting), and a variety of other tough calls. These challenges may go in the other direction too, as when an apparently more invasive attempt at preserving health may actually offer greater palliative and functional benefit for the person at the end of life (see Chapter 11). Reframing the challenge as "maximizing function and well-being" broadens the goals of public health but is critical, we would argue, in the case of aging populations.

Another way to frame the question is to ask how well public health's concern for people with disabilities subsumes the needs of older people. Are current approaches to disability a reasonable model for public health approaches to aging (or for thinking about aging more generally)? In this approach, aging can be seen as an accumulation of disabilities, and public health would accordingly aim to reduce the probability of disability at every age and lessen its impact on the quality of life. As we examine sources of disability in old age (in later chapters devoted to physical, cognitive, and affective function), the relevance of disability will become apparent. The difference between current public health approaches to disability and aging viewed as an accumulation of disabilities may lie in the type and generality of disability in old age (produced, for example, by slowing across multiple physiological domains) and the challenge of separating primary sources of disability and secondary conditions related to such disability among older people.

To think through these issues in light of population aging, it is helpful first to return to the elements of public health. "Health promotion" refers to activities that are not specific to any particular diseases but contribute to lowering the likelihood of disease. For example, maintaining a healthy weight, getting regular physical activity, eating a balanced diet, maintaining cognitive vitality, and managing stress would all be considered health promotion activities. These activities reduce the risk of disease and offer more immediate benefits for function. At the community level, cleaning up toxins in a neighborhood and putting in a park or walking paths would also be considered health promotion activities because they allow health-promoting behaviors, such as physical activity. Mounting evidence suggests that older adults benefit from health promotion activities, just as middle-aged and younger adults do. The gain is in lower risk of future disease and more immediate benefit in function.

"Disease prevention" includes primary, secondary, and tertiary efforts. Primary prevention efforts seek *to arrest disease processes by reducing or eliminating risk factors for disease.* Efforts of this kind include vaccination (for flu and pneumonia and now zoster), drug therapies (statins, anti-inflammatory agents, chemoprophylaxis for heart disease and possibly dementia), smoking cessation, physical therapy "prehabilitation," and assistive technology (hip protectors, grab bars, and other environmental modifications to prevent falls, for example).

Secondary prevention involves *early detection and treatment of disease to minimize morbidity and risk of disability.* These efforts involve increasing appropriate screening to detect disease at an early, asymptomatic stage. Examples of screening include checks for bone mineral density for osteoporosis, glucose metabolism for diabetes, cognitive assessment for dementia, mental health assessment to detect depression, and hypertension screening.

Tertiary prevention seeks *appropriate disease management to reduce disability.* Examples of tertiary prevention include education to support patient self-care, telemedicine to monitor clinical chemistries or heart rhythm, "lifeline" devices that allow elders to report medical emergencies, podiatry in diabetics, inhalers for pulmonary disease, and perhaps most critically a single medical provider to coordinate care.

These health promotion and disease prevention goals have been extended to people with congenital or degenerative conditions who may already face disease and disability. Here, the public health goal is to minimize the risk of "secondary conditions," conditions that may come about as the result of disability. For example, the Centers for Disease Control and Prevention (CDC) *Healthy People 2010* states:

> The health promotion and disease prevention needs of people with disabilities are not nullified because they are born with an impairing condition or have experienced a disease or injury that has long-term consequences. People with disabilities have increased health concerns and susceptibility to secondary conditions. Having a long-term condition increases the need for health promotion that can be medical, physical, social, emotional, or societal. (CDC, 2009)

How do we apply disease prevention and health promotion goals to the older adult with frailty, dementia, or terminal illness? Promoting function is a major goal of *Healthy People 2010,* which explicitly aims to increase years of healthy life, that is, disability-free years. This emphasis is carried forward in the draft vision for *Healthy People 2020,* which seeks "a society in which all people live long and healthy lives." This vision is echoed in the CDC *State of Health and Aging in America 2007,* which adopts the goal of increasing "the numbers . . . who live longer, high-quality, productive, and independent lives."

Yet, when one looks specifically at elder-specific public health recommendations beyond clinical prevention services, these documents do not say much about promoting function. The *State of Health and Aging in America 2007* offers the following additional calls to action: (a) increase physical activity among older adults by promoting environmental changes, and (b) encourage people to communicate their wishes about end-of-life care. The *Healthy People 2020* Older Adult Workgroup suggests a variety of additional goals and indicators that could be considered:

■ Increase the quality of life for those with multiple chronic illnesses
   ▲ Measure frequency and intensity of community supportive services
   ▲ Measure participation in self-management programs
   ▲ Measure use of Medicare prevention benefits and health utilization services
■ Increase the percentage of individuals reporting good physical functioning
   ▲ Measure frequency and type of exercise, including regular physical activity, vigorous physical activity, strength and endurance, flexibility, walking for transportation, bicycling for transportation
■ Decrease the rate of pressure ulcers and physical restraints in nursing homes
■ Decrease preventable hospitalizations of individuals receiving home health care
   ▲ Measure efficiency and effectiveness of transition between levels of care

These are extremely important advances in setting goals for public health and aging. They take us beyond the use of clinical prevention services and a narrow focus on disease prevention to health promotion in the fullest sense as maximization of function and well-being. However, they do not fully connect with the supportive services older adults also need for maximization of function and which, to date, have not made a bridge to public health. We turn to these in Chapter 3.

SUMMARY

Definition of Public Health and Aging. Public health and aging uses the methods and materials of public health to promote healthy aging—that is, to ensure conditions that promote the development and maintenance of optimal physical, cognitive, affective, and social well-being and function in later life. In addition to promoting primary and secondary prevention in old age, and facilitating older adults' adaptation to disease and disability, a central goal for public health and aging is to ensure conditions in the first 50 years of life that will predispose people to live a healthy second 50 years.

Defining Aging. Chronological aging is the passage of time, whereas biological aging or "senescence" involves maturation of cells and physiological systems. Senescence reflects changes that are age dependent, whereas disease represents changes that are age associated because of longer exposures to risks. In practice, senescence and disease are often difficult to distinguish, although public health interventions are currently more readily implemented to address the latter.

Types of Older Adult and Public Health Goals. It is useful to identify different types of "old age." Prominent types in geriatric care include the robust, frail, demented, and dying elder, as well as the compensating, adaptive elder. Just as the goals of medical care will be different for each type of elder, so too will the goals of public health. In the case of robust elders, the majority of whom have some chronic disease, public health goals include preventing frailty and disability. The public health goal for the frail elder is to maximize function. This typically takes two forms: environmental modification to reduce task demand, and rehabilitation to increase capacity and adapt spared abilities. The public health goals for the elder with dementia include excellent supportive care, support of informal caregivers, and, when possible, physical and cognitive remediation. For the dying patient, public health goals include a good death for both patient and family. To support compensation, the allied health specialties are critical.

How the First 50 Years Matter for Health in the Second 50 Years. It is difficult to study the ways in which health and risk behaviors in the first half of life may affect health in the second 50 years. Grip strength illustrates well the unity of the life span with respect to risk factors and later health outcomes. This is a measure of general muscle strength, easily obtained with a hand dynamometer. Grip strength in midlife is related to prenatal environment, and grip strength in midlife is related to disability in late life. These investigations represent a rare case in which a single important risk factor or health indicator has been investigated across the whole life span and related to outcomes at different points in the life span.

Successful vs. Healthy Aging. Rowe and Kahn suggested that successful aging consists of three elements: absence of disease and the risk factors for disease; maintenance of physical and cognitive abilities; and engagement in productive activities. About 20%–33% of older adults meet this definition. In contrast, the aim of public health and aging is healthy aging, that is, ensuring the conditions that allow older adults to develop and maintain optimal physical, mental, and social well-being and function across disease states and across the life span.

The Domains of Public Health and Aging. In practice, the field of public health and aging encompasses a wide variety of programs, services, and research activities. Some are aimed at health promotion and disease prevention in later life and others at self-management among those who have already developed chronic disease. Behavioral interventions that complement clinical care are of interest as are enhancements of the social context of older adults, including those geared to people living in residential or skilled nursing care settings. Development of quality indicators for particular kinds of aging experiences and settings, such as dementia care, nursing home residence, assisted living, home care, and end-of-life care, are important contributions. Programs to promote independence, through use of assistive technologies, and to maximize functioning and well-being more generally also fall in the purview of public health and aging.

Aims of Public Health in an Aging Society. In an aging society, where an increasing share of the population survives into older ages, traditional public health goals may be too narrow to meet the needs of the aged population. Instead, the aim of public health in an aging population is to maximize function and well-being of older adults irrespective of the level of disease or disability.

2 Population Aging: Demographic and Epidemiologic Perspectives

Chapter 1 defined public health's mission as promoting the conditions under which a population can be healthy (IOM, 2002). Although many individuals experience loss of health and functioning as they age, *populations* that age do not necessarily experience worsening health. To comprehend this paradox requires an understanding of what it means for a population to age, under what conditions this phenomenon occurs, and the implications of population aging for a population's health and for the aims of public health.

Population aging occurs when the age distribution of the population shifts toward older ages. The fields of demography and epidemiology offer complementary perspectives on this process. Demography is the study of population dynamics; and an increasingly important subfield, referred to as the demography of aging, emphasizes determinants and consequences of a population's age structure shifting toward older ages (Preston & Martin, 1994). Like demography, epidemiology is a population-focused science, but it emphasizes the distribution of diseases in populations, along with their causes and consequences. The subspecialty known as the epidemiology of aging has a distinctive focus on diseases among older populations (Satariano, 2006). Here, we provide both demographic and epidemiologic perspectives on critical aspects of population aging.

MEASURES OF POPULATION AGING

Projections based on the last Census suggest that in 2010, approximately 40 million people in the United States will be aged 65 or older, accounting for about 13% of the U.S. population (U.S. Census Bureau, 2004a). Over 6 million Americans, 2% of the total population, will be age 85 or older. The centenarian population—individuals ages 100 or older—reached 50,000 in 2000 (Hetzel & Smith, 2001), and given current mortality rates this figure is projected to nearly double approximately every 10 years (Krach & Velkoff, 1999). The median age, defined as the age at which half the population is older and half younger, will be about 37 in 2010. Compared with the world's "oldest" countries (with at least 10% of their population age 65 and older), the United States ranked 41st in 2006 (see Table 2.1). At the top of the list are Japan, Italy, Germany, and Greece, all with at least 19% of the population aged 65 and older.

Table 2.1

POPULATION OF COUNTRIES WITH AT LEAST 10% OF POPULATION AGE 65 AND OVER, 2006

		65 AND OVER	
REGION OR COUNTRY	TOTAL	NUMBER	PERCENT
Japan	127,464	25,535	20.0
Italy	58,134	11,450	19.7
Germany	82,422	16,018	19.4
Greece	10,688	2,027	19.0
Spain	40,398	7,170	17.7
Sweden	9,017	1,588	17.6
Belgium	10,379	1,809	17.4
Bulgaria	7,385	1,279	17.3
Estonia	1,324	228	17.2
Portugal	10,606	1,822	17.2
Austria	8,193	1,401	17.1

(Continued)

Table 2.1

POPULATION OF COUNTRIES WITH AT LEAST 10% OF POPULATION AGE 65 AND OVER, 2006 (*Continued*)

| REGION OR COUNTRY | TOTAL | 65 AND OVER | |
		NUMBER	PERCENT
Croatia	4,495	754	16.8
Georgia	4,661	768	16.5
France	60,876	9,998	16.4
Latvia	2,275	373	16.4
Ukraine	46,620	7,628	16.4
Finland	5,231	846	16.2
United Kingdom	60,609	9,564	15.8
Slovenia	2,010	315	15.7
Switzerland	7,524	1,171	15.6
Lithuania	3,586	554	15.5
Denmark	5,451	828	15.2
Hungary	9,981	1,518	15.2
Serbia	10,140	1,544	15.2
Belarus	9,766	1,462	15.0
Norway	4,611	683	14.8
Romania	22,304	3,275	14.7
Luxembourg	474	69	14.6
Czech Republic	10,235	1,481	14.5
Bosnia and Herzegovina	4,499	647	14.4
Netherlands	16,491	2,349	14.2
Russia	142,069	20,196	14.2
Malta	400	55	13.7
Montenegro	692	95	13.7
Canada	33,099	4,407	13.3
Poland	38,537	5,128	13.3
Uruguay	3,432	455	13.3
Australia	20,264	2,649	13.1

(*Continued*)

Table 2.1

POPULATION OF COUNTRIES WITH AT LEAST 10% OF POPULATION AGE 65 AND OVER, 2006 (*Continued*)

| REGION OR COUNTRY | TOTAL | 65 AND OVER | |
		NUMBER	PERCENT
Hong Kong S.A.R.	6,940	890	12.8
Puerto Rico	3,928	504	12.8
United States	298,444	37,196	12.5
Slovakia	5,439	653	12.0
New Zealand	4,076	481	11.8
Iceland	299	35	11.7
Cyprus	784	91	11.6
Ireland	4,062	470	11.6
Virgin Islands (U.S.)	109	12	11.2
Armenia	2,976	332	11.1
Macedonia	2,051	225	11.0
Moldova	4,326	465	10.7
Argentina	39,922	4,244	10.6
Cuba	11,383	1,206	10.6
Martinique	436	46	10.6

From Federal Interagency Forum on Aging-Related Statistics, 2006.

Such statistics suggest that the United States has a sizeable population living into what has traditionally been considered old age; however, these statistics say little about whether the population is aging. Demographers define population aging as a *shift in the age distribution of the population toward older ages.* The phenomenon is most often measured by increases in the percentage of the population reaching old age, but can also be captured by changes in a population's distribution across age groups (illustrated by age and sex in a population "pyramid") and by changes in ratios of the older to younger population ("age-dependency" or "support" ratios). By all three standards, the U.S. population is aging and has been for over a century, but the pace has accelerated over the past several decades.

Although some demographers have argued against use of a chronological age to indicate late life (Robine & Michel, 2004), reaching the threshold of normal retirement age—in the United States still age 65 for those born before 1938—is most often synonymous with reaching old age. At the turn of the century only 3 million people—less than 4% of the total population—were age 65 (Federal Interagency Forum on Aging-Related Statistics, 2008). Today, approximately 13% are considered old, and by 2030 the proportion of people in the United States aged 65 and older will approach 20% of the total population (Table 2.2). Other age cutoffs indicate a similar increase. For example, the percentage of the total population aged 85 or older is projected to reach 2.6% (nearly 10 million) in 2030 (U.S. Census Bureau, 2004a).

Population pyramids for the United States in 2010 and 2030 are shown in Figure 2.1. The pyramids depict the number of men (left) and women (right) in millions in each 5-year age group, ordered from lowest to highest. By comparing shapes across the two pyramids, the shifting age distribution toward older ages is readily apparent. These age-sex pyramids are perhaps less of a pyramid than an emerging rectangle or pillar, a typical shape for countries that have already undergone the demographic transition, in which a regime of high mortality and fertility is replaced by

Table 2.2

ESTIMATES AND PROJECTIONS OF THE NUMBER AND PERCENTAGE OF THE U.S. POPULATION AGES 65 AND OLDER AND 85 AND OLDER: 2000–2050 (U.S. CENSUS BUREAU, 2004A)

| YEAR | 65 AND OVER | | 85 AND OVER | |
	NUMBER	PERCENT	NUMBER	PERCENT
2000	35.0	12.4	4.2	1.5
2010	40.2	13.0	6.1	2.0
2020	54.6	16.3	7.3	2.2
2030	71.5	19.6	9.6	2.6
2040	80.0	20.4	15.4	3.9
2050	86.7	20.6	20.9	5.0

one of low mortality and fertility (see below). The left-hand figure has a bulge in the center, with age groups between 45–49 and 60–64 clearly the most populous. These age strata correspond to the aging baby boom generation, people born in the years 1946–1964. Lower fertility after this period, which continued over the next three decades, has led to fewer people at younger ages and hence absence of a wide base for the pyramid. By 2030, the pyramid will be even more rectangular, with age groups 65 and older nearly as populous as the nonelderly age groups. Projections of developed countries portend that by 2040 the pyramid shape will begin to invert as the age group 80 and older outnumbers all other age groups (Kinsella & He, 2009).

Both pyramids also show the strong preponderance of women over men in later life. Among people aged 65 and older, the sex ratio (number of women for each man) is 1.4; for people aged 85 and older it is 2.5, and for people 100 and older it is 4.0. This asymmetry affects living arrangements and marital status in important ways, leaving older women more likely to live alone, depend on children when frail, and enter assisted living and nursing homes at higher rates than men (for further discussion of long-term care, see Chapter 9).

A shift in age structure is also occurring in many less developed countries. Figure 2.2 shows the projected transformation in age structure underway in Pakistan for the years 2000, 2025, and 2050. In the 25 years separating the first two panels of the figure, the proportion of the population aged 65 and older will rise from 4.1% to 5.6%, 5.8 to 12.0 million people. In this period, life expectancy will also rise from 61.1 to 69.8 years. The major engine of this demographic transformation is declining fertility. In the same period, the number of births per 1,000 women will decline from 32 to 6; and completed fertility will drop from 4.6 children per woman to 2.3 (U.S. Census Bureau, International Data Base, 2002). With fewer children born, the base of the age-sex pyramid shrinks and the mean (or median) age of the population must rise, because people already alive continue to age. If this trend continues, as is expected, most of the world's countries will eventually have an age distribution shaped more like a pillar and less like a pyramid (Kinsella & He, 2009).

Aggregating across the strata of the pyramid gives the size of the older (aged 65 and older) population, or the combined young (ages 0–18) and older populations, relative to people of working age (ages 18–64). These so-called "support" ratios do not actually measure dependency, either in health or economic terms. In fact, only a minority of people

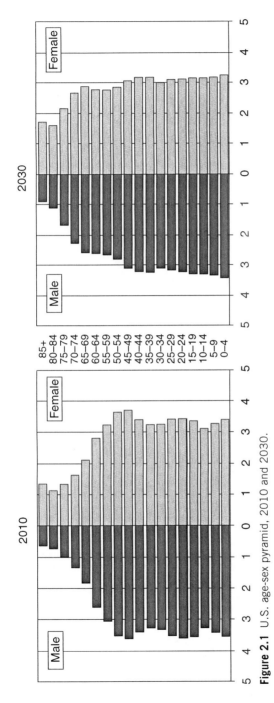

Figure 2.1 U.S. age-sex pyramid, 2010 and 2030.

Source: From "Population Projections. Interim Projections Consistent With Census 2000. Population Pyramids and Demographic Summary Indicators for U.S. Regions and Divisions," by U.S. Census Bureau, 2004b. Retrieved March 23, 2008 from http://www .census.gov/population/projections/52PyrmdUS1.pdf and http://www.census.gov/population/projections/52PyrmdUS3.pdf.

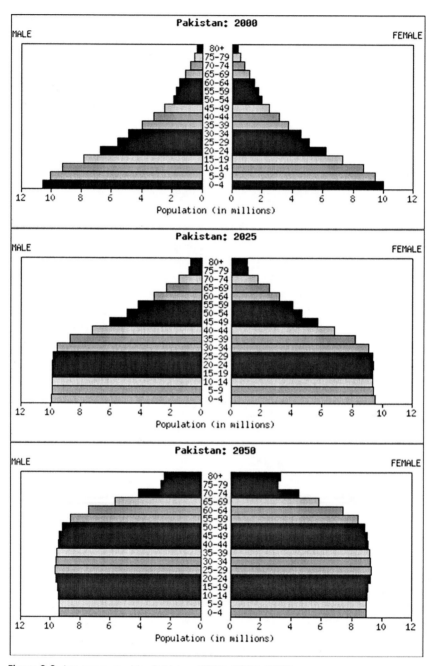

Figure 2.2 Age-sex pyramids, Pakistan, 2000, 2025, 2050.

Source: From http://148.129.75.3/ipc/www/idbnew.html (U.S. Census Bureau, International Data Base).

aged 65 and older, about 20%–25%, can be considered dependent, at least according to need for help in one or more of the personal self-maintenance activities, or ADLs (bathing, dressing, grooming, feeding, using toilet), and this proportion has declined over the past few decades (Spillman, 2004). Increasingly, people aged 65 and older delay retiring, provide intergenerational transfers of resources to their children aged 18–64, and contribute to child-rearing support for grandchildren. Instead, these ratios are more useful for providing insight into the age distribution of the population. Shifts in the elderly support ratio, in particular, indicate population aging. The elderly support ratio, obtained by dividing the number of elderly people per 100 working age population, was 21 for the United States in 2008 (Kinsella & He, 2009) and is projected to be 37 by 2030 (Kinsella & Velkoff, 2001).

Demographers have long recognized that the number of people in any given age group is influenced by births (or new entrants into an age group), deaths (or aging out of a given age group), and net migration (moving in or out of the geographic area of interest). Population aging cannot be attributed to high or low levels of fertility, mortality, or migration but to changes in such rates. The long-term downward trend in birth rates (the higher fertility of the baby boom cohorts notwithstanding) was the dominant factor driving population aging through the first half of the 20th century in the United States. During the 1980s, however, reductions in mortality at older ages were the dominant factor shaping population aging (Preston, Himes, & Eggers, 1989). Long-term shifts in birth and death rates are known more generally as the demographic transition.

THE DEMOGRAPHIC TRANSITION

The demographic transition is a model that describes sweeping changes that populations undergo from high to low rates of deaths and births (Population Reference Bureau, 2004). The model was initially developed based on data from the 19th century in Western Europe. It characterized the population's transition as an ordered sequence of four stages (Figure 2.3). In the first stage, a population has high birth rates, high death rates, and hence little or no population growth. The first stage is exemplified by agrarian, nonindustrialized societies, which historically averaged 35–45 deaths and births per 1,000 people. A population undergoing the second stage is characterized by high birth rates and falling death rates at younger ages as living conditions and nutrition improve, and hence rapid population growth. In the third stage, birth rates begin to decline while death rates remain low. As a result, population growth slows and the population begins to age.

The final stage was initially thought to consist of very low and relatively constant birth and death rates, and consequently very low or no population growth and a constant age distribution. Industrialized, urban societies in the 1980s, for example, with fertility and mortality rates of approximately 10–15/1,000, were thought to have reached the final stage (Mausner & Kramer, 1985). However, even "old" populations have experienced continued declines in mortality rates at older ages (see below), raising the possibility of a different fourth stage. In such a regime, birth rates are low and old-age death rates continue to decline, leading to low population growth, but, importantly, a continued shift toward older ages, or population aging.

The Demographic Transition and Declining Death Rates

The mortality side of this transition is clearly seen for death rates in Sweden over three centuries, summarized by Horiuchi (2003). Data for this

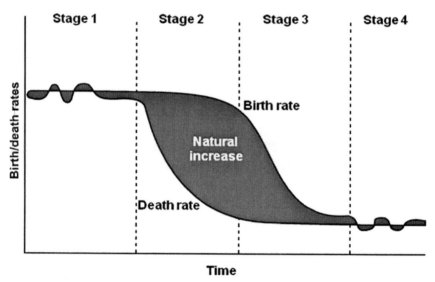

Figure 2.3 The demographic transition.

Source: From Population Reference Bureau, www.prb.org/LP/training_manual/DemoTrans.ppt. Reprinted with permission.
Note: Naturral incresase is produced from the excess of births over deaths.

comparison are not easily available, because the comparison requires nearly 300 years of continuous, complete mortality data on a national scale. Sweden is one of the few countries with vital registration systems that have collected such data. Figure 2.4 shows death rates for three cohorts of Swedish women, the first born in 1751–1755, the second in 1876–1880, and the third in 1951–1955. The figure (which graphs mortality on a logarithmic scale) shows little difference in mortality risk for the first two cohorts. Mortality is well over 10% per person-year in the first 1–2 years of life, reaches its nadir (<1%) at about age 10, hovers around 1%–3% until age 35 or so, and then climbs exponentially (i.e., doubling every 7 years or so).

The mortality risk is completely different for the third birth cohort (1951–1955), born 100 years later. Mortality in the perinatal period for this cohort is <1%, the mortality nadir is again around age 10 (as it is in all human populations), but is well under 1/1,000, and mortality risk does not reach 1% until age 60 or so. At every age, except perhaps when people reach their eighties, mortality for the most recent birth cohort is vastly lower than it is in the prior cohorts.

It is useful as well to plot the distribution of deaths by age for the three cohorts. Figure 2.5 shows what proportion of deaths occurred at each age across the life span. For the 18th and 19th century birth

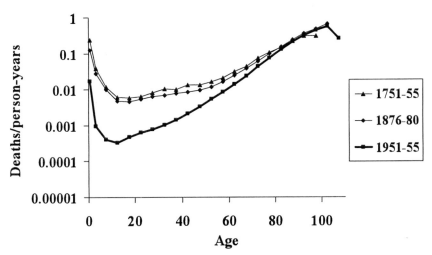

Figure 2.4 Death rates by age for Swedish females, three centuries.

Source: Prepared by Shiro Horiuchi, using Human Mortality Database (2003), http://www.mortality.org.

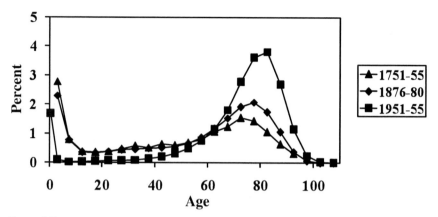

Figure 2.5 Distribution of ages at death: three cohorts of Swedish women, three centuries.

Source: Prepared by Shiro Horiuchi, using Human Mortality Database (2003), http://www.mortality.org.

cohorts, a relatively high risk of death prevails at all ages. Certainly, there are modes at both very young and very old ages, but high numbers of people are also dying at all ages across the life span. With the more recent 20th century birth cohort, the age distribution of deaths is quite different. Here, deaths are concentrated at the oldest ages, as shown in a large shift to the right in the distribution of deaths. The vast majority of deaths now occur in people over age 60.

If we add an even more recent birth cohort and plot its age distribution at death, as Figure 2.6 does, we see that this trend continues into our own era. The age distribution of death for Swedish women born 1996–1999 is pushed even further to the right and is even more clearly unimodal. Almost all deaths are concentrated in later life, with a mode above age 80.

These data should be kept in mind when examining the declining death rate in late life in the past half century. Although mortality rises with age, such that the annual risk of death approaches 15% for people in their early eighties, between 1950 and 2000 the rate of death for people over age 80 has actually declined. Declines in mortality for people aged 85 and older between 1950 and 2000 across a number of countries are shown in Figure 2.7. Between 1950 and 1990 death rates declined from 170 to 90 per 1,000 in the oldest old (Vaupel, 1997). Stratifying by age and plotting death rates by year shows that death rates fell even for people aged 90 and 95.

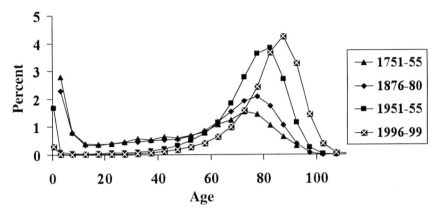

Figure 2.6 Age distribution of ages at death for Swedish females, selected periods, 1990s cohort.

Source: Prepared by Shiro Horiuchi, using Human Mortality Database (2003), available at http://www.mortality.org or www.humanmortality.de

Why should death rates among the oldest old population be declining? Some of the decline is probably due to medical advances applied specifically to the diseases of the very old. More of the decline is probably due to improvements in health and living conditions over the whole life course. The latter changes appear to have allowed a subset of people with some kind of long-life genetic endowment— "longevity genes"—to reach old age. While this genotype must have always been present in a subset of the human population, only in the 20th century have health and living conditions improved to the point where accidental mortality (such as death from trauma or infection) has been controlled well enough for substantial numbers to reach later life.

Will mortality rates continue to decline and life span continue to increase? The answer is hotly debated and depends in part on whether human populations have a limit to their life span—that is, a limit on the maximum number of years that can be lived—and, if so, whether humans have begun to reach such limits. Olshansky, Carnes, and Cassel (1990) have demonstrated that mortality rates would have to decline dramatically to very low levels for life expectancy to exceed 90 years in the 21st century. In contrast, Vaupel's findings that death rates for the oldest old have decreased over time and that mortality rates actually decelerate at approximately age 80, seem to suggest that continued declines are possible.

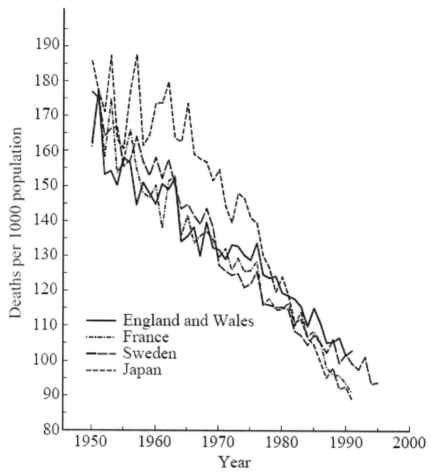

Figure 2.7 Mortality reductions in people aged 80 and older.

Source: From "The Remarkable Improvements in Survival at Older Ages," by J. W. Vaupel, 1997. *Philosophical Transactions of the Royal Society of London. Series B, Biological Sciences, 352,* 1799–1804; Figure 2, p. 1800.

The Demographic Transition and Increasing Life Expectancy

As mortality rates shift, populations experience changes in life expectancy. According to the National Center for Health Statistics, life expectancy at birth in the United States has nearly doubled in the past century to nearly 78 years in 2004 (Arias, 2007). Not everyone alive or born in 2004 can expect to live to this age. Instead, life expectancy is a hypothetical summary measure calculated by use of a demographic tool called the life table. The life table is a model of what would happen to a hypothetical birth cohort if age-specific death rates for a given period were to remain constant and were to apply throughout the experience of the entire generation.

Although we cannot give a full description of life table functions here, life expectancy cannot be fully understood without at least a basic familiarity with the life table. Essentially, the life table model applies the mortality risk prevailing at a given time to a hypothetical birth cohort, typically 100,000 in size. Mortality rates for each age (or age group, if abridged) are then applied to the cohort. An unabridged life table for the United States in 2004 (Arias, 2007) is shown in Table 2.3.

The function nqx is simply the mortality rate (proportion dying) for each age group in that year. Plotting nqx on the ordinate and age on the x-axis reveals the bathtub or j-shaped curve typical of mortality for human populations: a small but sharp upturn in the perinatal period, a decline that reaches its nadir at ages 5–15, and a slow but steady increase after this age.

The function l_x is the number of people entering each age interval; by convention, the starting number, or radix, is usually 100,000. The number of people entering each age interval reflects the number of deaths in the prior interval. The survival curve, or proportion of the population surviving to each age, is traced out by the l_x column. Fifty percent of the cohort is still alive at age 81.

The function ndx is the number of people dying in each age interval. If we multiply the mortality rate (nqx) by the number of people entering each age interval (l_x), we obtain ndx, the number of deaths. The number of people dying in each age interval is subtracted from the total and yields the number of people surviving to enter the next interval.

The function $_nLx$ is the number of person-years lived by the cohort in each age interval. The total number of person-years is the product of l_x and the number of years that define the age interval (1 year in a standard life shown in Figure 2.3; 5 years in an abridged life table). In calculating nLx we need to make an assumption about the timing of death. Did people die at the beginning or end of the age interval? This assumption clearly affects the total person-years contributed by the cohort in the age interval. By convention, we assume that people die in the middle of the age interval, except for the 0–1 age interval, which demands more sophisticated treatment because most deaths are concentrated near the time of birth.

Table 2.3

LIFE TABLE FOR THE TOTAL POPULATION: UNITED STATES, 2004

AGE	PROBABILITY OF DYING BETWEEN AGES X AND X+1 $Q(X)$	NUMBER SURVIVING TO AGE X $L(X)$	NUMBER DYING BETWEEN AGES X AND X+1 $D(X)$	PERSON-YEARS LIVED BETWEEN AGES X AND X+1 $L(X)$	TOTAL NUMBER OF PERSON-YEARS LIVED ABOVE AGE X $T(X)$	EXPECTATION OF LIFE AT AGE X $E(X)$
0–1	0.006799	100,000	680	99,403	7,783,712	77.8
1–2	0.000483	99,320	48	99,296	7,684,309	77.4
2–3	0.000297	99,272	29	99,257	7,585,013	76.4
3–4	0.000224	99,243	22	99,232	7,485,755	75.4
4–5	0.000188	99,220	19	99,211	7,386,524	74.4
5–6	0.000171	99,202	17	99,193	7,287,313	73.5
6–7	0.000161	99,185	16	99,177	7,188,119	72.5
7–8	0.000151	99,169	15	99,161	7,088,943	71.5
8–9	0.000136	99,154	14	99,147	6,989,781	70.5
9–10	0.000119	99,140	12	99,134	6,890,634	69.5
10–11	0.000106	99,129	11	99,123	6,791,500	68.5
11–12	0.000112	99,118	11	99,112	6,692,377	67.5
12–13	0.000149	99,107	15	99,100	6,593,264	66.5
13–14	0.000227	99,092	23	99,081	6,494,164	65.5
14–15	0.000337	99,070	33	99,053	6,395,084	64.6

Age						
15–16	0.000460	99,036	46	99,014	6,296,031	63.6
16–17	0.000579	98,991	57	98,962	6,197,017	62.6
17–18	0.000684	98,933	68	98,900	6,098,055	61.6
18–19	0.000763	98,866	75	98,828	5,999,155	60.7
19–20	0.000819	98,790	81	98,750	5,900,327	59.7
20–21	0.000873	98,709	86	98,666	5,801,578	58.8
21–22	0.000926	98,623	91	98,577	5,702,911	57.8
22–23	0.000960	98,532	95	98,484	5,604,334	56.9
23–24	0.000972	98,437	96	98,389	5,505,850	55.9
24–25	0.000969	98,341	95	98,294	5,407,460	55.0
25–26	0.000960	98,246	94	98,199	5,309,166	54.0
26–27	0.000954	98,152	94	98,105	5,210,967	53.1
27–28	0.000952	98,058	93	98,012	5,112,862	52.1
28–29	0.000958	97,965	94	97,918	5,014,850	51.2
29–30	0.000973	97,871	95	97,824	4,916,932	50.2
30–31	0.000994	97,776	97	97,727	4,819,109	49.3
31–32	0.001023	97,679	100	97,629	4,721,382	48.3
32–33	0.001063	97,579	104	97,527	4,623,753	47.4
33–34	0.001119	97,475	109	97,420	4,526,226	46.4
34–35	0.001192	97,366	116	97,308	4,428,805	45.5

(Continued)

Table 2.3

LIFE TABLE FOR THE TOTAL POPULATION: UNITED STATES, 2004 (*continued*)

AGE	PROBABILITY OF DYING BETWEEN AGES X AND X+1 Q (X)	NUMBER SURVIVING TO AGE X L (X)	NUMBER DYING BETWEEN AGES X AND X+1 D (X)	PERSON-YEARS LIVED BETWEEN AGES X AND X+1 L (X)	TOTAL NUMBER OF PERSON-YEARS LIVED ABOVE AGE X T (X)	EXPECTATION OF LIFE AT AGE X E (X)
35–36	0.001275	97,250	124	97,188	4,331,497	44.5
36–37	0.001373	97,126	133	97,059	4,234,310	43.6
37–38	0.001493	96,993	145	96,920	4,137,250	42.7
38–39	0.001634	96,848	158	96,769	4,040,330	41.7
39–40	0.001788	96,690	173	96,603	3,943,562	40.8
40–41	0.001945	96,517	188	96,423	3,846,959	39.9
41–42	0.002107	96,329	203	96,227	3,750,536	38.9
42–43	0.002287	96,126	220	96,016	3,654,308	38.0
43–44	0.002494	95,906	239	95,787	3,558,292	37.1
44–45	0.002727	95,667	261	95,537	3,462,506	36.2
45–46	0.002982	95,406	284	95,264	3,366,969	35.3
46–47	0.003246	95,122	309	94,967	3,271,705	34.4
47–48	0.003520	94,813	334	94,646	3,176,738	33.5
48–49	0.003799	94,479	359	94,300	3,082,092	32.6

49–50	0.004088	94,120	385	93,928	2,987,792	31.7
50–51	0.004404	93,735	413	93,529	2,893,864	30.9
51–52	0.004750	93,323	443	93,101	2,800,335	30.0
52–53	0.005113	92,879	475	92,642	2,707,234	29.1
53–54	0.005488	92,404	507	92,151	2,614,592	28.3
54–55	0.005879	91,897	540	91,627	2,522,441	27.4
55–56	0.006295	91,357	575	91,070	2,430,814	26.6
56–57	0.006754	90,782	613	90,475	2,339,744	25.8
57–58	0.007280	90,169	656	89,841	2,249,269	24.9
58–59	0.007903	89,512	707	89,159	2,159,428	24.1
59–60	0.008633	88,805	767	88,422	2,070,269	23.3
60–61	0.009493	88,038	836	87,621	1,981,848	22.5
61–62	0.010449	87,203	911	86,747	1,894,227	21.7
62–63	0.011447	86,291	988	85,798	1,807,480	20.9
63–64	0.012428	85,304	1060	84,774	1,721,683	20.2
64–65	0.013408	84,244	1130	83,679	1,636,909	19.4
65–66	0.014473	83,114	1203	82,513	1,553,230	18.7
66–67	0.015703	81,911	1286	81,268	1,470,718	18.0
67–68	0.017081	80,625	1377	79,936	1,389,450	17.2
68–69	0.018623	79,248	1476	78,510	1,309,513	16.5

(Continued)

Table 2.3

LIFE TABLE FOR THE TOTAL POPULATION: UNITED STATES, 2004 (*continued*)

AGE	PROBABILITY OF DYING BETWEEN AGES X AND X+1 $Q(X)$	NUMBER SURVIVING TO AGE X $L(X)$	NUMBER DYING BETWEEN AGES X AND X+1 $D(X)$	PERSON-YEARS LIVED BETWEEN AGES X AND X+1 $L(X)$	TOTAL NUMBER OF PERSON-YEARS LIVED ABOVE AGE X $T(X)$	EXPECTATION OF LIFE AT AGE X $E(X)$
69–70	0.020322	77,772	1580	76,982	1,231,004	15.8
70–71	0.022104	76,191	1684	75,349	1,154,022	15.1
71–72	0.024023	74,507	1790	73,612	1,078,673	14.5
72–73	0.026216	72,717	1906	71,764	1,005,060	13.8
73–74	0.028745	70,811	2035	69,793	933,296	13.2
74–75	0.031561	68,776	2171	67,690	863,503	12.6
75–76	0.034427	66,605	2293	65,458	795,812	11.9
76–77	0.037379	64,312	2404	63,110	730,354	11.4
77–78	0.040756	61,908	2523	60,646	667,244	10.8
78–79	0.044764	59,385	2658	58,056	606,597	10.2
79–80	0.049395	56,727	2802	55,326	548,542	9.7
80–81	0.054471	53,925	2937	52,456	493,216	9.1
81–82	0.059772	50,987	3048	49,463	440,760	8.6
82–83	0.065438	47,940	3137	46,371	391,297	8.2
83–84	0.071598	44,803	3208	43,199	344,925	7.7

84–85	0.078516	41,595	3266	39,962	301,727	7.3
85–86	0.085898	38,329	3292	36,683	261,765	6.8
86–87	0.093895	35,037	3290	33,392	225,082	6.4
87–88	0.102542	31,747	3255	30,119	191,690	6.0
88–89	0.111875	28,491	3187	26,898	161,571	5.7
89–90	0.121928	25,304	3085	23,761	134,673	5.3
90–91	0.132733	22,219	2949	20,744	110,912	5.0
91–92	0.144318	19,270	2781	17,879	90,168	4.7
92–93	0.156707	16,489	2584	15,197	72,289	4.4
93–94	0.169922	13,905	2363	12,723	57,092	4.1
94–95	0.183975	11,542	2123	10,480	44,369	3.8
95–96	0.198875	9,419	1873	8,482	33,889	3.6
96–97	0.214620	7,545	1619	6,736	25,407	3.4
97–98	0.231201	5,926	1370	5,241	18,671	3.2
98–99	0.248600	4,556	1133	3,990	13,430	2.9
99–100	0.266786	3,423	913	2,967	9,440	2.8
100 or over	1.00000	2,510	2510	6,473	6,473	2.6

From "United States Life Tables, 2004," by E. Arias, 2007. *National Vital Statistics Reports* (Vol. 56). Hyattsville, MD: National Center for Health Statistics. Retrieved May 15, 2009, from http://www.cdc.gov/nchs/data/nvsr/nvsr56/nvsr56_09.pdf.

The function T_x is the sum of nLx. It is the total number of person-years lived by the birth cohort in the given age interval and in all subsequent ones. Thus, the T_x entry in the first row of the life table is the sum down the column of all nLx entries and gives the total number of person-years lived by the birth cohort, 7,783,712 years. The second row T_x value shows that cohort members who survived the first year of life lived a total of 7,604,389 years. People who survived to age 85 lived a total of 261,765 person-years in this and subsequent years until the last person died.

If we divide T_x by l_x in any given age interval, we obtain e^x, life expectancy at a given age. Thus, life expectancy at birth for the U.S. population in 2004 was 7,783,712/100,000, or 77.8 years. Life expectancy at age 50 was 30.9 years, and at age 80, 9.1 years.

Life expectancy at a given age, then, is simply the total number of person-years lived by persons reaching that age, divided by the number of people reaching that age. Life expectancy at birth (usually called simply "life expectancy") is the total number of person years lived by a birth cohort divided by the number of people in the cohort. It is the average number of years a person can expect to live—with, we must hasten to add, all the assumptions that go into the life table model. The major assumption in these models is a fixed mortality schedule; the models assume that prevailing mortality rates do not change over the lifetime of the cohort. They also assume a fixed birth cohort, with no loss or gain to migration.

How then does life expectancy (at birth) change with the demographic transition? In the first stage of the demographic transition, life expectancy is low, typically age 20–30. As mortality rates begin to fall at younger ages, life expectancy increases to the 30–50 range. In stage 3, as death rates reach very low rates, life expectancy exceeds age 50 and may reach as high as age 70. In stage 4, if death rates continue to drop at advanced ages, life expectancy can reach age 80 and beyond.

THE EPIDEMIOLOGIC TRANSITION AND SHIFTING CAUSES OF DEATH

Whereas the demographic transition emphasizes shifting birth and death rates, the epidemiologic transition, a theory first proposed by Omran in the 1970s, focuses on causes of death as a population shifts from high- to low-mortality regimes. (For more on mortality and how causes of death are identified, see Chapter 10.) The stages of the epidemiologic transition correspond directly to the first three stages of the demographic transition, but the emphasis is on causes of death and the speed of change may vary. Stage 1 (high birth and death rates) was deemed the age of "pestilence and famine." Infectious and parasitic diseases such as pneumonia and influenza, tuberculosis, diarrhea, and enteritis dominated this period (along with deaths due to war, famine, malnutrition, and complications of childbirth). Stage 2 (falling death rates at younger ages and high population growth) was dubbed the "age of receding pandemics" and characterized by the emergence of degenerative diseases, notably heart disease, as a major cause of death. In stage 3 (declining birth rate, low death rates, and very low population growth), dubbed the "age of degenerative and man-made diseases" chronic degenerative diseases—heart disease, cancer, stroke, chronic obstructive pulmonary diseases—dominated as causes of death. Olshansky and Ault (1986) postulated the existence of a fourth stage, dubbed "the age of delayed degenerative diseases." In the proposed stage 4, the causes of death are similar to those in stage 3, but the age of death increases as a consequence of prevention and health promotion efforts.

Although not explicitly recognized by Omran's original theory, the epidemiologic transition also results in a fundamental shift in the morbidity profile of adults. As populations enter the 3rd and 4th stages of the transition, the prevalence of chronic conditions increases, although they may be less debilitating (Manton, 1989). In the United States, as in most developed countries, the two most common chronic conditions—arthritis and hypertension—are not among the most common causes of death (Table 2.4).

WHY POPULATION AGING MATTERS

According to demographers, "population aging will be one of the most important social phenomena of the next half century" (Preston & Martin, 1994). In the United States, population aging over the next few decades will be keenly felt in all major social institutions. Families will undoubtedly change in terms of composition and dynamics, work and retirement will be transformed, and the country's major social transfer programs—Social Security and Medicare—will be strained without major changes in financing or eligibility. Two additional consequences, the shifting health care needs of the population and the emergence of an oldest old population, are especially germane for public health.

Table 2.4

MOST COMMON CAUSES OF DEATH VS. MOST PREVALENT CONDITIONS

Cause of death	Prevalent conditions
Heart disease	Hypertension
Cancer	Arthritis
Stroke	Heart disease
COPD	Cancer
Unintentional injuries	Diabetes
Diabetes	COPD/Asthma
Alzheimer's disease	Stroke

From http://www.cdc.gov/nchs/products/pubs/pubd/hestats/finaldeaths04/finaldeaths04
.htm and Older Americans 2008: Key Indicators of Well-Being.

Shifting Health Care Needs of the Population

For over three decades demographers have debated the implications of longer life for population health and health care needs. Gruenberg (1977) argued that longer life meant worsening health and warned of a pandemic of disease and disability. Fries' famous "compression of morbidity" hypothesis (Fries, 1980; Fries & Crapo, 1981) purported the opposite: as individuals, on average, lived longer and the population approached the limits to human life, the period of morbidity before death would be compressed into a shorter period. Manton (1989) offered a third perspective, dubbed "dynamic equilibrium," which explicitly recognized the complex interactions among morbidity, disability, and mortality processes. The three processes are interrelated so that interventions designed to affect one of the processes inevitably influence the other two as well. Years of life are gained through a combination of postponement of disease onset, reductions of severity of disease and speed of progression, and improved techniques for clinical management.

These differing perspectives can be illustrated with the World Health Organization's model (1981) of the relationship between morbidity, disability, and survival (Figure 2.8). The curves in the figure represent the proportion of the population surviving to each age without morbidity (or subclinical disability), disability, and death, respectively. The model assumes that the survival function from the 2004 life table holds and presents hypothetical curves for morbidity and disability under the assumption that these risks follow the pattern established for survival: an increasing, accelerating risk with age. Further, these risks are assumed to be nested: morbidity precedes disability, so that people develop disease before disability, and everyone with disability has passed through a period of morbidity. Similarly, states of disability, with varying duration, precede mortality.

In this model, the proportion of older people surviving to each age is shown in the outermost curve. In the figure, which is based on the 2004 life table described above, 50% of elders are still alive at age 81. The area under the survival curve indicates the total person-years lived by the cohort. Survival in this model is further partitioned according to functional status. The area under the remaining curves represent person-years spent by the population without morbidity (under curve C) and with morbidity but no disability (between curves B and C). Person-years lived with disability are represented by the area between the survival and disability curves (curves A and B).

Increases in life expectancy mean that the survival curve in Figure 2.8 is shifting upward and to the right. The key question is whether the disability curve is shifting in the same direction at the same pace. If the disability curve shifts at a slower pace than the survival curve, then an expansion of the number of person-years of disability will occur, and active life expectancy will decline as a share of life expectancy, as predicted by Gruenberg (1977). If the disability curve moves outward at a rate faster than the survival curve, person-years of disability across the life span will be reduced. Accordingly, active life expectancy will increase as a share of life expectancy, as predicted by Fries (1983). In contrast, Manton's

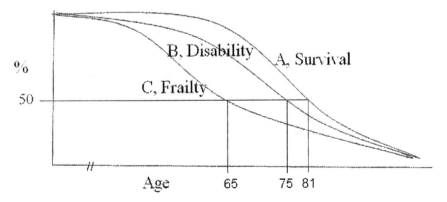

Figure 2.8 WHO model of observed survival and hypothetical morbidity and disability.

theory of dynamic equilibrium anticipates that all three curves will shift and change in shape with reduction in the incidence, prevalence, or severity of a disease. Thus, during one period a population may experience an expansion, and during another, a compression of morbidity. In fact, the evidence over the past 30 years for the United States is consistent with dynamic equilibrium, with expansion occurring during the 1970s and compression beginning in the 1980s (Crimmins, Saito, & Ingegneri, 1997a). As discussed in more detail in Chapter 5, evidence for more recent years is mixed, with some studies suggesting a continued compression and at least one finding a leveling off of active life expectancy.

Emergence of the Oldest Old in America

An additional consequence of population aging is the emergence of an "oldest old" population. The oldest old are typically defined as people aged 85 and older (Suzman, Willis, & Manton, 1992). Some of the characteristics of this group, now numbering 5.3 million (Federal Interagency Forum on Aging-Related Statistics, 2008), include:

- They are the fastest growing segment of older population in the United States; in fact, the United States will have the largest number of oldest old of any country in the next 50 years. This is a paradox because the United States will not have the most elderly, as defined by the proportion aged 65 and older.
- They are largely female (68% are women and 32% men), White, and widowed. Note, however, that people aged 65 and older are becoming increasingly more diverse racially. And women are twice as likely to be widowed as men (76% vs. 34%).
- In 2006, only 11% were living in poverty. This figure had declined steadily from 21% in 1982. The oldest old are also increasingly well educated. Educational attainment in this group has increased dramatically: 29.1% completed high school in 1985, and 63% of this age group is expected to have completed high school in 2015.
- Fewer women in this age group will be childless, compared with the young-old, although fewer will also have 5 or more offspring. This may affect the availability of family caregivers.
- The proportion of men aged 85 and older who are veterans is projected to increase from 33% in 2000 to over 60% in 2010.
- They are high consumers of supportive care. In 2005, 17% resided in a nursing home (a decline from nearly 25% in 1985) and an-

other 7% in community housing with services (sometimes called "assisted living"), such as meals, housekeeping, laundry, or medication management. Average annual Medicare costs were $22,000 per enrollee. Average nursing home costs were over $7,000.

■ Sixty-two percent of people age 85 and older have trouble hearing, 27% have trouble seeing, and 32% are edentulous, that is, have lost all of their natural teeth; 19% report depressive symptoms.

■ Thirty-eight percent of oldest old men and 56% of oldest old women are unable to perform common physical functions, such as stooping or walking 2–3 blocks. Forty-two percent report an activity limitation (difficulty with personal care activities such as dressing, bathing, or walking or activities necessary to live independently, such as doing housework, preparing meals, or managing money). Still, 66% rate their own health as good, very good, or excellent, and 10% engage in regular physical activity.

SUMMARY

Population Aging. Population aging is a *shift in the age distribution of the population toward older ages.* The phenomenon is most often measured by increases in the percentage of the population reaching old age, but can also be captured by changes in the population "pyramid" and by changes in ratios of the older to younger population ("age-dependency" or "support" ratios). By all three standards, the U.S. population is aging and has been for over a century, but the pace has accelerated over the past several decades.

Demographic Transition. The demographic transition is a model that describes sweeping changes that populations undergo from high to low rates of deaths and births. In the first stage, a population has high birth rates, high death rates, and hence little or no population growth. In the second stage, high birth rates are accompanied by falling death rates at younger ages as living conditions and nutrition improve, and hence rapid population growth occurs. In the third stage, birth rates begin to decline while death rates remain low; consequently, population growth slows as the population begins to age. In the fourth stage, the population experiences continued declines in late-life mortality and continued population aging.

Life Expectancy. Life expectancy at a given age is calculated from a life table. Life expectancy is the total number of person-years lived divided by the number of persons reaching that age. Life expectancy at birth is the average number of years a hypothetical person can expect to live under the assumption that that prevailing age-specific mortality rates do not change over the lifetime of a hypothetical cohort

Epidemiologic Transition. Whereas the demographic transition emphasizes shifting birth and death rates, the epidemiologic transition focuses on causes of death as a population shifts from high to low mortality regimes. Stage 1 was deemed the age of "pestilence and famine." Infectious and parasitic diseases, such as pneumonia and influenza, tuberculosis, diarrhea, and enteritis, dominated this period. Stage 2 is called the "age of receding pandemics" and is characterized by the emergence of degenerative diseases, notably heart disease, as a major cause of death. In stage 3, the "age of degenerative and man-made diseases," chronic degenerative diseases—heart disease, cancer, stroke, chronic obstructive pulmonary diseases—dominate as causes of death. Olshansky and Ault (1986) also postulated the existence of a fourth stage, "the age of delayed degenerative diseases."

Dynamic Equilibrium. The consequences of shifting disability and survival curves for health care needs are not clear and depend on the processes driving mortality declines. Several competing theories have been proposed to predict changes in population health as mortality declines. Evidence over the past 30 years for the United States has been most consistent with the theory of dynamic equilibrium, a theory that recognizes complex interconnections among morbidity, mortality, and survival curves (Manton, 1989). Expansion of active life expectancy occurred during the 1970s and a compression followed in the 1980s. More recent evidence is mixed with one study suggesting a continued compression and another suggesting no change overall despite shifting rates on onset, recovery, and mortality.

The Oldest Old. An additional consequence of population aging is the emergence of an "oldest old" population. The oldest old are typically defined as people aged 85 and older. They are the fastest growing segment of older population in the United States. They are largely female, White, and widowed. The percentage living in poverty in this group has declined, whereas the percentage completing high school has increased dramatically. Men in this age group are increasingly likely to be veterans. They are high consumers of supportive care and have high rates of functional loss. Still, 66% rate their own health as good, very good, or excellent, and 10% engage in regular physical activity.

3

The Aging and Public Health Systems: Building a Healthy Aging Network

"Healthy aging" is a focus of a number of professional and trade organizations, as well as advocacy groups, foundations, and research and training institutes. In the realm of academic medical and public health research, the Gerontological Society of America (GSA) and the Gerontological Health Section (GHS) of the American Public Health Association stand out as the primary organizations pursuing the aging and public health agenda. The two organizations are quite different. GSA covers aging from every angle, from geriatric medicine to representations of aging in literature, and consists of four sections (health sciences, behavioral and social sciences, social services research and planning, and biology of aging). GHS is one section among many in the American Public Health Association and is relatively small among these sections, as public health has historically focused most on maternal and child health, infectious disease, and environmental health. If one examines the annual meetings of the two organizations, it quickly becomes apparent that the two approach healthy aging in quite different ways, with different funding streams and, in many cases, different investigators. The focus at GHS mostly involves evidence-based interventions designed to promote physical activity, accessible communities, use of clinical preventive services, and other public health goals for older adults. The focus at GSA is more likely to involve mechanisms of function and disability in late life, randomized clinical trials, population-based and national studies, and policy.

This contrast is too sharp, because recent years have seen an increasing convergence between the two approaches, with investigators—and now policy makers as well (see below)—becoming increasingly aware of the need to bring together *aging services research* and *research on the mechanisms of health and aging* to develop the field of public health and aging. Yet the contrast between the two approaches is a reasonable place to begin because it reflects the larger division in the field between the focus on aging services, on the one hand, and health, on the other. This division, as we will see, is institutionalized in parallel systems of service delivery to promote healthy aging, one revolving around departments of health and one around area agencies on aging. The aging and public health system can be considered *bipolar* to the extent that the two have different funding streams, different legislative mandates, different national organizations and advocacy groups, different data systems, and little or no contact even in the same locality. Integrating these systems to develop a *healthy aging network* will be a challenge for the next decades and will likely result in streamlined service delivery, improved monitoring of population health, and better health for older adults. But we are not there yet by any means.

This chapter examines the two current systems of aging and public health. We take up the parallel workforces for older persons and current attempts to bring the two together. We present a case study to show how difficult it can be to conduct research across this divide. We then examine CDC and Administration on Aging (AoA) efforts to promote coordination around evidence-based public health interventions. We touch on the prominent role of the Center for Healthy Aging at the National Council on Aging and the CDC's Healthy Aging branch and Healthy Aging Research Network. We present a case study of the challenge of standardizing outcomes across different evidence-based interventions to promote healthy aging. We then present alternative community-level interventions and the challenges they pose to traditional public health approaches. We conclude with an example of community-wide estimation of the demand for aging services as a tool for public health planning.

PARALLEL "HEALTH CARE WORKFORCES" FOR THE AGED

The important Institute of Medicine report, *Retooling for an Aging America* (2008), focused on the health care workforce, defined as health care professionals, paraprofessional direct care workers, and unpaid family caregivers. The panel rightly focused on the striking shortfall between the health care needs of the rapidly growing population of elders and the health care workforce currently in place to meet these needs. Consistent with the greater prevalence of disability and chronic disease in later life, older adults are disproportionate consumers of health care resources. According to the IOM panel, older adults account for about 12% of the U.S. population, but 26% of physician office visits. This 12% of the population engages between a third and half of the health care workforce. For example, older adults make 47% of hospital outpatient visits with nurse practitioners and 35% of hospital stays. They use 34% of prescriptions and account for 38% of emergency medical service responses. The demands on the long-term care workforce are even more extreme. Approximately 90% of nursing-home users are over age 65; in addition, over 60% of older adults with disabilities residing in the community make use of long-term care services, most often help with transportation and household chores.

The IOM report goes on to show the inadequacy of current education, training, practice, and financing of public and private programs designed to meet these needs. The shortage of certified nursing assistants, home health care aides, and other paraprofessional direct care workers is clear and documented in surveys that show poor working conditions, minimal training, little room for advancement, and extraordinarily high turnover. But shortages in the professional health care workforce are also glaring. For example, the IOM reported that less than 1% of physician assistants, pharmacists, and nurses receive specialty training in geriatrics. Projections for the demand for case management and information and referral suggest that perhaps one third of social workers should receive geriatrics training, yet only 4% currently receive such certification (IOM, 2008). Geriatric medicine is similarly underresourced, with declining numbers of physicians even taking advantage of available geriatric fellowships.

This gap in care is well recognized, and the IOM report makes a strong case for strengthening this sector of the health care workforce. The prescience of the report in drawing attention to the vital role of unpaid family and community supports is also worth mentioning, because family caregivers are partners in elder care in virtually every medical setting and often the primary provider of services to elders with long-term care needs. This last point is worth further thought. Families are supported by the medical sector, described above, but also by an alternative workforce, which aims to maximize the functioning of older adults by providing the bulk of the meals, transportation, home modification, social visiting, daily monitoring, house cleaning, and medication management that families are unable to provide to elders with disabilities. These services come from the aging services sector, a loose network of nonprofit organizations and government agencies that often contract with nonprofits to deliver mandated services. Relevant government agencies include most centrally the 665 Area Agencies on Aging (AAA) in the United States that function at the level of the county (or, in some cases, groups of counties), but also the nation's 3,000 local health departments, as well as departments of public welfare and other government entities. Although not strictly part of the health care workforce, this loose and only partly coordinated network provides elders with services they would otherwise not be able to obtain on their own because of health limitations or lack of family, and in this sense can be considered a complementary workforce required by these elders if they are to age in place safely.

Taking the more narrow view of the health care workforce, the IOM report did not examine the aging services network, which from a public health perspective is at least as important as the health care professional and direct care paraprofessional workforce. We still lack a comprehensive account of this alternative, parallel supportive care sector. At this point, we have only a partial picture of the number and types of aging services providers, their division of labor and funding sources, and their capacity to meet the needs of elders in particular communities, let alone at a national level. Because of the lack of central reporting or accreditation of this mostly nonprofit sector, a national accounting of the aging services network would be much more difficult than studies of the more visible health care workforce. An IOM report of this type, however, would be very valuable. Until now only the state-level organization of aging services has been investigated. However, new efforts are underway to examine the activities of aging service providers, at least those providing similar services, across different communities.

The basic array of the aging services network is shown in Figure 3.1, drawn from the Aging States Project (Chronic Disease Directors, 2003). The figure shows fully parallel systems of elder care, one oriented around health and the other around aging services. The two do not touch (at least formally or by design) at any point, whether national, state, or local. The health silo begins with the CDC and includes 57 state health or territorial departments, 3,000 local health departments, and a variety of community organizations that deliver mandated services and serve as vendors to local health department efforts. The aging services silo begins with Administration on Aging (AoA) and includes 57 state units on aging, which in turn include 660 Area Agencies on Aging, and again a variety of community organizations (some 27,000) that deliver mandated services. The health and aging services systems are each well organized, with national organizations of their own at the state and county levels.

The separation of health and aging services must strike any student of public health as odd. Elders use aging services, in part, because health problems have brought about declines in their ability to carry out everyday tasks that are critical to maintaining residence in the community. Health and aging services would no doubt be delivered more efficiently if they were coordinated. Effective use of aging services for health promotion, medication management, or reduction of behavioral risk factors has immediate health consequences by stemming the need for hospitalization or emergency room care. Yet the two systems currently operate at arm's length and only slowly have begun to coordinate efforts. Research that attempts to breach the wall between the two is nearly impossible (see below for an example).

The lack of any good rationale for keeping these systems distinct is evident in the case of an older adult with activity limitations receiving services in the community. The elder unable to maintain a household independently may receive transportation support from a church-based volunteer caregiver agency (such as a local branch of Interfaith Volunteer Caregivers), home modification services from a nonprofit agency under contract with the local AAA, cleaning and cooking services from yet another AAA vendor or perhaps a nonprofit multiservices agency funded by a local United Way or some other philanthropy, clinical preventive services (such as immunization, falls prevention, cancer screening, or chronic disease management) through a local health department initiative, and finally housing services and social work support from yet other government agencies, such as a local housing authority or public welfare department. The organizational relationships between these entities and complex funding streams would, of course, not be apparent to an elder or a family; nor, at this point, are these providers able to track duplication of services easily or develop ways to streamline delivery.

ATTEMPTS TO BRIDGE THE PARALLEL SYSTEMS OF ELDER HEALTH SERVICE DELIVERY

The Aging States Project (Chronic Disease Directors, 2003), jointly carried out by the Association of State and Territorial Health Officials (from the health silo) and National Association of State Units on Aging (from

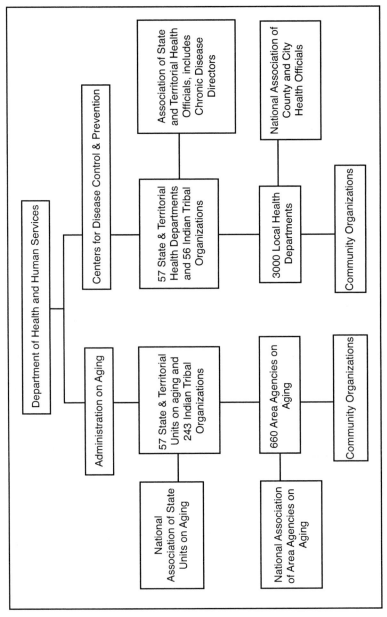

Figure 3.1 The aging services network and health network.

Source: From The Aging States Project: *Promoting Opportunities for Collaboration Between the Public Health and Aging Services Network*, by Chronic Disease Directors, National Association of State Units on Aging, 2003, p. 4; http://www .chronicdisease.org/files/public/aging_states_project.pdf.

the aging services silo), was designed to "promote opportunities for collaboration between the public health and aging services networks." It builds on earlier efforts that date back to 1994, when CDC, AoA, National Institutes of Health (NIH), American Association of Retired Persons (AARP), and the Gerontological Society of America first came together to discuss ways to link public health and aging services efforts. As part of the Aging States Project, state health departments and state units on aging were surveyed about their program priorities, activities, and funding. The survey was sent to directors of state entities and achieved good response (approximately 70% of state units on aging and 75% of state health departments participated).

The study found that state health departments and state units on aging address the health needs of older adults by use of different resources, approaches, and partners (Chronic Disease Directors, 2003; Lang, Benson, & Anderson, 2005). Each appears to focus on a different set of priorities, as shown in Figure 3.2. State health departments mainly provide programming involving clinical preventive services, such as cancer screening, immunization, and diabetes screening and treatment (with over 50% mentioning moderate-to-high involvement in these aging health issues). Nutrition, arthritis management, physical activity, and screening and treatment for cardiovascular disease are also priorities, although with somewhat lower health department involvement. By contrast, aging services network priorities center on a wider range of supportive services, such as information and referral for family caregivers, prevention of domestic violence, dementia care, legal issues, food security, transportation, access to prescriptions, and medication management support (with over 70% endorsing these as moderate-to-high priorities). Housing, financial resources, physical activity, and depression were also considered priorities by over 50% of state aging units.

Similarities in focus across the two systems are also notable. The aging services network was not limited to supportive services, such as transportation or caregiver referral, but instead actively provided disease management and health promotion programming, including evidence-based programs to identify depression, promote physical activity, and address medication management. Likewise, health department programming was not strictly limited to disease prevention. Health departments also supported programming designed to address nutrition, physical activity, and arthritis self-management. In fact, the two systems touch or overlap far more than one would expect, given their different funding-driven priorities and legislative mandates.

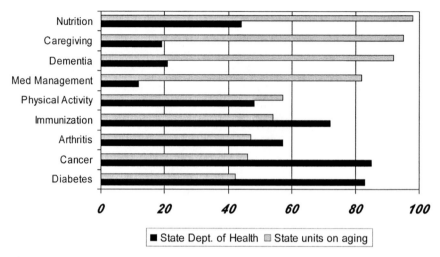

Figure 3.2 Priorities of state units on aging and state departments of health.

Note: Bars indicate percentage of responding agencies reporting moderate to high involvement in health promotion activity

Source: From The Aging States Project: *Promoting Opportunities for Collaboration Between the Public Health and Aging Services Network,* by Chronic Disease Directors, National Association of State Units on Aging, 2003, p. 4; http://www.chronicdisease .org/files/public/aging_states_project.pdf.

Part of the reason for this overlap is a change in the language of the Older Americans Act in 1992, which authorized the AoA to consult with the CDC on disease prevention and health promotion services. Title III-D of the Act essentially established a statutory basis for collaboration between public health and aging services (Chronic Disease Directors, 2003). Thus, beginning in 1992, the Older Americans Act added health promotion and disease prevention to its mandate, which already included funding for state and county units on aging (III-A, III-B), community services (such as senior centers, III-B), congregate and home-delivered meals (III-C), and later the National Family Caregiver Support program (III-E). With the change in Title III-D, state units on aging and county areas on aging were able to fund screening and risk assessments, nutrition counseling and education, physical fitness and activity programs, injury prevention, depression screening, medication management services, and even counseling for use of Medicare preventive health services.

This change should allow greater coordination between the aging and health services networks within communities, yet results from the

Aging States Project suggest many missed opportunities for coordination. The report concluded that "most states have a fragmented and limited approach to addressing the health needs of older adults," and that "one cause of this fragmentation is the lack of collaboration between state agencies that are responsible for assuring healthy residents and those that are responsible for aging adults." But it is hard to know how much of the underdelivery of services to older adults, itself difficult to measure, is due to lack of coordination and how much is due to simple underinvestment of resources in both sectors. For example, despite recognition of cardiovascular health as a key program priority by a majority of respondents from both state units on aging and state health departments, neither sector reported intensive programming in this area (Lang et al., 2005), suggesting funding limitations. On the other hand, it is likely that state health department initiatives to boost receipt of clinical preventive services (such as zoster or pneumococcal vaccination) would reach more elders if these efforts took advantage of existing area agency-on-aging networks. The broader problem may be absence of a clearly defined role for state health departments in promoting the health of older adults (Chronic Disease Directors, 2003), but perhaps greater coordination with the aging services network would help define such a role.

One conclusion from the Aging States Project remains especially timely: the current separate networks of aging and health services do not adequately meet the needs of elders and do not effectively leverage resources in the two sectors. The need for a "healthy aging network" to replace or bridge the current systems is clear.

The Challenges of Bridging the Aging Services and Health Department Networks: A Case Study

In an attempt to use routinely collected health department data for surveillance of elder neglect and abuse one of us (SA) accidentally ran afoul of this organizational separation of "health" and "aging," described above. Elder abuse and neglect is common (with prevalence ranging from 2% to 10% in community prevalence surveys) (Dyer, Goodwin, Pickens-Pace, Burnett, & Kelly, 2007; Lachs & Pillemer, 2004) and is significantly associated with poor outcomes, including mortality (Lachs, Williams, O'Brien, Pillemer, & Charlson, 1998). (See Chapter 7 for further treatment of elder abuse and neglect.) We thought it might be valuable to examine public health monitoring of housing violations as a way to identify severe elder neglect or abuse. We reasoned that elders with cognitive, physical, or psychiatric limitations would be less likely to maintain homes adequately, and that as a result housing violations reported to local health departments might serve as an indicator of elder neglect in communities. We completed a data-sharing agreement with an urban health department and obtained a de-identified dataset of housing violations over a 3-year period. In fact, we determined that the housing violations division of the health department was the only division that had contact with a sizable number of elders and routinely collected age information.

The dataset included an indicator for whether residents were over age 65, the census tract for the residence, and a text field for the inspector's report on the nature of the violation. Eliminating noncommunity housing (for example, violations involving institutions, backyards, and pools) left a sample of 3,319 housing violations, of which 229 involved elder residences. Of the 229 cited elder residences, 57% involved elders living alone. The high proportion living alone is impressive, given Census reports of singleton residences for 20% of older men and 38% of older women (Federal Interagency Forum on Aging-Related Statistics, 2008). We were thus encouraged to pursue this line of investigation.

Housing inspector reports in the database ranged from single-sentence reports to detailed accounts. We initially coded any mention of 54 housing problems, which we later collapsed into 11 different categories: HVAC (heating, ventilation, air conditioning), windows/doors, animals, air quality, electrical wiring, water/sewage, gas, fire hazards, poor housekeeping, structural problems, or other. Interrater reliability between two raters for a random set of 100 inspection reports was excellent (*kappa* = 0.91). We noted any mention of the 11 different sources of housing problems, so that a single inspection report could have multiple problems recorded. The "poor housekeeping" category included reports of clutter, garbage accumulation, and poor living conditions. It is illustrated well by one inspection report, which read, "Elderly people living in junked conditions; can't see the windows due to accumulation."

We compared younger-age and older households to determine whether the likelihood of types of housing violation differed. In fact, households with residents over age 65 were more likely to be cited for poor housekeeping: 31.9% of elder housing violations involved poor housekeeping, compared with 22.4% in non-elder households ($p < .001$). Elder households were less likely to be cited for electrical or structural problems ($p < .05$). Within elder residences, the proportion with poor housekeeping reported by inspectors did not differ according to whether elders lived alone, as couples, or with other nonelderly adults.

Across census tracts, the number of nonelder residences cited for housing violations was significantly correlated with indicators of low socioeconomic status, such as the number of vacant dwellings and median value of housing stock. In the case of elderly households, the number of housing violations per census tract was not significantly correlated with either (or any) socioeconomic status (SES) indicator.

Together, these results suggested that housing violations, routinely recorded by health departments, could be a potentially useful indicator of elder neglect or health limitation severe enough to interfere with household maintenance. A more adequate test of the value of monitoring housing violations for this purpose would be to determine whether elders cited for housing violations also come to the attention of adult protective services, which is often called in for cases of potential neglect. Adult protective services, however, is an agency within the local area agency on aging. To determine the proportion of elders cited for housing violations who also received an intervention from adult protective services would require getting two datasets, and the two different networks, to talk to each other.

We failed. We asked the state unit on aging, represented by the state ombudsman, to take our health department data on housing violations, match it to adult protective services data, and determine the number of older adults who appeared in both databases. This request was rejected. The statements from the state ombudsman are revealing. The first response claimed confidentiality strictures as the reason for rejecting our request:

> This is in response to your below email requesting personal information on consumers who are in Pennsylvania's Adult Protective Services (APS) system. Unfortunately, the protective services files and any other information collected during investigations are kept confidential as noted in Pennsylvania Code Title 6, Aging §§15.101 through 15.106. Therefore, we cannot provide you with any personal information on consumers who have received protective services in Allegheny County. We apologize we could not be of any further assistance, and wish you success in your project. Thank you again for contacting our offices.

Not one to give up so easily, we reminded the ombudsman that an aggregate proportion measure would be acceptable and would not require breach of confidentiality. The second request was rejected on the grounds of inability to match data fields, incompatible data systems, and possibly the amount of work involved in matching on address text fields:

> Dr. Albert, we are unable to provide you with a number based on the information you are providing in your excel sheet. In fiscal year 2005–06, the Department of Aging protective services program migrated into a new database system (OMNIA Interviewer and SAMS). This new system resulted in a complete reformation of the way protective service data had been collected over the preceding years. Specifically, it utilizes unique identifiers such as name, date of birth, and social security numbers for consumers receiving protective services. Because there are no unique identifying data for comparison between your list and the consumers in our database, there is no way to ensure the consumers are the same. Setting aside the inherent errors in entry of text data, using strictly address information could cause misidentification of consumers and incorrect results. Because of this, we are unable to produce the data you are requesting for your study. We hope that the above information is helpful, and thank you for contacting us. Good luck with your project.

This experience is valuable for showing the difficulty of crossing between aging services and health networks. We were limited by our data-sharing agreement to strictly de-identified data; hence, matching to another data system would indeed be difficult. In fact, absence of a common identifier within the aging services network itself has made tracking individuals across service venues difficult and has only recently been remedied with the implementation of a common Web-based data system (Social Assistance Management Software, SAMS). To attempt to merge data across different systems, even with an honest broker arrangement and with the expertise required, would be difficult. But this limitation should lead us to ask why a common identifier is not available in the different data systems and why no one has taken steps to make it possible to track people across the two systems.

Thus, we were not able to determine how many of the elders with housing violations in one local department of health database also appeared in the corresponding adult protective services database of a local area agency on aging. Other investigators have apparently been able to access adult protective services data, but we are unaware at this point of research that has successfully crossed the divide between health departments and aging services networks and managed to merge data systems.

These organizational divisions clearly interfere with efforts to promote healthy aging.

EFFORTS TO DEVELOP HEALTHY AGING NETWORKS

Improving the health of older adults is a CDC priority, as indicated in *Healthy People 2010* objectives to increase life expectancy and reduce disability in old age. "CDC promotes the use of effective preventive measures to make healthy aging a reality for older adults" (CDC, 2007). The CDC's Healthy Aging program, set within the National Center for Chronic Disease Prevention and Health Promotion, has developed a program of research and partnerships that begins with the premise that "poor health is not an inevitable consequence of aging." To this end, CDC has increasingly joined forces with the AoA to promote physical activity, better nutrition, and tobacco cessation among older adults. More recent efforts support disease management in the case of diabetes, heart disease, and arthritis and seek to increase uptake of preventive services available through Medicare, such as immunization and cancer screening. CDC's injury prevention program has begun to address the high rate of injury among seniors and falls prevention. Finally, CDC has supported a Healthy Aging Network (HAN) within its Prevention Research Centers program. The HAN mission "is to better understand the determinants of healthy aging in older adult populations; to identify interventions that promote healthy aging; and to assist in the translation of such research into sustainable community-based programs throughout the nation."

Still, these efforts go only so far. The testimony of one CDC director to the U.S. Senate in 2003 suggests some frustration: "To a certain extent, it is as if we have not fully engaged in applying public health practice to older populations. . . . The aging network is looking to public health for science-based health promotion and disease prevention strategies that are tested and proven effective" (J. S. Marks, CDC, Testimony: U.S. Senate, May 19, 2003). However, in the intervening years, evidence suggests that major progress has, in fact, been made to bring the health and aging services networks together to forge the healthy aging network mentioned earlier. The role of CDC and AoA in this effort is clear, but the supporting role of nongovernmental entities, such as the National Council on Aging, advocacy organizations, and foundations (especially Atlantic Philanthropies, Hartford, and Robert Wood Johnson), must also be recognized. These efforts are quite recent, with the Aging States Project in 2003 a key milestone.

One explicit effort to connect state aging services networks and health department efforts is a series of partnerships funded through the State-Based Examples of Network Innovation, Opportunity, and Replication (SENIOR) program, a joint CDC and AoA program. The focus of these small grants is to foster relationships between aging and public health establishments in states willing to build bridges across the divide. Efforts initially focused on coordinating activity to promote physical activity, nutrition, use of Medicare preventive services, and other standard health department programs. Later years saw collaboration around evidence-based health promotion and disease prevention projects. With this new focus, state organizations were required to adopt specific programs (clinical preventive services, physical activity, and chronic disease self-management) with a strong evidence base. Later efforts added other evidence-based programs, such as oral health, falls prevention, and depression screening. By 2007, 28 states or territories had received funding through this mechanism, a small but important advance in bridging the gap between health promotion and aging services at the state level. Of course, these small grants ($10,000–$15,000), which are designed solely for coordinating health and aging services pale in comparison with Medicare spending for prevention activity (see Chapter 4). Still, the program has helped states develop larger comprehensive plans for promoting healthy aging (for example, New Jersey's *Blueprint for Healthy Aging* and Oregon's *Healthy Aging in Oregon's Counties*, 2009) and statewide coalitions to support healthy aging.

The next step in this process of integration appears to involve standardization of measures and outcome assessment as part of the implementation of such evidence-based interventions. NCOA's Center for Healthy Aging has played a key role in working with CDC and AoA to promote use of evidence-based programming in these efforts and to develop standard tools and benchmarks. Thus, states participating in the projects are required to collect the demographic features of participants in a standard way. Common protocols for enrollment and tracking are also required, and standardized codebooks and data collection are in place. Most critical from the perspective of prevention science is the move to standardize the recording of outcomes, a difficult challenge for programs that implement interventions differently or apply these interventions to different target populations (see below for a case study of this challenge). Grantees were also encouraged to use a common framework to assess the scope, reach, and sustainability of their efforts, RE-AIM (*R*each into the target population, *E*fficacy or effectiveness, *A*doption by target settings or institutions, *I*mplementation—consistency of delivery of intervention, *M*aintenance of intervention effects in individuals and populations over time) (www.re-aim.org).

Evidence-based interventions are defined as those proven to bring about desired outcomes in randomized trials or other high-quality research designs. These often need to be translated into programs suitable for a particular community or target population while retaining fidelity to the core components of the original intervention. This translation is also challenging, and NCOA's Center for Healthy Aging has developed guidelines for such evidence-based health promotion (NCOA, 2006a). Some of the evidence-based programs adopted by CDC/AoA grantees include the following (NCOA, 2006b):

- *Chronic disease self-management programs:* Chronic Disease Self-Management Program (Lorig et al., 1999); Healthy Changes: A Community-Based Diabetes Education and Support Program; and Women Take PRIDE in Managing Heart Disease (Janevic et al., 2004).
- *Care management programs:* Healthy IDEAS: Evidence-based Disease Self-Management for Depression and Program to Encourage Active Rewarding Lives for Seniors, PEARLS (Ciechanowski et al., 2004; Unutzer, Patrick, Marmon, Simon, & Katon, 2002b); Community-Based Medication Management Intervention (Stewart, Pearson, & Horowitz, 1998); and Healthy Moves for Aging Well.
- *Physical Activity programs:* Active Start; and EnhanceFitness (Ackermann et al., 2003; Wallace et al., 1998).
- *Nutrition programs:* Preventive Nutrition Education for Cardiovascular Disease (Luepker et al., 1996); and Project SIEN (for diabetes).
- *Fall prevention programs:* A Matter of Balance; and Step by Step: Thoughtful Fall Prevention.

Other evidence-based interventions are also available and will likely be introduced with this mechanism in other grant cycles. These include Active Choices (King, Baumann, O'Sullivan, Wilcox, & Castro, 2002), Strong for Life (Etkin, Prohaska, Harris, Latham, & Jette, 2006; Jette, et al., 1999), EnhanceWellness (Leveille et al., 1998; Phelan et al., 2002),

Fit and Strong! (Hughes et al., 2004), and Prevention and Management of Alcohol Problems in Older Adults (Fleming, Manwell, Barry, Adams, & Stauffacher, 1999). Results from these efforts remain to be seen, but first results (made available in 2008) suggest that the programs have been successfully implemented, with efforts to standardize measures and record data completed.

THE CHALLENGES OF STANDARDIZING MEASUREMENT IN HEALTHY AGING INTERVENTIONS: A CASE STUDY

The NCOA experience with evidence-based interventions for healthy aging gives a hint of the challenges of standardizing measures. Along with the move to use evidence-based interventions, funders are increasingly demanding standardized accounting of the populations served, the services delivered, and the extent to which outcomes are met. This demand can be challenging to the small nonprofit agency without a background in evaluation research. It can also be a challenge to the funding agency, which, if it insists on such measures, must work with grantees to develop a common set of measures that agencies can reasonably collect.

When funded agencies offer different interventions and serve different populations, these challenges are magnified even further. This was the situation for a recent grant award to five agencies by a local United Way agency as part of their "vulnerable seniors" programming. The agencies offered different programs (chronic disease self-management, enhanced information and referral, home modification, case management in low-income senior housing, and enhanced home-delivered meals using community volunteers) and served populations that only partly overlapped (frail older persons in the community, elders with chronic conditions who attend senior centers, middle-aged adults with disabilities living in low-income subsidized senior housing). The programs also differed in their length of time with elders and amount of personal contact. What kinds of measures could plausibly be collected to provide standardized indicators of populations served or outcome?

A first decision involved the level of data agencies should collect. Should they collect individual-level data, with common data forms across the agency programs? Or should the agencies instead provide aggregate indicators, with data collection left up to each agency? In a series of planning meetings involving grantees, the funding agency, and an external evaluator, all agreed that individual-level data were ideal but not practical in this case. Collecting such data would raise confidentiality issues and questions of informed consent, and would also not be feasible in programs that did not have the regular contact with elders required for detailed interviews. Aggregate data offered the advantage of more flexible reporting but required careful selection of indicators and risked lower quality data. Team discussions led to a compromise position in which agencies would report findings for selected aggregate indicators but use common data collection forms and shared definitions of key indicators.

Tables 3.1 and 3.2 show the consensus aggregate indicators developed for the project. Some indicators were mandatory, others optional. Mandatory indicators were considered basic and applicable to all programs and represent a minimum data requirement. Optional indicators were in many cases specific to programs and were to be completed only for programs that had these indicators as additional outcomes. An innovation in this effort was a requirement that agencies provide indicator data quarterly in a Web-based application. Program success would be gauged by improvement in outcomes relative to national and regional benchmarks, as well as improvement in target populations over the course of the project.

Agencies were required to provide two indicators of consumer health: (a) self-rated health, using a standard elicitation, and (b) ADL status, as indicated by disability severe enough to qualify for nursing home placement, that is, two or more disabilities or eligibility based on state or county criteria. For outcomes, the funder made a distinction between the "preferred outcome," "increasing the number of frail and vulnerable seniors or adults with disabilities who remain safely in their homes or in a least restrictive community-based setting," and intermediate outcomes that support the preferred outcome. These include greater access to services, improvements in health, and greater use of prevention services. Common outcomes required of all agencies included the proportion of clients remaining in the community or transitioning to different levels of supportive care, the proportion declining in ADL, and the proportion with hospital or emergency department admissions. Optional outcomes covered much greater ground and were specific to particular programs.

These common outcomes represent the solid core of aging services interventions. They link health and aging services explicitly. In fact,

Table 3.1

VULNERABLE SENIORS: AGGREGATE SOCIODEMOGRAPHIC AND HEALTH INDICATORS

Demographics—total no. of client services for reporting period	
Total no. of clients served by the program in reporting period	**All**
Total no. of new clients served	**All**
Total no. of caregivers served	Optional
No. of clients served who are nursing home eligible (as determined by county/state aging or have 2 or more ADL deficits)	**All**
No. of clients served who have only one ADL limitation	Optional
No. served with at least one IADL limitation	Optional
Number served with mobility limitations	Optional
No. of clients at each level of self-assessed health status	**All**
No. who lived alone	**All**
No. who live with others but lack a responsible caregiver in household	**All**
Gender	**All**
Race/ethnicity	**All**
Client zip code	**All**
Age: 18–24 25–34 35–44 45–54 55–59 60–64 65–74 75–84 85+	**All**
Family income: Receiving medical assistance (< 200% poverty level)	**All**
Family income: <100% of poverty level, 100%–300%, >300%	Optional

the preferred outcome—aging safely in place or in the most integrated and nonrestrictive setting—represents a key outcome for the healthy aging network. Providing the services elders need to support health or remediate health deficit should allow them to age well in their communities. Because seniors overwhelmingly endorse the desire to age in their homes, and because communities also benefit when elders remain in their homes, the focus on allowing elders to age in place should be a central outcome of community health promotion efforts.

Table 3.2

VULNERABLE SENIORS: AGGREGATE PROGRAM OUTCOMES

PREFERRED: Increase the no. of frail and vulnerable seniors or adults with disabilities who remain safely in their homes or in a least restrictive community-based setting

No./% of clients who maintain noninstitutional status	**ALL**
No./% who relocated to nursing homes (long-term care facilities)	**ALL**
No./% who became nursing-home eligible during period (as determined by county/state definition or 2+ ADLs)	optional
No./% who relocated to other settings appropriate for level of care (i.e., assisted living, family)	optional
No./% of clients who maintain stable housing (no evictions, pass inspections)	optional
No./%. of clients who attain service plan goals	optional
No./% of clients who completed training sessions	optional

SUPPORTING OUTCOMES for Supportive Services: Increase the no. of low-income seniors or adults with disabilities that have greater access to subsidized programs such as rent rebates, appropriate levels of housing, tax abatements, and Supplemental Security Income

No./% of clients who are referred to supportive services	optional
No./% of eligible clients who are enrolled in benefits	optional
No./% whose housing expense is within the recommended expense to income ratio	optional

SUPPORTING OUTCOMES for Functional Status: Increase the no. of frail seniors and adults with disabilities that have adequate/improved nutritional, health, and/or functional status

No. of clients who report/demonstrate maintained or improved ability to function independently in everyday life (i.e., in the area of activity limitations or IADLs)	**All**
No. of total hospital admissions among all program clients during reporting period	**All**
No. of total emergency room visits among all program clients during reporting period	**All**
No./% of clients who maintained or improved protective factors (domains include physical, social, mental, and economic status)	optional

(Continued)

Table 3.2

VULNERABLE SENIORS: AGGREGATE PROGRAM OUTCOMES (*Continued*)

No./% of clients who attain service plan goals	optional
No./% who maintain or improve physical and mental health (fatigue, nutritional status)	optional
No./% who complete an assessment of physical/mental health status	optional
No./% who have regular medical visits/communication with physicians	optional
No./% of clients who have immediate/emergency medical needs addressed	optional
No./% of clients who report positive changes in physical activity	optional
No./% of clients who have control over type II diabetes	optional
No./% of clients who have control over high blood pressure	optional

SUPPORTING OUTOMES for Prevention: Increase the no. of vulnerable and frail seniors or adults with disabilities that receive necessary safety checks, home modifications, immunizations, and preventative health screenings

No./% of clients who eliminate a safety hazard from their home	optional
No./% of clients who use needed safety devices	optional
No./% who have falls at home	optional
No./% who report decreased isolation	optional

PROMOTING HEALTHY AGING: ALTERNATIVE COMMUNITY-BASED APPROACHES

As we have seen, nonprofit agencies, funded by area agencies on aging, departments of health, or other sources, provide the bulk of supportive and health services elders require for healthy aging. These services are mostly addressed to more vulnerable elders with health needs; but, as described earlier, recent trends suggest a growing interest in providing disease prevention and health promotion services through the same networks. An entirely different approach to prevention is the direct outreach to elders to teach principles of healthy aging and to empower seniors themselves to obtain preventive health services. This approach gets away from the one-disease or one-problem–one-intervention focus of most evidence-based interventions, and instead stresses a whole-person approach to healthy aging. This is the focus of a University of Pittsburgh program, the 10 Keys™ to Healthy Aging (Bayles et al., 2008).

The 10 Keys are 10 targets for healthy aging, each designed to reduce a risk factor for one or more chronic diseases, as shown in Table 3.3. Each of the keys has a strong clinical evidence base and involves health behaviors or preventive medical care within the reach of informed, community-dwelling elders. Information on the 10 Keys is available now as a printed course guide and in Web modules (http://www.healthyaging. pitt.edu). The University of Pittsburgh Center for Healthy Aging also teaches courses in the 10 Keys, in which elders are certified as "Health Ambassadors" who spread the message of health promotion through their social networks. These courses are offered in a variety of settings, including lifelong learning programs on college campuses, senior centers, subsidized low-income senior housing, churches, workplaces, and alumni organizations. More recently, health care providers and aging services providers have found the training useful for their interaction with seniors.

The 10 Keys approach has its origins in a population-based study. In 2002, the University of Pittsburgh Center for Healthy Aging conducted assessments on a sample of 544 people, 217 men and 327 women, with an average age of 74.5 years. One group received counseling on risk factors and an intensive healthy lifestyle intervention that included

Table 3.3

10 KEYS TO HEALTHY AGING

1. Prevent bone loss and muscle weakness
2. Control lipids (low-density lipoprotein-cholesterol <100 mg/dl)
3. Control systolic blood pressure to less than 140 mmHg
4. Regulate diabetes; blood glucose to less than 100 mg/dl
5. Be physically active at least 2½ hours per week
6. Stop smoking
7. Maintain social contact at least once a week
8. Participate in cancer screening
9. Combat depression
10. Get regular immunizations

nutritional advice and an exercise program to increase physical activity, muscle strength, and mobility. The other group received counseling and follow-up on risk factors only. The intervention was offered weekly for 6 months. All participants had access to a health counselor and were monitored for 2 years.

The survey revealed that a majority of these elders were below prevention targets for colorectal cancer screening, cholesterol reduction, hypertension management, and physical activity. In addition, the healthy lifestyle intervention developed for this effort was not adequate to produce significant differences between groups. One may reasonably conclude that health promotion programs, even if reasonably delivered and based on good science, may not have their desired effects unless they are more firmly anchored in the community. Recognizing the need for behavior change, becoming aware of health practices, seeing others practice prevention, and taking ownership of preventive care must be continually reinforced where people live, in their daily round of social contacts and in regular tasks, if prevention is to become routine practice.

To put prevention into communities in this way is difficult. The elders targeted by the 10 Keys program are active and may not attend senior centers. They are, on the whole, not limited functionally and so may not perceive the need for prevention or lifestyle modification. To reach these elders, the Center for Healthy Aging developed a program model based on education and empowerment, which sought to demystify health promotion and old age and reinforce the message that illness is not an inevitable part of aging. The aim was to offer a flexible program in health promotion that could spread virally through communities through a growing cadre of trained health ambassadors. The Health Ambassador program is a certificate course for individuals who want to help promote and support healthy aging in their communities. A certificate is awarded to volunteers who complete the 12-hour training. Health Ambassadors are expected to:

- Make 10 Keys presentations throughout the community (churches, alumni groups, community organizations, etc.)
- Assist in the recruitment of new Health Ambassadors
- Be a positive advocate for healthy aging in the community, demonstrating a personal commitment to the 10 Keys and modeling preventive behavior
- Learn basic health assessment skills, such as keeping exercise logs, measuring blood pressure, and understanding basic nutrition counseling messages

■ Become knowledgeable about preventive health screenings (bone density, mammogram, colonoscopy)

The Health Ambassador class schedule is shown in Table 3.4. The health promotion training is now a 120-page manual written at an 8th grade level. Although it is not a requirement of Ambassador training, participants are encouraged to undergo cholesterol and glucose blood draws and hypertension screening. This service is provided as part of Ambassador training. Approximately 80% of Ambassador trainees agree to venipuncture. The protocol in place refers participants to their medical providers when values are abnormal. Ambassadors accept the idea that practicing prevention is the key to credibility and adequate self-education. Over 300 Health Ambassadors have been trained to date.

Initial efforts with the first cohort of 120 Ambassadors show great promise both in meeting prevention targets for participants and in developing community outreach for this effort. Ambassadors have found the program very useful and empowering. As one woman has said, "After almost 87 years I still am learning things about my own body and now I understand the information well enough to share it with others." Two-year follow-up with this first cohort of Ambassadors demonstrates (a) high retention of prevention knowledge, as indicated by questionnaire; (b) continued involvement in Ambassador outreach efforts; and (c) maintenance or increases in prevention services obtained from physicians.

After training, Ambassadors agree to conduct outreach in monthly presentations. They keep a log of such activity. Our McKeesport group's outreach in a month shows the broad reach of people when they mobilize naturally occurring networks. In one month, 10 Ambassadors made 14 presentations in venues ranging from a quilting group to a business school alumni association.

A related approach to direct community health promotion is to organize communities themselves to seek improvements in public health. In 2004–2006, The University of Pittsburgh Center for Healthy Aging developed a community-organizing approach to health promotion in the setting of low-income senior high rises managed by a county housing authority. Using a community-based participatory research model, the Center facilitated development of Blue Ribbon Health Panels (BRHPs) at each of 12 different senior high rises. The BRHPs were community councils convened to generate community involvement in health promotion. Each high-rise building has an active tenant council with elected officers, which was the basis for the

Table 3.4

CLASS SCHEDULE: 10 KEYS TO HEALTHY AGING

Class 1

Orientation to the CHA Ambassador Program: Aging in America, history of the 10 Keys; Ambassador qualities and program goals.

Keys to Activity: Definition of activity and benefit to health and well-being. Identify present levels of activity, common barriers, and motivation techniques.

Class 2

Blood Pressure Basics: Anatomy of blood vessels, the heart, and controllable risk factors. View a brief video displaying the blood path and the effects on the vessel when blood pressure measurement occurs.

Bone Loss and Muscle Weakness: Role of muscles and bones in body. View a brief video displaying normal bone appearance and osteoporosis. Importance of bone density testing, physical activity, nutrition. Muscle strengthening and fall prevention.

Class 3

Smoking: Smoking as an addiction, principles of smoking cessation.

Social Contact: Benefits of maintaining social contact as we age, opportunities for isolated individuals.

Class 4

Cancer Prevention: Nature of cancer, importance of regular screening for early detection. Tour or video of colonoscopy and mammogram.

Combat Depression: Depression as an illness, symptoms and referral.

Class 5

Get Shots: Immunization, value of record keeping.

Lower Low-Density Lipoprotein-Cholesterol: The role of reading labels, knowing portion sizes, and the value of lipid-lowering drug therapy.

Class 6

Prevent and Control Diabetes: Diabetes and prediabetes. Importance of nutrition and activity; blood glucose, HA1C.

Review: Review all materials; importance of follow-up education sessions; review mentorship "alumni" program.

efforts to develop BRHPs. Tenant councils met monthly to address issues of community concern and were a natural starting point for this effort. Councils typically met in a community room that residents used as a public space for gatherings, and working groups also met in this setting. The Center succeeded in developing BRHPs at each site, with a signed memorandum of agreement from tenant council presidents. Each BRHP, consisting of 5–10 residents, met monthly with a member of the project team.

Once constituted, the BRHP identified a number of community health issues and action plans. The summary of BRHP quarterly activity for six sites, shown in Table 3.5, gives a sense of the health issues raised by the panels and steps they evolved to address these concerns. The summary shows the wide variety of health concerns raised by BRHP members, which ranged from repainting of pedestrian crosswalks in front of a high rise to the need for floor captains to look in on residents with disabilities, depression, and cognitive impairment. The BRHPs met these challenges with highly creative solutions: obtaining hand-me-down exercise equipment for a common room, connecting with a local food bank to set up a special service for high-rise residents, and arranging for fire department personnel to give a presentation.

Given that participants were all volunteers without formal community-organizing training, and given the few resources available to the BRHPs, their accomplishments were impressive. The research team facilitated meetings and suggested avenues for obtaining contacts or making inquiries but otherwise let the panels proceed as they thought best. The biggest challenge was to keep residents focused on health issues rather than standard building maintenance, although these are often related. For example, it quickly became clear that efforts to promote walking and physical activity would have little effect in a building that residents perceived as unsafe or which lacked reasonable sidewalks or pedestrian crosswalks. Similarly, recommendations to increase fruit or vegetable consumption were unlikely to be successful if residents lacked transportation to stores or if stores in low-income neighborhoods did not stock fresh foods.

In fact, this community-based effort suggested that professional public health goals and community or lay public health goals do not always correspond. As shown in Table 3.6, we can draw a rough correspondence between the two, but community goals stress the social context for adequate health promotion, something the public health community often

Table 3.5

RESULTS OF BLUE RIBBON HEALTH PANEL EFFORTS: SIX SITES

Site 1

Concerns about difficulty of evacuation in event of fire. Addressed by having safety officer present on fire safety information and survey to determine which residents would like a door decal indicating disability.

Site 2

Concern to find resources to aid seniors in grocery shopping. Addressed by gathering information on subsidized transportation, drafting an information flier, and distributing to residents.

After several contacts made with borough and state representatives, borough has committed to repainting pedestrian crosswalk in front of the building.

Site 3

The BRHP conducted a walk-through to meet with residents and document physical environment issues.

Site 4

Connected with a local agency and food bank office to set up a meeting where available food bank services were introduced. A new priority issue has been identified (i.e., getting blood work drawn on site) along with potential solutions. The previous priority issue was addressed by having the unused adjacent tennis court reduced in size, allowing the residents to park in the new spaces.

Site 5

The BRHP has worked on getting exercise equipment transferred to the community room. In addition, the BRHP has received "in-kind" donations of equipment from several outside sources, including residents' family members. The BRHP requested the services of an exercise physiologist to provide introductory sessions on how to use the equipment properly.

Site 6

Concern that frail residents were not "being looked in on." Site once had floor captains who were responsible for checking on the status of residents and sending get well and sympathy cards. Former floor captains and new ones agreed to the job effective immediately. All floors now have floor captains.

neglects. The BRHPs suggested that public health goals in this setting would be best realized in the context of changes in their social environment, notably development of floor captain systems, food pantries, enhanced security, effective use of common rooms, regular meetings with building managers, and contact with local government officials. This is an important lesson for public health efforts in the community.

Table 3.6

HEALTH PRIORITIES OF BLUE RIBBON HEALTH PANELS COMPARED WITH 10 KEYS OBJECTIVES

10 KEYS OBJECTIVES	COMMUNITY PANEL OBJECTIVES
Glucose <100 mg/dl	On-site blood draw
Physical activity	Exercise equipment on site
Low-density lipoprotein <100 mg/dl	Access to fresh fruit, vegetables in food bank
Bone health	***
Social contact	Social visiting and check in for impaired residents
Cancer screening	Diversity in diet

ESTIMATING AGING SERVICES NETWORK CHALLENGES IN THE COMMUNITY

The nonprofit agencies that provide most aging services depend on volunteers, yet few local statistics on the availability or need for volunteers are readily available. Instead, those engaged in this area of public health and aging must piece together existing information by using the best assumptions possible as a way to estimate need for aging services and the ability of communities to provide volunteer time for these services. One of us (SA) developed such a model using population projections in Pittsburgh, PA. The model requires many simplifying assumptions, some of which are highlighted here to illustrate how "real world" data must be applied creatively—but with caution—in coming up with statistics that adequately describe public health and aging issues. Sometimes there is no option but to rely on data that are not meant to be applied to your population, but with proper caveats and assessment of direction of bias, it is still possible to learn a great deal.

To estimate the demand for volunteer services among vulnerable elders, the modeling began with projections of the size of the vulnerable elder population over the next 20 years. Complete population projections for the county over this time period are available (University Center on Social and Urban Research [UCSUR], 2005). Regional figures are most appropriate because of flows in population between the city center and surrounding suburbs.

Elder demand for aging services support through volunteering is estimated as the number of older persons multiplied by the proportion living alone without family involvement (15% and 20% by age band, 65–74 and 75 and older, respectively) times the proportion with IADL limitations (6.4% and 18.3% by age band). This calculation yields a count of older persons by age range who can be considered vulnerable and in need of volunteer services. Table 3.7, lower panel, shows the demand for volunteer hours in 2005.

Vulnerability is based on concurrent disability and relative isolation. Disability prevalence draws upon estimates of age-specific limitations in the IADLs (difficulty with household competencies) from national estimates derived from *Health US, 2007* (National Center for Health Statistics [NCHS] 2008). Although national estimates are gross, data sources that allow disaggregation by locality are also limited. Census data (2000) become out of date quickly, the American Community Survey for Pittsburgh offers estimates closer in time but does not provide data on IADL limitations, and the Behavioral Risk Factors Surveillance System (BRFSS) offers excellent disaggregation (down to the census tract or telephone area exchange) but suffers from low response. None are ideal; consequently, investigators needed to choose carefully and justify this choice of data.

The IADLs cover the need for help with cooking, shopping, filling prescriptions, doing light housework, using the telephone, managing money, and related activities. These are a plausible indicator of disabilities that can be addressed by volunteers and have been associated with transition to more severe limitations in ADLs (difficulty in personal self-maintenance activities, such as bathing, dressing, using the toilet, and feeding oneself). IADL limitations also are associated with the need for social contact, because they imply activity outside the home has been curtailed. For isolation, the model assumes that 15%–20% of elders live alone and do not have strong connection to family or neighbors. This estimate is based on the prevalence of elders who live alone in the community, which is approximately 30%–40% of older persons, depending on the locale (Arias, 2007). It is reasonable to assume that approximately half of these elders lack a family nearby and have weak neighbor ties.

The model also assumes that older people in this situation require 2 hr/day of help over the year. This estimate is based on the hour commitment required to perform household tasks, check in, and transport an elder outside the home.

Table 3.7

CALCULATION OF YEARLY AGGREGATE VOLUNTEER HOUR SUPPLY AND VULNERABLE ELDERLY HOUR DEMAND, 2005: BASE MODEL

SUPPLY	N	TOT VOL %[a]	COM %	ELD VOL %[b]	VOL_N	MED_HR	HR_YR
25–34	128,784	0.354	0.124	4.4	5,653	43	243,083
35–44	176,140	0.4	0.103	4.0	7,256	62	449,932
45–54	198,477	0.412	0.119	4.9	9,730	66	642,241
55–64	140,824	0.29	0.157	4.6	6,411	72	461,644
65–74	93,524	0.22	0.161	3.5	3,312	115	380,951
75+	114,343	0.195	0.157	3.1	3,500	72	252,044
					35,866		2,429,896

DEMAND[c]	N	ALONE %	IADL %	N, ELDERS	2 HR DAY^{-1} YR^{-1}
65–74	94,084	0.15	0.064	903	659,792
75+	120,870	0.2	0.183	4,424	3,231,617
				5,327	3,891,409
				Vol/Elderhours[d]	**0.62**

[a]Population estimates for Allegheny County, 2005, taken from UCSUR (2005), Table 1. On the volunteer supply side, potential volunteers aged 65–74 and 75 and older adjusted by removing vulnerable elders.

[b]Total volunteer rates by age taken from *Pittsburgh Volunteer Trends, Volunteering in America, Cities, 2007*. Corporation for National and Community Service. Elder volunteer prevalence by age calculated as proportion volunteering for social-community service × total proportion volunteering. Rates of elder volunteering range from 3% to 5% in each age group. Number of volunteers is then calculated by applying this rate to number in age bands. Yearly hours are calculated as number of volunteers × median yearly hours, inflated to median of 70 for Pittsburgh. These are summed to yield the aggregate yearly supply of elder volunteer hours.

[c]Elder demand for volunteering calculated as number of older persons × proportion living alone without family involvement (15% and 20% by age band) × proportion with IADL limitations (6.4% and 18.3% by age band). Age-specific IADL limitations (difficulty with household competencies) taken from *Health US, 2007* (NCHS, 2008, Table 58). Volunteer need assumed to be 2 hr/day over year. Age-specific yearly hour need summed over age bands to yield aggregate hours of volunteer need.

[d]Sufficiency of volunteers calculated as ratio of aggregate volunteer hour supply to vulnerable elder hour demand. Ratio of 1 or greater indicates elder need met. Ratio less than 1 indicates shortfall. In 2005, by this calculation, 52% of elder volunteering need was met.

Both modeling assumptions can be challenged. It is always suspect to use national data to derive local estimates. If there is something different about the local area, national estimates can introduce potentially large biases. Likewise, assuming that all seniors need the same amount of daily volunteer support time is crude. Yet specifying these parameters is useful for pointing out data limitations and for suggesting the need for sensitivity analyses, in which these assumptions are altered to see how model estimates change.

With these assumptions, the number of vulnerable elders in each age band is multiplied by the 2 hr/day for the year to yield an estimate of age-specific yearly volunteer hours need. This is the basic model. An alternative scenario for elder volunteer demand was also developed, in which a combination of additional family care, elder financial resources, and in-home paid services cut the proportion of older persons requiring volunteer services by 25%.

A fully worked out calculation for the basic scenario in 2005 is shown in Table 3.7. In 2005, approximately 5,300 elders (2.5% of elders) required volunteer effort. In the aggregate, they would require 3.89 million hours over the year if each received 2 hr/day of volunteer time. In the more favorable alternate scenario, 3,995 elders (1.9%) would require volunteer effort for a total of 2.92 million hours of volunteer time over the year. These calculations assume no residential group settings for senior care, so that each elder would receive volunteer time one person at a time. Again, although this assumption simplifies calculations, it neglects an important variant in living arrangements, which, if large, would bias estimates.

As shown in Figure 3.3, assuming no change in the definition of vulnerability, this aggregate yearly demand for volunteer hours is expected to decline through 2015 and then pick up, given current projections of a declining but increasingly older population through 2015 and then an increasing older population through 2025. Demand for volunteer hours is anticipated to be 3.73 million in 2010, 3.67 million in 2015, 3.87 million in 2020, and 4.35 million in 2025. In the alternate scenario, demand for volunteer hours will be 2.80, 2.75, 2.90, and 3.26 million, respectively, over the same years.

Estimating the supply of volunteer hours for vulnerable elders required another set of calculations, again pieced together from various sources under varying assumptions. Supply calculations began again with Allegheny County population projections. Total volunteer rates by age are from *Pittsburgh Volunteer Trends, Volunteering in America,*

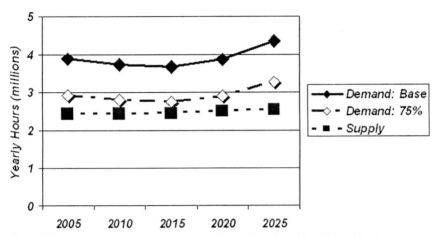

Figure 3.3 Projected volunteer demand and supply: vulnerable elders, Allegheny County, 2005–2025.

Note: "Demand: 75%" represents a more favorable scenario in which elders needing volunteer hours in each year are reduced by 25% because of alternative support hours provided through a combination of additional family care, elder financial resources, and in-home paid services. Even in this scenario, 11%–22% of elder volunteer need in each year goes unmet.

Cities, 2007 prepared by the Corporation for National and Community Service (2007). This gives the prevalence of volunteerism by age group, which ranges from 20% to 40%. The proportion volunteering for "social/ community service" is used as a proxy for senior volunteerism, because figures for elder volunteering are not available. This seems reasonable because it is intermediate between the highest volunteer venues (religious organizations) and other venues with lower volunteer involvement, but it could over- or underestimate the true levels. Multiplying these first two estimates, yields an estimate of age-specific elder volunteering, which ranges from 3% to 5% for different age bands. Applying this proportion to the number of people in each age group, yields an estimate of the number of volunteers to vulnerable elders. Median yearly hours for each age group are available from *Volunteering in the United States, 2007* (Bureau of Labor Statistics, 2007) and are inflated to capture the median of 70 hr/year of volunteer time reported for Pittsburgh in a Corporation for National and Community Service city-by-city analysis. These are summed to yield the aggregate yearly supply of elder volunteer hours.

The fully worked out example for the volunteer pool in 2005 is also shown in Table 3.7, upper panel. In 2005, about 36,000 volunteers in

Allegheny County provided 2.43 million volunteer hours for vulnerable elders.

Projecting to future years requires calculating volunteer prevalence among older adults, removing elders who cannot volunteer because they themselves need such services. Building this factor into the model shows that the aggregate supply of volunteer hours in Allegheny County is estimated to be 2.42 million in 2010, 2.45 million in 2015, 2.50 million in 2020, and 2.55 million in 2025.

That these estimates are projections, not true forecasts, in that they only show how assumptions about current processes or trends, if carried forward, will lead to change in aggregate supply and demand of volunteer time. The further out one projects, the less reliable the estimate. The projections are dynamic only to the extent they account for change in population (for which there exist reasonable estimates). Other factors, such as change in volunteerism by age group, or change in rates of disability and recovery, or change in living arrangements and care delivery, are all absent. Here again, modeling, even if primitive, is useful for clarifying the parameters to be included and the limitations in available data.

Recall that, in Chapter 2, we described the old-age dependency ratio as a measure of population aging: that is, the proportion of older adults in the population divided by the number of adults, in general, ages 18–64. This measure has sometimes been used to suggest crudely how many older adults there are per potential caregiver. Paralleling these calculations, the notion of "sufficiency of volunteers" can be calculated as the ratio of the aggregate volunteer hour supply to aggregate vulnerable elder hour demand. A ratio of 1 or greater indicates that the hours of care are sufficient so that elder needs can be "met." (Note that the ratio does not say anything about how well they are being met or the quality of the volunteer hours.) In this case, ratios less than 1 indicate a shortfall in volunteer aggregate hours. In 2005, by this calculation, ample volunteer hours were available to meet 62% of needed hours in the base scenario. In the more optimistic alternative scenario, available volunteer hours were available for 83% of hours of elder need.

Projecting forward, as shown in Figure 3.3, the volunteer sufficiency ratio increases steadily through 2015, moving from 0.62 (2005) to 0.65 (2010) and then to 0.68 (2015), showing a slight closing of the gap driven mainly by the declining elder population. In 2020 and 2025 the trend reverses, first to 0.65 and then to 0.59. In other words, given current trends in population, only about two thirds of the vulnerable elder demand for volunteer services is ever met and the proportion met will begin to decline after 2015 (see Table 3.3).

Under the alternative scenario with fewer older persons requiring volunteer effort, available volunteer hours meet 86% (2010), 89% (2015), 86% (2020), and 78% (2025) of elder volunteer need. Thus, even in the more favorable scenario, 11%–22% of elder volunteer need goes unmet.

For the base model, the most potent way to close the gap is to increase the number of people providing volunteer services for the older persons by about half. This would mean going from about 36,000 volunteers in 2010 to 50,000, a 14,000-person increase, and would immediately bring the supply of volunteer hours in line with projected elder demand. Alternatively, the gap could be closed by increasing the median yearly hours provided by these volunteers, increasing it to about 100 hours per year. This seems more challenging given that one large obstacle to volunteerism, mentioned again and again in community surveys, is perceived lack of time. Alternatively, and perhaps more realistically, we could seek to increase both the number of volunteers and the yearly hours they contribute. In this case, one would need to increase the number of volunteers by 15%–20% and seek as well to increase median hours per year to 80–85.

Yet another way to close the volunteer sufficiency gap is to reduce elder demand. This can be modeled by reducing the prevalence of IADL limitations, decreasing the proportion of elders who are isolated, or both. National studies suggest that reductions in IADL limitations have been taking place, with approximately a 2% decline per year between 1990 and 2005 (Schoeni, Freedman, & Martin, 2008.). This level of improving elder health would not change demand to a great extent, however. Combining expected health improvement with reductions in isolation would have a larger effect, but data are unavailable on the extent to which such isolation may be declining.

Although the specific estimates and targets depend heavily on the assumptions specified earlier, such assumptions are not unreasonable, given the data currently available, and parameters can be refined as new data become available. These initial estimates, although challenging to piece together, allow us to see what kind of changes in elder volunteerism or elder demand for aging services will be necessary to close the sufficiency gap.

SUMMARY

Parallel "Health Care Workforces" for the Aged. Families are supported by the medical sector in providing care to vulnerable seniors, but also by an alternative workforce that provides the bulk of services families are unable to provide to disabled elders. Help with meals, transportation, home modification, and many other facets of elder care come from the aging services sector, a loose network of nonprofit organizations and government agencies. The health and aging services sectors at present operate as parallel systems without effective integration. Because elders need aging services, in part, because of health needs, this lack of integration represents a great inefficiency that has only recently been addressed by joint CDC and AoA statewide efforts.

Attempts to Bridge the Parallel Systems of Elder Health Service Delivery. It is hard to know how much of the underdelivery of services to older adults, itself difficult to measure, is due to lack of coordination and how much is due to simple underinvestment of resources in both sectors. Still, the Aging States Project suggests that the two systems do not effectively leverage resources and makes a compelling case for a "healthy aging network" to replace or bridge the current systems. An effort to bridge local department of health housing violations data with adult protective services data from a local area agency on aging shows the difficulty of moving between the systems.

Efforts to Develop Healthy Aging Networks. CDC, AoA, and the National Council on Aging have begun to push toward integration with a focus on evidence-based interventions that link health and aging services, such as falls prevention or exercise programs offered in senior centers. These interventions often need to be translated into programs suitable for a particular community or target population, a challenge in itself. Along with the move to use evidence-based interventions, funders are increasingly demanding standardized accounting of populations served, services delivered, and the extent to which outcomes are met. Developing feasible indicators and benchmarks is an important challenge to the field.

Promoting Healthy Aging: Alternative Community-Based Approaches. An entirely different approach to prevention is direct outreach to elders to teach principles of healthy aging and to empower seniors themselves to obtain preventive health services. This approach gets away from the one-disease focus of most evidence-based interventions and instead stresses a whole-person approach to healthy aging. These interventions are less developed, but also offer promise.

Estimating Aging Services Network Challenges in the Community. Area agencies on aging project service needs in their yearly plans and budgets, but these are rarely used for research or public health planning. A community-wide accounting of the supply and demand of volunteer hours available each year for vulnerable elders suggests how programs might be targeted. However, local statistics that bridge public health and aging are often difficult to obtain. Instead, those engaged in public health and aging must piece together existing information by using the best assumptions possible as a way to estimate need for services. Such models require many simplifying assumptions along the way, and often involve the creative—but cautious—application of data from state or even national resources to the local level. Indeed, sometimes there is no option but to rely on data that are not meant to be applied to your population, but with proper caveats and assessment of bias, it is still possible to learn a great deal. Assessment of bias is critical in piecing together data from different sources.

4   Chronic Disease in Older Adults

Prevention has been identified as a key element of healthy aging, yet a substantial number of older adults are living with one or more chronic diseases. This chapter provides an introduction to common population-based measures of chronic illness and disease. Verbrugge and Patrick (1995) define chronic conditions as "long-term diseases, injuries with long sequelae, and enduring structural, sensory, and communicative disorders." They add, "their defining aspect is duration. Once they are past certain symptomatic or diagnostic thresholds, chronic conditions are essentially permanent features for the rest of life. Medical and personal regimens can sometimes control but can rarely cure them."

We also review the current state of health promotion and disease prevention aimed at older adults, including which preventive services are currently recommended for older adults and how scientific evidence is used in the process of setting these recommendations. A third section discusses the Medicare program and its role in financing preventive services. A final section offers an overview of existing chronic disease management programs.

COMMON POPULATION-BASED MEASURES
OF ILLNESS AND DISEASE

Prevalence

One of the most common measures of illness and disease is referred to as disease prevalence. If you want to understand at a point in time, what a "snap shot" of the population looks like, you are probably interested in prevalence. Point prevalence refers to the number of persons who have a particular disease among the population at a given point in time. Most of the time true point prevalence is not available, because large surveys and epidemiologic studies take place over a period of time. Instead, epidemiologists count the number of people with illness (the numerator) and divide it by the average population during the study period (the denominator), yielding a measure of period prevalence. Prevalence measures in general give a useful cross section of what is happening, but the measure is influenced by at least two processes: the chance among those who do not have the condition of developing it (incidence) and the duration of the condition among those who develop it. The latter is a function of the probability of surviving with the condition and recovering from it.

Figure 4.1 shows reports of prevalent chronic conditions for men and women for 2005–2006 from the National Health Interview Survey, ordered from most to least prevalent. Note that, like most surveys, participants are asked whether a doctor ever told them they had a particular condition. For many conditions that approach is a reasonable way to ascertain prevalence, but for some conditions that are known to be underdiagnosed, such as diabetes or hypertension, these estimates will likely be lower than the true prevalence.

Although older men and women have a similar (within 2 percentage points) prevalence of hypertension, stroke, asthma, chronic lung disease, and diabetes, there are several important differences: women report higher levels of arthritis and depressive symptoms, whereas men report higher levels of heart disease and cancer.

Not shown in Figure 4.1 are important differences by race and ethnicity. According to the most recent chart book on older Americans prepared by the Federal Interagency Forum on Aging-Related Statistics (2008), in 2005–2006, among people age 65 and over, the prevalence of hypertension and diabetes was higher for non-Hispanic Blacks than for non-Hispanic Whites: 70% vs. 51% for hypertension and 29% vs. 16% for diabetes. Hispanics also reported higher levels of diabetes than

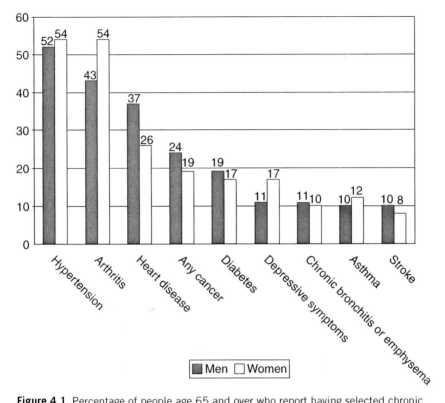

Figure 4.1 Percentage of people age 65 and over who report having selected chronic conditions, by sex, 2005–2006.

Source: From *Older Americans 2008: Key Indicators of Well-Being,* by Federal Interagency Forum on Aging-Related Statistics, March 2008. Washington, DC: U.S. Government Printing Office.

non-Hispanic Whites (25% vs. 16%), but similar levels of hypertension (54% and 51%, respectively) and lower levels of arthritis (40% vs. 50%).

Incidence

In contrast to prevalence, the incidence rate provides a measure of new events that occur during a specified period of time among a population at risk for getting the disease. Incidence rates are especially useful in establishing risk factors linked to the onset of conditions and for understanding whether prevention efforts are reducing the onset of new cases.

The difference between the numerator in a prevalence estimate and in an incidence rate is relatively straightforward: instead of including everyone with the condition in the numerator, as is done in calculating prevalence, only *new* cases found during the specified period of time are counted in the numerator for calculating incidence.

The denominator in an incidence rate also differs conceptually from that found in prevalence calculations. The denominator for an incidence rate ideally should exclude individuals who already have the condition of interest, because they are not at risk for becoming a new case. For rare conditions, this adjustment does not make much difference, but for common chronic conditions, like hypertension, heart disease, arthritis, and even some forms of cancer, these adjustments may be important. Because the incidence rate is calculated over a time period, the number of people at risk for developing a condition is likely to change over time. Sometimes the population at risk at the beginning of the period is used and then the rate is called a cumulative incidence rate. In other cases, the population that is at risk at the midpoint is used to represent the average size population that is at risk. If people are observed for different follow-up periods, the denominator may be expressed in terms of "person-time" units. That is, individuals contribute to the denominator, for instance, one month for each month they are alive, in the study, and have not contracted the condition. All new cases are then divided by this person-time denominator.

In practice, large surveys that monitor individuals at regular intervals (say, every 2 years) do not provide a true incidence rate. Instead, one can get an estimate of onset between waves if one limits calculations to those who did not have the condition at first contact, and reports the percentage that are alive, and report having the condition at follow-up. Onset differs from a true incidence rate because individuals who die or are lost from the study are not included in the calculations, but it is a reasonable approximation over short periods of time for conditions with relatively low mortality. For higher mortality conditions, onset calculations will probably be lower than true incidence.

Table 4.1 shows by sex the percentage of adults age 55 and older who reported having one of six common chronic conditions in 2002 and the percentage who reported a new condition in 2004 (among those without the condition in 2002). Consistent with the statistics from the National Health Interview Survey, women report higher levels of arthritis and whereas men report higher levels of heart problems. However, gender patterns are different in Table 4.1 than in Figure 4.1. Why might this be the case?

Two obvious possibilities come to mind. First, the populations are defined differently (65 and older in Figure 4.1 vs. 55 and older in Table 4.1).

Table 4.1

PERCENTAGE OF 55 AND OLDER POPULATION REPORTING CHRONIC CONDITIONS IN 2002, AND PERCENTAGE REPORTING ONSET OF CONDITION IN 2004, BY SEX

CONDITION	MEN		WOMEN	
	PREVALENCE: % REPORTING CONDITION IN 2002	*2-YEAR ONSET:* % REPORTING ONSET OF CONDITION IN 2004 (AMONG THOSE WITHOUT CONDITION IN 2002)	*PREVALENCE:* % REPORTING CONDITION IN 2002	*2-YEAR ONSET:* % REPORTING ONSET OF CONDITION IN 2004 (AMONG THOSE WITHOUT CONDITION IN 2002)
High blood pressure	50.2	10.2	52.5	12.3
Arthritis	49.8	11.2	64.8	15.2
Heart problems	27.1	6.3	21.9	5.4
Diabetes	17.9	3.5	15.0	3.3
Cancer	13.4	3.5	13.6	2.4
Stroke	8.3	1.9	7.7	2.1
No. in 2002	6,580	—	8,794	—

Analysis of the 2002 and 2004 waves of the Health and Retirement Study adapted from "Neighborhood Associations With Chronic Disease Prevalence and Onset in Later Life," by V. A. Freedman, I. B. Grafova, R. F. Schoeni, & J. Rogowski, November 16–20, 2007a. Paper presented at the annual meeting of the Gerontological Society of America, San Francisco, CA.

Second, and more subtle, the two surveys have different definitions of cancer. The National Health Interview Survey asks: "Have you EVER been told by a doctor or other health professional that you had . . . Cancer or a malignancy of any kind?" Whereas the Health and Retirement Study asks: "Has a doctor ever told you that you have cancer or a malignant tumor, excluding minor skin cancers?" It is possible that the exclusion of skin cancer results in a different pattern by gender. Because men are more likely than women to develop skin cancer, leaving minor skin cancers out of the calculations tips the scale toward women.

Another pattern evident in Table 4.1 is that high blood pressure and arthritis are the most prevalent conditions, but also have the highest rates of onset in this population, with higher rates of prevalence and onset reported by women than men. In contrast, diabetes, cancer, and stroke have much lower rates of onset (in the 2%–4% range over the 2-year period), with women reporting fewer onsets of diabetes and cancer, but not stroke.

It is noteworthy, based on Table 4.1, that greater onset does not always mean greater prevalence. In the case of cancer (excluding minor skin cancers), for example, men have a higher percentage experiencing onset (3.5% vs. 2.4%), but a similar, or slightly lower, prevalence than women (13.4% vs. 13.6%). Why might this be? The populations and definitions are the same, so we must consider other explanations. Recall that prevalence is influenced not only by incidence, but also by survival. The pattern we see for cancer suggests that men are not surviving as long with cancer as women are.

COMPARING PREVALENT, DEBILITATING, AND HIGH-MORTALITY CONDITIONS

To this point, we have focused on the most commonly reported chronic conditions. However, the most prevalent conditions among older adults are not necessarily the most debilitating, nor are they necessarily likely to result in death. An important distinction then is among conditions that are common, those that are debilitating, and those that are most likely to result in death. Table 4.2 shows the top six conditions falling into each category. The first two columns are based on analysis of the 2004 National Health Interview Survey (NHIS). Note that omitted from the NHIS analysis were two relatively debilitating conditions: unintentional injuries (such as hip fractures) and cognitive conditions such as Alzheimer's disease and related dementias. The last column comes directly from death certificate data, which are discussed in more detail in Chapter 10.

The only condition common to all three lists is diabetes. It is not only highly prevalent (17% in 2004) but also fairly debilitating (18% of those with diabetes in 2004 reported having an activity limitation). And in 2004 diabetes was the 6th leading cause of death. In contrast, hypertension and arthritis are highly prevalent but do not make the top six debilitating or common causes of death. Other conditions, such as stroke and lung conditions, are debilitating and have high mortality, but they are not prevalent enough to make the top-six list.

Why are these distinctions important? If the goal of public health is to prevent the onset of or to detect early highly prevalent chronic conditions (primary and secondary prevention), the six most prevalent conditions make excellent targets. At the other extreme, programs like Nixon's "war on cancer" are appropriate if the goal is to maximize life expectancy. However, if the aim is to maximize functioning, then conditions appearing in the middle of Table 4.2 become important to target: mental distress and hearing limitations, for example, do not appear on either of the other two lists, but clearly are important in maximizing the functioning and well-being of older adults.

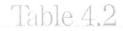

Table 4.2

SIX MOST PREVALENT, MOST DEBILITATING, AND MOST COMMON CAUSES OF DEATH IN THE 65 AND OLDER POPULATION

MOST PREVALENT CONDITIONS[a]	MOST DEBILITATING CONDITIONS[b]	MOST COMMON CAUSES OF DEATH[c]
Hypertension	Mental distress	Heart disease
Arthritis	Stroke	Cancer
Heart disease	Vision limitation	Stroke
Cancer	Hearing limitation	Lung conditions
Diabetes	Diabetes	Alzheimer's disease
Vision Limitation	Lung conditions	Diabetes

[a,b]Freedman et al. (2007a), based on National Health Interview Survey.
[c]Center for Disease Control. National Vital Statistics System, National Center for Health Statistics. 10 Leading causes of death by age group, United States—2004.

COMORBIDITY, MULTIMORBIDITY, AND SELF-CARE

In later life, most adults do not have a single chronic condition. The term comorbidity, sometimes also called multimorbidity, is the presence of two or more health conditions in the same individual. The experience of having multiple conditions can lead to a long list of unfavorable outcomes, including mortality, poor functioning, and increased use of health care (see Gijsen et al., 2001, for a review of consequences). There are several common approaches to measuring comorbidity (John et al., 2003) including counts of conditions, weighted indices that take disease severity into account, examination of the proportion of the population with a condition who have a second condition, and analysis of measures of association and whether patterns and levels are greater than what would be found owing to chance (if conditions were independent).

In the United States, 35% of adults between ages 65 and 79 and more than 70% of adults ages 80 and older have more than one chronic condition (Fried, Ferrucci, Darer, Williamson, & Anderson, 2004b). Per capita annual medical expenditures double with each additional condition up to three, and persons with four or more chronic conditions on average have more than 12 times the medical expenditures of someone with one condition (Wolff, Starfield, & Anderson, 2002). Because of out-of-pocket medical expenses associated with treatments for chronic disease, comorbidity leads to significant wealth depletion in later life, especially for unmarried older adults (Kim & Lee, 2006).

We know very little about specific patterns of multimorbidity in the older population. Recent data from Sweden suggest that in older persons with multimorbidity, there exists co-occurrence of specific types of diseases beyond chance (Marengoni, Rizzuto, Wang, Winblad, & Fratiglioni, 2009). That is, there seem to be a higher probability than just due to chance of reporting clusters of circulatory conditions, clusters of cardiopulmonary conditions, and both mental health and musculoskeletal conditions.

Today, older individuals who have multiple conditions are expected to participate in the management of their conditions. An older adult with hypertension may be encouraged to have his or her pressure checked between visits to the physician, perhaps with a home monitor or at a local drug store. If he or she also has diabetes, that person will need to check his or her blood sugars, potentially several times a day, and follow a diet to help keep his or her glucose stable. If the person has another common condition, congestive heart failure, he or she may also be asked to follow a low-salt diet and weigh him- or herself daily. We know very little about how well patients manage these tasks in the face of multiple conditions. It is likely that family members—spouses and other people living with the patient or even children who live nearby—may play an important supportive role, but little research to date has focused on this topic.

What is known is that, because of shifts that took place many years ago in the educational system and in policies that provided education to soldiers returning from the Second World War, the older population today is better educated than it was just a few decades ago. This means that they may have more skills with which to manage their conditions. The concept of *health literacy*—the degree to which individuals have the capacity to obtain, process, and understand basic health information and services needed to make appropriate health decisions (CDC, *Healthy People 2010, 2009*)—has gained attention in recent years. People who have limited health literacy may have difficulty with a variety of self-care tasks, including finding providers and services, filling out forms, accurately sharing a medical history, taking medications according to directions, and following other instructions from providers for managing health conditions. Health literacy is different from literacy in that it encompasses skills that are needed to make treatment and self-care decisions. An individual who is literate (can read) but has a low health literacy might have difficulty finding and evaluating the credibility of health information, assessing risks and benefits of health care decisions, calculating the amount of a prescription to take, or understanding test results.

Health literacy may be measured in three domains: the ability to search, comprehend, and use information from a continuous text source ("prose"); the ability to search, comprehend, and use information from a noncontinuous text source like a bus schedule ("document"); and the ability to identify and perform calculations by using numbers found in printed materials ("quantitative"). According to the Federal Interagency Forum on Aging-Related Statistics, the health literacy of older adults in each of these areas is improving. In 2003, only 23%, 27%, and 34% of older adults had below basic prose, document, and quantitative health literacy skills, respectively (see Figure 4.2), whereas the figures in 1992 were 33%, 38%, and 49%, respectively.

Nevertheless, health literacy in later life remains a significant challenge. In 2003, 60%–71% of people age 65 and over had below basic or basic health literacy skills, depending on the measure. It is not surprising

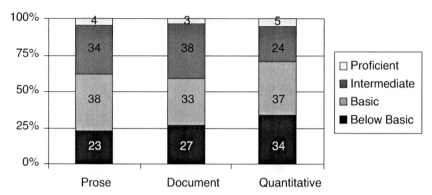

Figure 4.2 Percentage of people age 65 and over who demonstrate proficient, intermediate, basic, and below basic health literacy: 2003.

Source: From *Older Americans 2008: Key Indicators of Well-Being,* by Federal Interagency Forum on Aging-Related Statistics, March 2008. Washington, DC: U.S. Government Printing Office.

that limited health literacy increases with age, and is more common among minority populations, those with fewer economic resources, fewer years of education, and cultural or language barriers.

THE STATE OF HEALTH PROMOTION AND CHRONIC DISEASE PREVENTION FOR OLDER ADULTS

The idea of primary prevention in late life still strikes some people as strange. We have been unable to identify any comprehensive treatment of the subject. Even the field of "preventive" or "interventional geriatrics," which is further along, is still relatively new. In fact, efforts toward this end are underway in a number of fields, from neuroscience to occupational therapy, and continued progress toward primary prevention in late life is reported nearly weekly. Still, no comprehensive account is available.

In this section, we review current recommendations for older adults made by the U.S. Preventive Services Task Force (USPSTF). At this point, the Task Force does not provide separate guidelines for adults aged 65 and older but rather offers "adult health" guidelines. Indeed, there are so few recommendations that apply to older adults that they can be summarized in a single table. Here, we review the source and nature of these recommendations and how research was used in the process.

The U.S. Preventive Services Task Force

First convened by the U.S. Public Health Service in 1984, and now sponsored by the Agency for Healthcare Research and Quality, the USPSTF is the leading independent panel of private-sector experts in prevention and primary care in the United States. The panel's job is to conduct rigorous, impartial assessments of the scientific evidence for clinical preventive services. The range of services is unusually broad and covers screening, counseling, and preventive medications and procedures. The USPSTF's recommendations are considered the "gold standard" for clinical preventive services.

Initially published in 1989 as the Guide to Clinical Preventive Services, the USPSTF has made periodic updates (e.g., 1996). The current guide (2008) is available on the Web at http://www.ahrq.gov/clinic/pocketgd08/. The process by which these recommendations are made involves several steps: reviewing the existing evidence base, estimating the magnitude of the benefits and harms for each preventive service, reaching a consensus about the net benefit for each preventive service, and issuing a recommendation. The recommendation is made in the form of a grade from A to I, whereby A means strongly recommended, B means recommended, C means there is no recommendation for or against, D is a recommendation against, and I indicates insufficient evidence on which to base a recommendation. Of the 40 or so screen recommendations relevant to older adults, nearly half involved insufficient evidence. The remaining recommendations (5 strongly recommended, 8 recommended, and 10 interventions which are explicitly recommended *against* as of the 2008 report) are shown in Table 4.3.

Use of Evidence in Setting Recommendations

It would not be unusual for a student to wonder, at this point, just how does the task force decide that a particular preventive service should receive a "D" grade? To understand how research is used to determine a recommendation, one needs to have an appreciation for the concepts of reliability, validity, power, and diagnostic utility of screening. We turn to each of these concepts now.

Reliability is the extent to which a measurement instrument yields consistent results when repeated multiple times. Think of getting on a scale several times in a row: does the scale always read the same value? If so that scale is reliable. Another analogy that is helpful when thinking

Table 4.3

RECOMMENDATIONS, U.S. PREVENTIVE SERVICES TASK FORCE, 2008

STRONGLY RECOMMENDED (A)

1. Clinicians discuss aspirin chemoprevention with adults who are at increased risk for coronary heart disease
2. Clinicians screen adults aged 18 and older for high blood pressure
3. Clinicians routinely screen men aged 35 years and older and women aged 45 years and older for lipid disorders and treat abnormal lipids in people who are at increased risk of coronary heart disease
4. Clinicians screen men and women 50 years of age or older for colorectal cancer
5. Clinicians screen all adults for tobacco use and provide tobacco cessation interventions for those who use tobacco products

RECOMMENDED (B)

1. One-time screening for abdominal aortic aneurysm (AAA) by ultrasonography in men aged 65 to 75 who have ever smoked
2. Screening mammography, with or without clinical breast examination (CBE), every 1–2 years for women aged 40 and older
3. Screening adults for depression in clinical practices that have systems in place to ensure accurate diagnosis, effective treatment, and follow-up
4. Screening for type 2 diabetes in adults with hypertension or hyperlipidemia
5. Intensive behavioral dietary counseling for adult patients with hyperlipidemia and other known risk factors for cardiovascular and diet-related chronic disease
6. Clinicians screen all adult patients for obesity and offer intensive counseling and behavioral interventions to promote sustained weight loss for obese adults
7. Women age 65 and older and women age 60–64 who are at increased risk of osteoporotic fracture be screened routinely for osteoporosis
8. Women whose family history is associated with an increased risk for deleterious mutations in BRCA1 or BRCA2 genes be referred for genetic counseling and evaluation for BRCA testing

RECOMMENDED AGAINST (D)

1. Routine use of tamoxifen or raloxifene for the primary prevention of breast cancer in women at low or average risk for breast cancer
2. Routinely screening women older than age 65 for cervical cancer if they have had adequate recent screening with normal Pap smears and are not otherwise at high risk for cervical cancer

(Continued)

Table 4.3

RECOMMENDATIONS, U.S. PREVENTIVE SERVICES
TASK FORCE, 2008 (*Continued*)

3. Routine use of combined estrogen and progestin for the prevention of chronic conditions in postmenopausal women

4. Routine screening for ovarian cancer

5. Screening for pancreatic cancer in asymptomatic adults

6. Routine screening for bladder cancer in adults

7. Routine screening for peripheral arterial disease (PAD)

8. Routine screening for testicular cancer in asymptomatic adolescent and adult males

9. Use of beta-carotene supplements, either alone or in combination, for the prevention of cancer or cardiovascular disease

10. Routine use of aspirin and nonsteroidal anti-inflammatory drugs (NSAIDs) to prevent colorectal cancer in individuals at average risk for colorectal cancer

about reliability is playing a game of darts. Hitting the same spot on the board over and over would mean you have reliable aim. Reliability is relatively easy to demonstrate or refute and, in general, takes the form of assessing how closely aligned (or correlated) are multiple measures of the same phenomenon.

Validity is a much harder concept to demonstrate. Validity is the extent to which a measure accurately reflects the concept that it is intended to measure. Think of the scale described above. It gives you the same value every time you get on, but is that scale showing you 5 pounds lighter than you are? If so, the scale may be reliable, but it is not valid. Invoking the dart board image, you may be hitting the same spot over and over again with the darts, but are you hitting the bull's eye (which in this case represents what you truly wish to measure)? If you are hitting the bull's eye, you have a valid and reliable measurement tool. Note a scale can be reliable but not valid (a scale that always shows you weigh 5 pounds less than you do), but a valid scale must always be reliable.

There are different types of validity that become important in assessing the validity of a research study. Internal validity is the extent to which conclusions can be drawn from the study sample about relationships among variables measured in the study. For a study to have internal validity its measures must be both valid and reliable. In addition, the study must be designed in such a way that one can compare individuals who received a preventive service with those who did not, and such comparisons must be valid over time—that is, the groups must be comparable before the service and nothing else but direct consequences of receiving the service should be different between the two groups after the services are given. Groups typically are made to be comparable through the process of randomly selecting who receives the treatment, but even randomized trials can have threats to internal validity if follow-up differs between the treatment and control groups.

Even if a study has excellent internal validity, there still may be threats to drawing conclusions beyond the study sample. External validity refers to whether such conclusions can be drawn more generally and depends on whether the sample was drawn probabilistically or if it relied on volunteers who did not look like people who would actually use the service in the real world. External validity also depends on whether all groups of interest are represented. A study of 40–59-year-olds, for instance, does not necessarily have external generalizability to older adults. Likewise, studies of men may not generalize to women, and studies that exclude minorities may not apply to groups that have not been represented.

A related concept that is important for the task force to set its recommendations is the notion of *power*. The power of a trial is the probability you will detect a meaningful difference, or effect, if one really exists. The larger the sample size, the more power a trial will have. Another way to define power is in terms of probabilities—in this case, the probability of NOT making an error in which you say there is no effect when there actually is one. This is the probability of not making a type II error, or falsely rejecting the null. By convention, most studies are designed to have a power of at least .80 or higher to detect clinically meaningful differences, so that type II errors will be minimized.

Finally, we turn to the *diagnostic utility of screening*. One of the best treatments diagnostic utility we have found was by T.-W. Loong in the *British Medical Journal* (2003). Here, we provide a brief summary, but we urge the reader to review the visual aids in Loong (2003). Imagine a hypothetical population in which 25% of the population has a disease. Twenty-five percent is the disease prevalence. Now imagine you have a screening test and you screen the entire population and find that 20% test positive for the disease. The *sensitivity* of your screening test is calculated as follows: among those with the disease, what percent test positive? The sensitivity tells you an important piece of information— were you able to identify when someone had the disease that they actually have it. Subtracting the sensitivity from 100% yields the false-negative rate—the extent to which you say someone does not have the disease when they actually do. Sensitivity and false-negative rates are only one way to evaluate your instrument. You also need to know the *specificity* of your screening test: among those without the disease, what percent test negative? The specificity tells you whether your test goes too far and identifies people as having the disease when they really do not have it. In fact, 100% minus specificity gives you the false-positive rate. Both sensitivity and specificity are considered to be "disease-denominator" measures—in the first case, people with the disease are in the denominator, and in the latter, people without the disease are in the denominator. The advantage of disease-denominator measures is that they are not sensitive to the prevalence of the disease. So you can use sensitivity and specificity with rare and common conditions alike.

There are two additional ways to evaluate your screening test. You can look among those who test positive and ask, what percentage truly have the disease? This is called *positive predictive value.* You can also look among those who test negative and ask, what percentage truly do NOT have the disease? Not surprisingly, this is called *negative predictive value.* Together these are referred to as "test-denominator" measures. Unlike disease-denominator measures, positive and negative predictive value change depending on the prevalence of the disease. For example, the rarer the disease, the lower the positive predictive value will be.

Now that we have covered all the basic concepts, we can turn to the question of under what circumstances does the USPSTF assign a "D" recommendation (recommend against)? A "D Grade" is given if:

- The condition has a low prevalence and the screen misses people with the condition, that is, has a low sensitivity or a high rate of false negatives.
- There is limited evidence that early treatment improves outcomes. Even if a screening tool has excellent sensitivity and specificity, if intervening early does not improve health outcomes, a preventive service may receive a "D" rating.
- There is harm that comes from a false positive (100% minus specificity). A range of harms may be considered from actual risks associated with the procedure to the experience of unnecessary anxiety.

Case Study of Breast Cancer Screening

Let's take a look at a specific example of how a recommendation is set. In 2008, the USPSTF recommended: screening mammography, with or without clinical breast examination (CBE), every 1–2 years for women aged 40 and older. The rationale for the recommendation follows:

Rationale: The USPSTF found fair evidence that mammography screening every 12–33 months significantly reduces mortality from breast cancer. Evidence is strongest for women aged 50–69, the age group generally included in screening trials. For women aged 40–49, the evidence that screening mammography reduces mortality from breast cancer is weaker, and the absolute benefit of mammography is smaller, than it is for older women. Most, but not all, studies indicate a mortality benefit for women undergoing mammography at ages 40–49, but the delay in observed benefit in women younger than 50 makes it difficult to determine the incremental benefit of beginning screening at age 40 rather than at age 50.

The absolute benefit is smaller because the incidence of breast cancer is lower among women in their 40s than it is among older women. The USPSTF concluded that the evidence is also generalizable to women aged 70 and older (who face a higher absolute risk for breast cancer) if their life expectancy is not compromised by comorbid disease. The absolute probability of benefits of regular mammography increase along a continuum with age, whereas the likelihood of harms from screening (false-positive results and unnecessary anxiety, biopsies, and cost) diminish from ages 40–70. The balance of benefits and potential harms, therefore, grows more favorable as women age. The precise age at which the potential benefits of mammography justify the possible harms is a subjective choice. The USPSTF did not find sufficient evidence to specify the optimal screening interval for women aged 40–49. (USPSTF, 2002)

In a report prepared for the task force and subsequent peer-reviewed article, Humphrey and colleagues (2002a, 2002b) searched the Controlled Trials Registry, medical literature databases, and reference lists of articles found to compile a list of randomized, controlled trials of screening with death from breast cancer as the outcome. The authors abstracted information about the patient population, the study design, issues of study quality, data analysis, and findings at each reported length of follow-up. They then rated each study in terms of internal validity, with good meaning all criteria were met and the study's findings were likely to be correct; fair meaning there were important but not major flaws so that the study was possibly valid; and poor indicating there were major flaws with the results likely to be invalid. Seven criteria were used for rating the studies:

1. The intervention was clearly defined
2. All important outcomes were measured
3. Data were appropriately analyzed according to how participants were initially assigned (also called "intention to treat" analysis)
4. The treatment and control groups that were initially assembled were demonstrated to be comparable, for example, through randomization, by showing equal distribution of confounders and similar mortality rates prior to the intervention
5. The treatment and control groups were equally maintained over time, through, for example, high adherence, low crossover from one group to another, and low contamination of information from one group to another
6. Low, nondifferential loss to follow-up across treatment and control groups
7. Valid and reliable measures applied equally in treatment and control groups

Humphrey and colleagues identified eight trials, seven of which were rated as "fair." The reasons for fair ratings varied. For instance, the Health Insurance Plan Study took place from 1963 to 1966, so its findings, although valid for that time period, are not necessarily relevant to the equipment in use today. Four Swedish trials all had issues with randomization and some had issues with measuring the outcome (death from breast cancer). Two Swedish (Malmo) trials were perhaps the best designed, one focusing on women ages 45–69 and the other on women ages 70–74, but still were deemed only "fair." The sensitivity and specificity of the trials rated as fair are summarized in Table 4.4.

Overall, the studies suggested that 77%–95% of cases with breast cancer are correctly identified as having cancer with 1-year screening. The rate is lower for women in their forties and lower for 2-year screening intervals. In terms of specificity, 94%–97% of cases without breast cancer are correctly identified as not having cancer. In other words, 3%–6% of those who did not have breast cancer are incorrectly screened positively (false-positive rate). The test-denominator measures (not shown), suggested that the positive predictive value ranged from 2% to 22%. That is, 2%–22% of cases with positive ("abnormal") results were found to have cancer upon further evaluation, and 12%–78% of cases

Table 4.4

SENSITIVITY AND SPECIFICITY OF STUDIES EVALUATING BREAST CANCER MAMMOGRAPHY FOR WOMEN IN THEIR 40s

| STUDY (AGES) | SENSITIVITY | | SPECIFICITY |
	1-YEAR INTERVALS	2-YEAR INTERVALS	
Health Insurance Plan of Greater New York (HIP) (40–64)	NR	NR	—
Malmo, Sweden (45–69 / 70–74)	.92 / .81	—	.97
Swedish 2-County (40–74)	.95	.86	.96
Stockholm, Sweden (40–64)	.86	.68	.95
Canadian National Breast Screening Study-1 (40–49)	.77	.56	.94
Canadian National Breast Screening Study-2 (50–59)	.88	.56	—

From "Screening for Breast Cancer," by L. L. Humphrey, B. K. S. Chan, S. Detlefsen, & M. Helfand, 2002a, *Systematic Evidence Review No. 15*. Prepared by the Oregon Health & Science University (Practice Center under Contract No. 290-97-0018). Rockville, MD: Agency for Healthcare Research and Quality.

with positive ("abnormal") results were found to have cancer on biopsy. The positive predictive value increased with age.

What about effects on mortality? Four Swedish trials compared two to six rounds of mammography with usual care among 50–74-year-olds. They found a 9%–32% reduction in risk for death from breast cancer, but this result was significant in only one of the four trials. When the results were combined across studies (in a "meta-analysis"), the relative risk of dying for those who screened compared with those who did not was 0.84 (95% confidence interval 0.77–0.91), a statistically significant reduction. Of seven trials including 40–49-year-old women, five showed a benefit, but only one had sufficient power to show statistically significant results and only after many years (11–19) of follow-up. Combining the results in a meta-analysis resulted in a relative risk of mortality from breast cancer of 0.85 (95% confidence interval 0.73–0.99) after 14 years. The benefit appears to increase with longer follow-up.

Although the USPSTF is the leading panel evaluating preventive services in the United States, it is worth noting that not all scientists agree. Another view of the breast cancer trials that appeared in the *Lancet* (see Gotzsche & Olsen, 2000; Olsen & Gotzsche, 2001; and related commentaries) is instructive in this regard. The authors reviewed the same body of evidence and found that the practice of assigning breast cancer diagnoses was not blinded to researchers involved in the studies. So they chose to focus on deaths from all causes rather than deaths from breast cancer. They also focused exclusively on the Malmo and Canadian (CNBSS) studies, and chose to exclude the remaining trials as not having adequate validity. When only the Malmo and CNBSS studies were considered, the effect of screening on all causes of mortality was zero. Moreover, the incidence of mastectomies and lumpectomies was 30%–40% higher in screening groups compared with groups of every study done after 1970. The authors concluded that 40 unnecessary surgeries were conducted for every 10,000 women screened and that mammographic screening for breast cancer was unjustified.

The ensuing debate depicted the state of evidence-based medicine in crisis (Goodman, 2002). Others have suggested that there are flaws, albeit minor, in all of the trials, but nevertheless six show significant breast cancer mortality reduction for women who underwent screening (Jackson, 2002). In 2009, after reviewing the evidence again, the USP-STF changed course and recommended against screening for women ages 40 to 49 and for screening every two years for women ages 50 to 74. They also concluded there was insufficient evidence to recommend for or against screening for women ages 75 or older. Perhaps the moral of this story is that we need well designed clinical trials *before* recommendations for preventive services are made. This may also help explain why it is so important that the USPSTF have and maintain a rating of "I" (insufficient evidence).

Older Adults and the Influenza Vaccine

Research suggests great benefit in a number of clinical preventive services but perhaps none greater than influenza vaccination. In a comparison of older adults who were vaccinated compared with those who were not over two flu seasons, Nichol et al. (2003) showed great reductions not just in hospitalization for pneumonia, but also hospitalization for stroke and cardiac disease. The reduction in risk and the number needed to treat to gain this benefit are shown in Figure 4.3.

Older adults who were vaccinated faced a much lower risk of mortality as well. This analysis is complicated by lack of a randomized,

Generalized Benefit of Influenza Vaccination

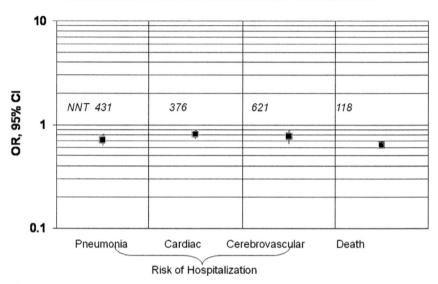

Figure 4.3 Generalized benefit on influenza vaccination.

Source: Nichol (2003).

controlled design (it would be unethical today not to vaccinate older people and people with chronic disease), and the investigators recognized that people who accept vaccination are different from those who do not. Vaccine acceptors are likely to be more proactive in health behaviors, but in this case were older and likely to have more chronic conditions as well. Nichol et al. (2003) and colleagues adjusted for differences between the group and made a strong case for the benefits of vaccination. More recently, Nichol and colleagues (2007) found, among older adults in the community, that influenza vaccination was associated with significant reductions in the risk of pneumonia- or influenza-related hospitalizations and mortality over 10 seasons. They concluded that vaccine delivery to older adults should be improved.

Results such as these suggest that the yearly prevalence of flu vaccination among older adults—which ranges from 40% to 60%—needs attention. Recognizing the need to increase vaccination among the older population, the Vote and Vax project makes vaccination clinics available to older adults at polling places. In November 2008, the program delivered 21,434 influenza vaccinations at 331 locations in 42 states and the District of Columbia. The effort is unique in its targeting of older adults at polling places and its recognition that older adults are most likely to vote.

Notwithstanding this program's success, it is useful to ask, do the nation's current efforts go far enough? Would it be possible, for instance, to have standing orders for older adults, in which nurses or other health personnel are able to vaccinate whenever someone comes to an appointment and is not up to date on vaccination? Is an even more proactive approach possible, one that is modeled, for example, after the U.S. experience with folate supplementation in bread? Folate is now added to all bread in the United States because of its clear benefit in preventing neural tube defects and spina bifida. It would be an interesting exercise to explore the effects of making flu vaccine similarly available. What might the effects on health and functioning of older adults be from such a program, and how might health effects differ in both the short and long term and at the individual and population levels? We offer some further insights into how to evaluate and compare different types of intervention in Chapter 5. Here, we take up the more fundamental issue of how criteria for setting up public health programs differ from the kinds of preventive services guidelines we have just reviewed.

Criteria for a Public Health Program

The preventive services guidelines are made based on whether there is sufficient evidence that individuals will benefit. But what if we are setting up a public health program? Recall from Chapter 1 that clinical geriatrics and public health differ in important ways. Clinical geriatrics stresses medical management of chronic disease and rehabilitation in the face of disabilities related to these conditions. Wallace (2005) explains that unlike clinical geriatrics, public health and aging places emphasis on prevention, proactive measures to preserve and promote health, rather than on a reactive treatment of disease. Moreover, public health focuses on the population rather than individual, and its programs and policies therefore address the community as a whole. How then might the criteria for such public health programs differ from clinical guidelines?

New York State's Department of Health offers some insight into the issue. They have outlined a set of principles to help guide adoption of public health screening efforts in that state. The Web site (http://www. health.state.ny.us/diseases/chronic/discreen.htm) suggests that the following criteria must be met for a condition to be a target of screening programs:

- Life-threatening diseases and those known to have serious and irreversible consequences if not treated early
- Conditions for which treatment at earlier stages is more effective than treatment begun after the development of symptoms
- Conditions for which screening tools have adequate sensitivity and specificity
- Conditions for which screening is low cost, easy to administer, safe, imposes minimal discomfort on administration, and is acceptable to both patients and practitioners
- Conditions that are high enough in prevalence for the program to be cost-effective
- Conditions for which appropriate follow-up care is available

Note that the public health concerns extend beyond those identified by the USPSTF to include administrative concerns related to cost and cost-effectiveness, ease of administration, and the availability of follow-up care.

MEDICARE AND FINANCING OF PREVENTIVE CARE IN AN AGING SOCIETY

In Chapter 3, we introduced the aging and public health systems in the United States, and described critical areas of commonality between the Center for Disease Control's public health apparatus and the Administration of Aging's area agencies on aging. A main focus of these agencies is prevention of chronic disease and disability, whether through exercise or fall prevention programs, immunization efforts, chronic disease management techniques, or other health promotion efforts. Yet most medical care for older adults in the United States is not financed or provided through the CDC or AoA, but through the Medicare program operated by the Centers for Medicare & Medicaid Services (CMS). Here, we review the Medicare program, providing an historic perspective of its development, ways in which its focus has been shifting toward preventive efforts, and issues the program will face in light of the aging of the population.

Medicare's Basic Benefit Structure

In 2008, Medicare provided health care coverage to 45 million people (CMS, 2009). Eligibility for this program is determined by another federal program: Social Security. Medicare covers 38 million people ages 65 and older with Social Security old-age benefits. In addition, the program serves about 7–8 million people under age 65 who receive Social Security disability benefits (most after a 24-month waiting period). Another 100,000 or so persons with end-stage renal disease also receive Medicare. In 2007, benefits amounted to $462 billion, making Medicare the largest public health program in the United States.

Signed into law by President Johnson in 1965, Medicare's original goal of was to provide "mainstream acute health care—hospital, physician, and related services—to persons ages 65 and older" (Moon, 2006). President Johnson (Public Papers, 1965) described the program as follows:

> During your working years, the people of America—you—will contribute through the social security program a small amount each payday for hospital insurance protection. For example, the average worker in 1966 will contribute about $1.50 per month. The employer will contribute a similar amount. And this will provide the funds to pay up to 90 days of hospital care for each illness, plus diagnostic care, and up to 100 home health visits after you are 65. And beginning in 1967, you will also be covered for up to 100 days of care in a skilled nursing home after a period of hospital care.
>
> And under a separate plan, when you are 65—that the Congress originated itself, in its own good judgment—you may be covered for medical and surgical fees whether you are in or out of the hospital. You will pay $3 per month after you are 65 and your Government will contribute an equal amount.

Over the past four decades, Medicare has been amended numerous times, but the basic benefit structure has remained largely intact. Medicare *Part A* (Hospital Insurance) covers inpatient care in hospital stays, skilled (short-term) nursing home stays, and some hospice and home care services for beneficiaries meeting certain requirements. Part A is financed through payroll taxes, and therefore most beneficiaries do not pay a premium for this benefit. Persons ages 65 and older who did not work or did not pay enough Medicare taxes while they worked may purchase Part A (premiums were up to $423 per month in 2008).

Medicare *Part B* (Medical Insurance) covers doctors' services and outpatient care as well as therapists and some home care when these services and supplies are medically necessary. Through the years, some preventive services designed to maintain beneficiaries' health and keep certain illnesses from getting worse have been added to Medicare Part B (see below). Most people pay a monthly premium for Part B. Starting in January 2007, the amount of the premium became tied to income.

In 2008, for example, a beneficiary earning less than $82,000 per year ($164,000 if married) paid $96.40 per month whereas a beneficiary earning more than $205,000 per year ($410,000 if married) paid $238.40 per month. In addition, beneficiaries are responsible for a deductible (the first $135 in 2008) and coinsurance (a percentage of every claim, with the percentage depending on the type of service).

Together Parts A and B are sometimes referred to as "original" Medicare (in contrast to Part C, described below). Beneficiaries who choose original Medicare may also choose to purchase supplemental coverage. These supplemental policies are designed to fill the gaps in Part A and Part B coverage. The majority of Medicare beneficiaries in original Medicare have some sort of supplemental coverage. In 2006, approximately 43% received supplemental coverage from an employer; approximately 22% purchased a Medigap policy from insurance companies, which must conform to specific standards set by CMS; and another 20% (so-called dual eligibles) were also covered by the Medicaid program (Gold, 2008). Economists and policy makers have long argued that older adults who have such supplemental policies use more medical care services because they are not required to pay out-of-pocket Medicare's cost-sharing requirements, although the extent to which reduction in Medigap policies would save Medicare dollars has been subject to debate (Lemieux, Chovan, & Heath, 2008).

Beneficiaries have been able to choose to receive services through managed care organizations since 1976. Beginning in 1997, however, the Medicare + Choice program (now known as *Part C*, Medicare Advantage) was enacted. This program initially allowed beneficiaries to receive combined benefits from Parts A and B through Health Maintenance Organizations (HMOs). In more recent years the types of plans available through Medicare Advantage have expanded. Today, most beneficiaries have a choice among at least two of the following: HMOs; local and regional Preferred Provider Organizations (PPOs), in which enrollees have lower out-of-pocket costs if they use network-based providers; Private Fee-for-Service Plans, which do not have restrictions on providers that a beneficiary can use; Medical Savings Accounts, which allow beneficiaries to deposit funds into a checking account to cover medical costs; and Special Need Plans, designed primarily for beneficiaries eligible for both Medicare and Medicaid, those in institutions, and those with serious or chronic disabling conditions.

The percentage of beneficiaries choosing to enroll in Medicare Advantage options increased from less than 10% in 1995 to approximately

19% in 2008 (Congressional Budget Office [CBO], 2007a; Gold, 2008) and is projected to increase substantially in the coming decades (CMS, 2009). Approximately 60% of Medicare Advantage enrollees are still enrolled in HMOs, which may include all the preventive services covered by Medicare described above, plus prescription drugs, and additional benefits such as vision, dental, and hearing services, physical examinations, and health/wellness education.

Growing Emphasis on Prevention

When the Medicare program was established in 1965, preventive services were not covered. Through the years, Medicare has increased the number of preventive services that are made available to beneficiaries. Specifically, since 1980, the Medicare program has been amended several times to add coverage for certain preventive services. During the 1980s, coverage for pneumococcal (1981) and hepatitis B (1984) vaccination became covered. From 1990 to 2000, coverage was extended to influenza vaccination (1993); screening for vaginal (1990), cervical (1991), breast (1993), colon (1998), and prostate (2000) cancers; bone mass measurements (1998); and diabetes screening (1998). In 2002, glaucoma screening tests and medical nutrition therapy were added. More recently, we have witnessed the addition of a one-time "welcome to Medicare" physical examination, cardiovascular screening, diabetes self-management training, smoking and tobacco-use cessation counseling, abdominal aortic aneurysm screening, and health risk assessments. According to Nelson and colleagues (2002b), most states experienced increases in mammography and adult vaccinations during the 1990s.

Table 4.5 shows current rates of preventive service use among Medicare enrollees by various demographic and socioeconomic characteristics. Two points are noteworthy. First, only cardiovascular disease screening exceeds the 50% mark; all other preventive benefits are used at much lower rates. Second, minorities, especially African Americans, have lower rates of preventive service use than White beneficiaries.

Not shown in the table is Medicare's most recent benefit addition: the prescription drug coverage benefit known as Medicare Part D, which was added in January 2006. For beneficiaries in original Medicare, a separate drug plan may be purchased from private companies that provide coverage. Beneficiaries enrolled in Medicare Advantage often have a prescription drug benefit as part of their plan; if not, they may enroll in a free-standing prescription drug plan. Beneficiaries pay a

Table 4.5

RATES OF USE OF MEDICARE PREVENTIVE BENEFITS BY SEX, AGE, AND RACE/ETHNICITY, 2006

DEMOGRAPHIC	INFLUENZA IMMUNIZATION	PNEUMOCOCCAL VACCINATION	MAMMOGRAPHY	PAP TEST	PELVIC EXAMINATION	PROSTATE CANCER SCREENING	DIABETES SCREENING	CARDIOVASCULAR DISEASE SCREENING	BONE MASS MEASUREMENT	WELCOME TO MEDICARE VISIT
Male	41.1	5.7	N/A	N/A	N/A	19.7	9.4	54.6	2	5.3
Female	46.5	6.3	37.9	11	5.9	N/A	9.7	58.2	13.7	6.3
Under 65	20.3	3	24.9	13.3	5.6	8.8	8.6	37.8	4	0.6
65–74	44.3	7.1	48.9	15.1	8.5	24.6	9.6	62	10.3	34.5
75–84	54.3	6.3	39.1	8	4.7	22	10.1	63.2	10	0.6
85 and Over	49.7	6.7	40.3	10.5	6	23	9.8	61.1	9.7	31
Caucasian	47.2	6.3	39.4	11.3	6.3	21	9.4	57.5	9.1	6.9
African American	24.9	4.5	31.6	9.6	4.1	13.4	10.7	50.5	5.1	1.3
Hispanic	22.7	4.1	25.1	7.3	2.7	9.7	11.1	55.1	7.5	0.5
Asian/Pacific Islander	43.8	6.2	23.8	6.9	3.1	11.4	10.1	60.3	9.5	1.8
National Total	44.2	6	37.9	11	5.9	19.7	9.6	56.7	8.6	5.8

From Centers for Medicare & Medicaid Services. Retrieved from http://www.cms.hhs.gov/PreventionGenInfo/20_prevserv.asp#TopOfPage.

monthly premium for prescription drug coverage, which may vary with the type of coverage. Those with incomes less than 150% of the federal poverty limit are eligible for subsidies for the new Part D prescription drug program.

How does the prescription drug benefit work? Enrollees have expenses covered (often with a copayment amount that depends on the generic status of the medication) until they reach a prespecified covered amount. Beneficiaries then enter a period of noncoverage (called the "donut hole") until they spend a prespecified out-of-pocket amount. At that point, the beneficiary is responsible for a minimal copayment (in 2008, $2.25 for a generic, $5.60 for a brand-name drug, or 5% of the cost of the drug, whichever is greatest). Actual benefit designs vary widely and some have argued for simplification of the program through standardization (Hoadley, 2008).

Early evaluations of the prescription drug benefit program suggest that, despite the voluntary nature of the program and its complexity, approximately 90% of Medicare beneficiaries had a drug benefit in 2006 (Heiss, McFadden, & Winter, 2006). That is, of 43 million beneficiaries, approximately 39 million had prescription drug coverage by June 2006, and 22 million of these had coverage through Medicare Part D (Kaiser Family Foundation, 2006). It is noteworthy that the program did not result in "adverse selection" in which those needing more prescriptions sign up and "healthy" beneficiaries refused coverage. Nevertheless, sizeable numbers of older adults—4.4 million in 2006—remain without coverage (Kaiser Family Foundation, 2006).

Medicare's Fiscal Health and Disability and Disease Prevention

The annual report of the Medicare trustees projects the fiscal health of the Medicare trust funds. According to the 2009 report (CMS, 2009, p. 3), the HI trust fund (Part A) is not adequately financed over the next 10 years and will be exhausted in 2017. This is not the first time the Medicare trustees have found the short-range financial status of the HI trust fund to be inadequate. The short-term outlook for the HI fund has been considered unsatisfactory since 2003; however, the outlook for this fund deteriorated substantially as a result of the economic downturn in late 2008/2009.

Parts B and D, the report explains, are adequately financed over the next 10 years, in part, because premium and general revenue income for these programs reset each year to match expected costs. However, Part B solvency could be jeopardized if Congress continues to override physician fee reductions that have been built into projections (as they have from 2003 through 2009) while maintaining a "hold harmless" provision that restricts premium increases for most beneficiaries. Without these reductions, Part B will increase at a rate of approximately 8%–9% per year. The trustees also project that expenditures for Part D will increase at a rate of approximately 11% through 2018. Both programs are projected to grow much faster than the U.S. economy.

Can a shift toward preventive services help defray the future costs of Medicare? It is too early to tell for sure, but early evaluation of the prescription drug benefit suggests perhaps not. It appears that prescription drug use *increased* for seniors newly insured under Part D. Some argue that Part D coverage will reduce medical problems and hospitalization costs enough to offset a significant portion of its cost. However, reduced adherence to therapies by consumers who hit the gap may adversely affect health outcomes. A study by Raebel and colleagues (2008) suggests that medication adherence declines after beneficiaries reach the gap, but how this influences other medical care utilization remains unclear.

Notably, the trustees' projections do not take into account shifts in the health and functioning of the older population. Some researchers have asked, if late-life disability rates continue to decline (say, as the result of more spending on preventive care), could Medicare spending slow? Projections by researchers at the RAND Corporation provide some insight into this question. Using a microsimulation model, Goldman and colleagues (2005) project that total health care expenditures for Medicare beneficiaries will more than double between 2000 and 2030, growing 3% per year from $300 to $621 billion (in 1999 constant dollars). Further technological breakthroughs will greatly increase spending beyond these levels. Varying assumptions about future declines in the prevalence of late-life disability, however, do not appear to have a large effect on projected health care spending.

Why is growth in health care spending so robust in the face of assumptions about disability declines? One study of lifetime expenditures provides some clues. Lubitz and colleagues (2003) found that an individual reaching age 70 is likely to spend approximately $140,000 (in 1998 dollars) over his or her remaining lifetime, whether that individual reaches age 70 with functioning intact, with some limitations, or with severe disability. Based on this analysis, Lubitz and colleagues conclude, "Health promotion efforts aimed at persons under age 65 may improve the health and longevity of the elderly without increasing health expenditures" (p. 1048). Because cumulative spending for older adults over their remaining lifetimes is largely invariant to health status, it also follows that disability prevention efforts may improve the health and longevity of older adults without *decreasing* such expenditures.

Where, then, might cost savings emerge? Some have argued that the highly variable practice patterns observed across the United States—and the apparent lack of association between intensity of care and outcomes—suggests that there is much excess waste in the current chronic care system (Wennberg, Fisher, Skinner, & Bronner, 2007). The authors propose that savings—and improved care—could emerge by transitioning to a system of prospectively managed, cost-effective, and coordinated care, one in which medical providers are paid for their performance (so-called P4P) based on measurable cost-effectiveness outcomes. Such a system would require extensive investments in creating the research base to support evidence-based medicine, as well as investment in the technological infrastructure of the medical care system. Others have argued that investing in prevention and wellness programs could result in substantial cost savings; however, this will undoubtedly depend on careful choices about the types of prevention, the groups targeted, and the costs of such measures (Russell, 2009). A recent article in the *New England Journal of Medicine* underscores this point with a demonstration that the distribution of cost-effectiveness ratios is very similar for preventive measures and treatments (Cohen, Neumann, & Weinstein, 2008).

PROMOTING CHRONIC DISEASE MANAGEMENT IN LATER LIFE

Of the $1.9 trillion spent on personal health care in the United States in 2007, Medicare accounted for 22%, or $409 billion (Medicare Payment Advisory Commission [MedPAC], 2009). On average, Medicare spending per beneficiary is about $7,500, but the roughly 10% of Medicare beneficiaries who describe themselves as being in poor health incur approximately one-fifth (20%) of Medicare expenditures (MedPAC, 2009). In 2005, for example, per capita expenditures were $4,286 for those with excellent health, $8,346 for those with good or fair health, and $15,705 for those with poor health. An effective means of identifying this group at highest risk for medical care would be an important addition to the armamentarium of public health. As Boult and Pacala (1999) argue, "this dense concentration of morbidity and use of health-related services is unfortunate for those afflicted, but it offers hope for effectively focusing resources where they will do the most good."

Who is the high-risk senior? In ambulatory and hospitalized patients, one way to identify the high-risk elder is to identify factors associated with hospitalization (and repeated hospitalization). An effective tool for identifying the high-risk elder is the P_{ra}, the Probability of Repeated Admissions (Pacala, Boult, Reed, & Aliberti, 1997). The eight items of the P_{ra} reliably identify people with high likelihood of repeated hospital admissions. The items include self-rated health, hospital stays over the prior 12 months, number of physician visits in the prior 12 months, diabetes, heart disease (coronary heart disease, angina, myocardial infarction), gender, presence of a person "who would take care of you for a few days, if necessary," and age. Thus, a male with coronary artery disease, angina pectoris, diabetes in the past year, and a self-rating of only "fair" health faces a high risk for hospitalization. He meets five of the eight P_{ra} risk factors, and Pacala and colleagues have developed regression equation weights for combining the factors into a single-risk index. We could also add additional risk factors. If this person also has a medication regimen of five or more prescriptions and a medical condition that requires regular injections or catheter care, he would obviously be at even higher risk. The P_{ra} is useful for its identification of eight simple indicators that reliably identify high-risk elders.

Covinsky and colleagues (2006; Lee, Lindquist, Segal, & Covinsky, 2006) have developed risk indices for mortality and decline in competency in the ADLs. The goal in this effort was to develop very simple indices that do not depend on laboratory biomarkers or extensive assessments, which could thus be useful for a clinical management or interpretation of new conditions in older adults. Mortality over 4 years was significantly associated with a series of these independent risk factors, which included age, male gender, disease status (diabetes, lung disease, heart failure), low body mass index (<25), current smoking, and functional status (difficulty with bathing, walking several blocks, and pushing or pulling heavy objects). Each of the factors was weighted as 1 or 2 points (except age, which ranged from 1 to 7) and the presence of the risk factors was summed, yielding a composite score ranging from 0 to 23. Among older adults with scores of 0–5 on this index (the lowest quartile of risk), 4% died over 4 years. Among older adults in the higher quartile risk categories, mortality was 15%, 42%, and 64%, respectively.

A similar approach with respect to decline in ADLs yielded nine risk factors: age older than 80 years, diabetes, difficulty walking several blocks, difficulty bathing or dressing, needing help with personal finances, difficulty lifting 10 lbs, unable to name the vice president, falling in the past year, and low body mass index. A simple count of these risk factors was highly related to onset of need for help in ADLs. For example, less than 1% of people in this large sample without any risk factors developed ADL dependency over 2 years. In people with five or more risk factors, by contrast, incidence was 40%.

Once the high-risk elder is identified, how should this person's medical care be managed to maximize effective treatment and minimize disability? Three areas of progress in this area, offering major benefit to older people, include geriatric evaluation and management, self-management of chronic disease, and reduction in polypharmacy.

Geriatric Evaluation and Management

The core of geriatric evaluation and management (GEM) is comprehensive geriatric assessment. This assessment includes a medical, psychological, and functional assessment that is integrated to develop an overall plan for treatment and follow-up (Beswick et al., 2008; Boult & Pacala, 1999; Fletcher et al., 2004; Gravelle et al., 2007; Rubenstein, Stuck, Siu, & Wieland, 1991; Stuck, Egger, Hammer, Minder, & Beck, 2002). Interdisciplinary teams meet to establish a comprehensive care plan for each patient that takes into account the full picture of this person's medical risks, ongoing preserved abilities, personal resources, and preferences for care. GEM works best when the team making the care plan is also involved in its implementation; otherwise, recommendations from comprehensive geriatric assessment may go unfulfilled (Stuck, Siu, Wieland, & Rubenstein, 1993).

A meta-analysis of controlled clinical trials involving GEM showed that effects were stronger in inpatient than outpatient settings (Stuck et al., 1993). A number of randomized trials in inpatient settings have shown benefits for GEM in a variety of areas, such as improvement in diagnostic accuracy, reduction in disability risk, improvement in mental health, and reduction in nursing home admission and mortality. Elders in the treatment arms of these trials were more likely to report satisfaction with medical care, and their family caregivers also reported lower stress. Finally, some of the trials reported decreases in hospital and emergency department services. Although the interventions usually involve greater use of home care and other long-term care services, these expenses are balanced and, in some cases, offset by lower hospitalization costs.

However, GEM results must be interpreted cautiously, that is, in light of the particular program elements involved and specific outcomes (and time frame) assessed. In early randomized clinical trials assessing GEM in inpatients, one showed no benefit in mortality risk, disability, or health status over 12 months (Reuben et al., 1995). The 1-year mortality rate in the two arms of the study was approximately 25%, typical of the mortality risk in older people discharged from hospitals. A second study showed no benefit in survival, but significant reductions in disability risk and admission to long-term care facilities (Landefeld, Palmer, Kresevic, Fortinsky, & Kowal, 1995). However, the two studies are not truly comparable. The second study examined only the change from hospital admission to discharge, whereas the former study involved a full year of follow-up.

Improvements in discharge status, as shown in this second GEM program, should translate into longer term benefits. If they do not, as shown in the first trial, it may be because selection criteria in these trials do not always identify people likely to benefit (i.e., they may be too ill or, conversely, too healthy to show benefit), or because the trials take place in settings where control group participants already receive services and assessment protocols typical of GEM.

Table 4.6 shows key elements in the GEM program that successfully improved outcomes at hospital discharge. The program illustrates well how hospital care can be modified to promote appropriate discharge planning from the point of admission by use of the many resources required for such a focus. The hospital environment was remodeled to focus on readying the patient for the return home, the patient-centered care protocol stressed skills and interventions that patients would need to bring with them when they returned home, and the barrier between the hospital and home care was broken down through active involvement of case management teams.

GEM has also been applied outside the inpatient and ambulatory care setting. In a randomized, controlled trial of annual in-home GEM, Stuck and colleagues showed that a program of home visits by geriatric nurses, who consulted with geriatricians, reduced disability risk (12% vs. 22% in ADL) and nursing home admission (4% vs. 10%) over 3 years (Stuck et al., 1995). These benefits came with the additional cost of significantly more visits to physicians, but the total incremental cost of the program was very favorable, with a cost of approximately $6,000 for each

Table 4.6

INPATIENT GERIATRIC EVALUATION AND MANAGEMENT PROTOCOL

KEY ELEMENT	FEATURES
Prepared environment	Make hospital ward approximate adapted natural living conditions: carpeting, handrails, uncluttered hallways, large clocks, calendars; elevated toilet seats, door levers
Patient-centered care	Daily nursing assessment Nursing interventions to improve self-care, continence, nutrition, mobility, sleep, skin integrity, mood, cognition Daily multidisciplinary assessment
Planning for discharge	Emphasis on return to home Early involvement of case manager/social worker to develop appropriate discharge plan
Medical care review	Daily review of medications Protocols to minimize iatrogenesis

From "A Randomized Trial of Care in a Hospital Medical Unit Especially Designed to Improve Functional Outcomes of Acutely Ill Older Patients," by C. S. Landefeld, R. M. Palmer, D. M. Kresevic, R. H. Fortinsky, & J. Kowal, 1995. *New England Journal of Medicine, 332*, 1338–1344.

additional well (disability-free) year. Other in-home intervention studies have shown benefit with different program elements (i.e., preventive home visits without comprehensive geriatric assessment, one-shot comprehensive assessment with follow-up, telemedicine contact); thus, it is unfortunately not clear which element of the program was most responsible for the beneficial effect.

A less extensive application of GEM principles is visible in geriatric case management. In this approach, a specially trained case manager arranges social- and health-related services and coordinates these services across long-term care settings. Results from this approach to GEM, on the whole, have been favorable. One randomized assessment of geriatric case management to increase access to primary care did not show a benefit in hospitalization or quality of life (Weinberger, Oddone, & Henderson, 1996). This was a study of veterans with a variety of conditions. Studies involving other elderly patient groups, such as patients with congestive heart failure, have shown benefit (Rich et al., 1995).

The benefits of geriatric assessment in the case of older people with chronic disease are becoming clearer now that a number of randomized trials have been completed. It is sometimes difficult to compare results of such trials because of differences in patient populations, bundling of intervention elements, duration of follow-up, and outcomes. Still, Berwick and colleagues (2008) conducted perhaps the best research synthesis to date. Their meta-analysis suggests that significant benefit of these interventions can be realized in chronic disease populations, as shown in Figure 4.4.

Figure 4.4 shows that community-based care after hospital discharge was associated with significantly lower risk of nursing home admission and repeat hospitalization. Similar results were obtained for interventions involving general geriatric assessment, fall prevention programs, group education and counseling, and a composite of all such interventions. Combining results across interventions showed benefit for all care transition outcomes (nursing home admission, hospital admission, falling, and declines in physical function), but no reduction in mortality. Aggregation across these randomized trials involved outcomes from nearly 40,000 people in the intervention and control arms and nearly 90 randomized clinical trials.

It is noteworthy that this meta-analysis did not find the expected dose-response relationship, given these findings. That is, interventions with more intensive services, more involvement of health professionals, longer duration, or more clinical specialties involved did not offer greater

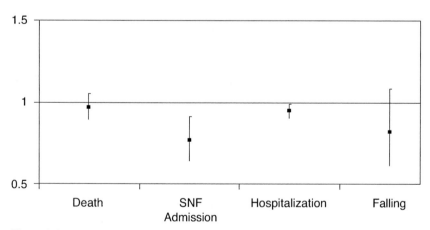

Figure 4.4 Meta-analysis: Community-based care after hospitalization. SNF, skilled nursing facility. Odds ratios and confidence intervals shown.

Source: After Berwick, et al., (2008).

benefit than less intensive forms of intervention. Thus, even short, less intensive home- and community-based services may offer great benefits to seniors.

2 Making Patients and Families Partners in Medical Care

Chronic disease is highly prevalent among older people, as we have seen. People aged 60 and older have a mean of over two chronic conditions, and these conditions account for the vast majority of health care expenditures (Hoffman, Rice, & Sung, 1996; Rothenberg & Koplan, 1990). Clinical and personal experience suggest that people differ in their capacity to manage the disability and symptoms typical of chronic disease. Some adapt well and maintain relatively active lifestyles, whereas others are less able to do so. Given these differences, it would be valuable to know what is involved in the successful management of chronic disease. Second, assuming these tasks can be identified, it would be valuable to know whether such skills can be taught. Finally, it would also be valuable to know whether disease management in this sense is associated with important health outcomes, such as physician utilization or hospitalization.

Recent research has examined the elements of effective chronic disease self-management. Lorig and colleagues (1999) identified 12 common features of successful disease self-management. These allow people to adapt to states of limited health and minimize the effects of disease on function. They include "recognizing and acting on symptoms, using medication correctly, managing emergencies, maintaining nutrition and diet, maintaining adequate exercise, giving up smoking, using stress reduction techniques, interacting effectively with health providers, using community resources, adapting to work, managing relations with significant others, and managing psychological responses to illness" (Lorig et al., 1999). These elements have been incorporated into a program of patient education, the Chronic Disease Self-Management Program (CDSMP), which has been used to teach patients with a variety of chronic conditions to manage symptoms well, to communicate effectively with health professionals, and to develop realistic appraisals of the health risks they face. Principles of this program include use of peer patient educators, mobilization of small groups of patients who develop joint problem-solving strategies, and a stress on self-efficacy, that is, development of weekly action plans with realistic goals and expectations of success. CDSMP is now considered an evidence-based model of self-management and may soon be tested in a Medicare demonstration effort.

A randomized trial of this model involving different chronic disease groups showed encouraging results for a variety of outcomes. One hundred eight CDSMP groups were convened for the 664 participants in the self-management treatment arm. Outcomes for these patients were compared with the experience of a waiting-list control group (n = 476) over 6-months of follow-up. Participants were drawn from people with a diagnosis of chronic lung disease, heart disease, stroke, or arthritis. People in the treatment arm completed a mean of 5.5 of 7 program sessions, showing effective delivery of the intervention, an important consideration in behavioral interventions of this type.

The trial showed significant benefit for CDSMP on a variety of outcomes, including health behaviors (self-reports of exercise, symptom management, effective communication with physicians), health status (self-rated health, disability, fatigue, and distress over health), and health service use (physician visits, hospitalization). These benefits were maintained over 2 years (Lorig et al., 2001) and were replicated when the control was offered the intervention. Comparing the CDSMP group with other samples assessed with a common measure of disability (HAQ, the Health Assessment Questionnaire) showed that CDSMP participants were more or less stable in disability scores, where other samples, matched for age and health status, declined.

These are impressive findings, and as a result CDSMP has been embraced by large HMOs, such as Kaiser Permanente, and by the National Health Service's (UK) Expert Patient program (AHRQ, 2002). Still, some caution is in order. Lorig and colleagues (1999) do not report participation rates in their initial randomization (i.e., how many patients randomly assigned to the intervention declined to participate). They do report that only 72% of controls agreed to enter the intervention when offered the chance to do so after the end of the initial 6-month trial. This suggests that the intervention group may have been enriched with more highly motivated participants, that is, people able to benefit from the program, or more motivated to self-manage their disease in any case. These selection effects are difficult to assess in behavioral trials.

CDSMP can also be faulted for ignoring a number of other factors that may be central to effective self-management. One is the availability of objective ways to monitor a chronic disease condition, such as urine or blood tests to identify hypoglycemia, as in diabetics. Access to these indicators allows patients to monitor and adjust medications or behaviors (Tattersall, 2002). Another factor is fostering effective partnerships between patients and health professionals. The "copy letter," in which physicians send patients a copy of their recommendations and the results of jointly planned care plans, is one way to build such partnerships. Finally, more needs to be done from the physician side, especially giving patients approval, or permission, to take a more active role in their care. Tattersall (2002) suggests that "many doctors and other healthcare professionals feel uncomfortable with the idea of empowering their patients."

In the case of some medical conditions, such as arthritis and diabetes, self-management has recently become the focus of randomized clinical trials that seek to determine whether patients trained in appropriate exercise, control of fatigue, adequate nutrition, stress reduction, and effective medication management manage symptoms more effectively. A large trial of an arthritis intervention showed benefit in patient mental health but not pain or physical function (Buszewicz et al., 2006). A smaller trial showed benefit for physical function (Heuts et al., 2005). Efforts to promote self-management and train "expert patients" have become widely adapted in the U.K. National Health Service as a promising way of reducing morbidity in chronic disease (www.expertpatients. nhs.uk). One interactive Internet-based self-management program to develop expert patients reported reductions in most symptoms and in health services utilization as well (Lorig et al., 2008). However, this effort did not involve a control group or a randomized design and should be interpreted in that light. More generally, a Cochrane Collaboration review of self-management education by peer leaders examined 17 randomized trials involving nearly 7,500 patients with chronic disease (Foster, Taylor, Eldridge, Ramsay, & Griffiths, 2007). The review found that lay-led self-management education promoted short-term reductions in pain, disability, fatigue, and depression, but it did not alter health care utilization.

Albert and colleagues explored self-management in osteoarthritis with reference to CDSMP guidelines for optimal self-management in a large biracial sample of Medicare beneficiaries (Albert, Musa, Kwoh, & Silverman, 2008). Lorig and colleagues recommend exercise, management of activity, and use of hot compresses on affected joints to manage pain and stiffness in osteoarthritis (Lorig et al., 2000). To operationalize this approach, the study considered optimal self-management to include at least two of the three behaviors. Only 20% practiced optimal self-management by this definition. Both White and African Americans who practiced optimal self-management reported significantly less pain than suboptimal self-managers, but other outcomes were not related to self-management competency.

Apart from promotion of effective self-management of chronic disease, it is also worth asking how older people actually manage chronic conditions. In fact, for the most disabled and oldest patients, management usually involves a patient-physician-family triad, rather than the traditional patient-physician dyad. Little is know about self-management behaviors in the home, or outside of contact with physicians or other health professionals. Up to one third of older people are accompanied by other family members in their physician consults (Silliman et al., 1996). Presumably, the patient's family plays an even larger role in management decisions beyond physician contact. This would be an important topic for future research on self-care.

Avoiding Inappropriate Medication Use and Managing Polypharmacy

Inappropriate medication use is a common problem in older people. One community-based study of people aged 75 and older found that 14% were using at least one inappropriate drug (Stuck et al., 1994), and a second study found a higher prevalence of 23.5% over a 1-year period (Willcox, Himmselstein, & Woolhandler, 1994). Forty percent of nursing home residents have been reported to receive one or more inappropriate drugs (Beers et al., 1992). "Inappropriate medications" in these studies are defined as drugs that should generally be avoided by older people, as specified in expert consensus panels. The drugs have all been shown to be ineffective or have been replaced by safer alternatives. For example, long-acting benzodiazepines (sedative-hypnotic agents) have been replaced by short-acting benzodiazepines with better side-effect profiles. The same is true for a number of antidepressant agents, antihypertensives, nonsteroidal anti-inflammatory agents, oral hypoglycemic agents, analgesics, dementia therapies, platelet inhibitors, muscle relaxants, and gastrointestinal antispasmodic agents (Stuck et al., 1994).

In these efforts to identify inappropriate medication use, the authors obtained valuable information on the prevalence of medication use in older people in general. In the sample of community-resident people aged 75 and older, medication use was fairly high. People were taking an average of 2.4 prescription and 2.4 nonprescription medications. A very small proportion, less than 5%, managed to avoid all medications, and about one third were taking six or more medications. The 14% of the sample taking at least one inappropriate drug were more likely to be older, on an antidepressant, and taking many medications (Stuck et al., 1994).

More recent prevalence surveys continue to show that at least one potentially inappropriate medication is prescribed for approximately 20% of elderly patients living in the community each year (Fialová et al., 2005; Hanlon et al., 2001). Although overuse (polypharmacy) and underuse are likely to account for a larger amount of avoidable morbidity in the elderly, studies have focused on potentially inappropriate medications because modifying prescribing behavior may be easier than addressing polypharmacy or underuse. In addition, the consequences of inappropriate medication use may be severe. In an analysis of pharmacy and medical claims from a large employee retiree database, we have shown that use of medications on "do not prescribe" lists is associated with elevated risk of hospitalization in analyses that control for sociodemographic status, medical status, and total use of medications (Albert, Colombi, & Hanlon, in press).

A distinction should be drawn between inappropriate and excessive use of medications on the one hand, and polypharmacy on the other (Stuck, 2001). Inappropriate or excessive medication use involves use of medications in which the harm exceeds the benefit, as described above. Polypharmacy, by contrast, is simply use of many medications, all potentially appropriate. It is a problem, however, because of the greater risk of adverse events associated with a greater number of medications, which is complicated further by interactions between medications (drug-drug interactions) and between medications and nonindicated medical conditions (drug-disease interactions). Also, the greater the number of medications, the less likely compliance, and, hence, the greater the risk that people will not take the medications they should be taking.

One operational definition of polypharmacy is regular use of four or more prescription medications. By this definition, approximately 50% of the oldest old meet criteria for polypharmacy. A challenge to geriatric care is to determine which medications are inappropriate, because it is possible for diseases to be poorly managed and symptoms undertreated even with an excessive number of medications. The following tests can be used to determine the appropriateness of medications: Is there an indication for the drug and is the drug effective for the condition? Is the dosage correct (taking into account changes in renal clearance and other features of pharmacokinetics and pharmacodynamics associated with aging)? Are there drug-drug or drug-disease interactions? Are directions for administering the drug reasonable for the patients, that is, is the patient likely to be able to take the drug according to directions and for as long as indicated? Does the drug duplicate an existing drug? Can the drug be replaced with something less expensive? (Stuck, 2001).

In pursuit of proper polypharmacy, physicians may have to take patients off medications as part of a comprehensive examination of medication profiles. It is much easier to add a medication than to remove one, but good management of patients may also require taking patients off drugs. Evidence suggests that physicians, like patients themselves, are reluctant to remove medications that have been prescribed for a long time. For example, in-home evaluations of medicine cabinets show a great number of expired and obsolete medications, stored just in case (Rubenstein et al., 1991). Likewise, with the passage of time, patients are likely to accumulate medications, with a comprehensive assessment of medications undertaken by physicians only when adverse events or a medical event requires it.

The rational management of polypharmacy is a major challenge of public health and aging. Some success in this effort will likely come from new partnerships between physicians and pharmacists (Weinberger et al., 2002), and from greater consumer awareness, and perhaps increased regulatory pressure.

SUMMARY

Prevalence and Incidence. Prevalence refers to the number of persons who have a particular disease among the population at a given point in time, whereas incidence refers to the number of new cases of a disease that occur within a specific time frame in a population that is at risk for developing the disease.

Prevalent vs. Debilitating vs. High-Mortality Conditions. If the public health goal is to prevent the onset of or to detect chronic conditions early in the process (primary and secondary prevention), highly prevalent conditions such as hypertension, heart disease, and arthritis make excellent targets. If the goal is to maximize life expectancy, targeting high-mortality conditions such as heart disease, cancer, and strokes is appropriate. However, if the aim is to maximize functioning, then conditions such as mental distress, strokes, and vision and hearing limitations, all of which can be highly debilitating, must be considered.

Managing Comorbidity and Multimorbidity. The experience of having multiple conditions can lead to a long list of unfavorable outcomes, including mortality, poor functioning, and increased use of health care.

Today, older adults are increasingly responsible for managing their chronic conditions. Although health literacy has increased over the past decade, 60%–71% of people age 65 and over had below basic or basic health literacy skills, and may have difficulty finding and evaluating the credibility of health information, assessing risks and benefits of health care decisions, calculating the amount of a prescription to take, or understanding test results.

U.S. Preventive Services Task Force. The USPSTF's recommendations are considered the "gold standard" for clinical preventive services. The USPSTF recommendation is made in the form of a grade from A to I, whereby A means strongly recommended, B means recommended, C means there is no recommendation for or against, D is a recommendation against, and I indicates insufficient evidence on which to base a recommendation. Of the 40 or so screen recommendations relevant to older adults, nearly half involved insufficient evidence (I). The remaining recommendations include 5 A's, 8 B's, and 10 D's. In setting recommendations the USPSTF considers issues of reliability, internal and external validity, diagnostic utility (including sensitivity, specificity, and positive and negative predictive values), and the power of a study design. The panel also considers which negative consequences might occur as the result of screening. Despite agreement that USPSTF is the "gold standard" for preventive services recommendations, there have been disagreements in the literature as to how to correctly interpret the evidence base.

Public Health Screening Program Criteria. Criteria for public health screening programs go beyond those identified by the USPSTF to include administrative concerns related to cost and cost-effectiveness, ease of administration, and the availability of follow-up care.

Prevention and Medicare. When the Medicare program was established in 1965, preventive services were not covered. Through the years, Medicare has increased the number of preventive services that are made available to beneficiaries. Specifically, since 1980, the Medicare program has been amended several times to add coverage for certain preventive services. In 2006 a prescription drug benefit was added. It is unclear whether these preventive efforts will result in cost savings in terms of the lower prevalence of chronic conditions. Projections suggest that even if disability prevalence were reduced, costs to the Medicare program would not be affected, because average lifetime costs would not be altered. Medicare is not adequately financed to meet its obligations over the next 10 years

Managing High-Risk Elders. A small share of "high-risk" elders are responsible for a disproportionately high share of medical care expenditures. Such high-risk elders are subject to repeated hospitalizations and can be identified with an eight-item scale called the Probability of Repeated Admissions (P_{ra}). Items include self-rated health, hospital stays over the prior 12 months, number of physician visits in the prior 12 months, diabetes, heart disease (coronary heart disease, angina, myocardial infarction), gender, presence of a person "who would take care of you for a few days, if necessary," and age. Once the high-risk elder is identified, this person's medical care should be managed to maximize effective treatment and minimize disability. Three areas of progress in this area, offering major benefit to older people, include geriatric evaluation and management, self-management of chronic disease, and reduction in polypharmacy.

5　Disability and Functioning

Disability and functioning are central outcomes for public health and aging. The prevalence of chronic disease increases with older ages, as does the development of senescent changes that lead to frailty. As such, older people are at risk for dropping below the thresholds of physical, cognitive, affective, and sensory functioning required for safe, independent, and efficient completion of everyday self-maintenance and domestic-related tasks and for participation in social and community life. Self-maintenance tasks include, the basic "activities of daily living": bathing, dressing, grooming, feeding oneself, and getting to and using the toilet. Domestic-related activities include getting groceries, preparing meals, cleaning clothes, and performing everyday household chores. Participation restrictions refers to reduced involvement for reasons related to functioning in major life activities such as working, volunteering, or caring for others, or in social or community activities, such as participating in organized activities or attending religious events.

As we will see, the term "disability" is not used consistently by those conducting research on aging or by those working in public health. In this chapter, we use disability as a broad term that encompasses reductions in physical, cognitive, affective, and sensory functioning, difficulty with self-maintenance and domestic-related tasks, and restrictions in the ability to participate in productive, social, and community life. When compensatory mechanisms (such as environmental modification, use of assistive technology, or other behavior adaptations) are unavailable or no longer suffice for completion of tasks that have become difficult, older adults may need the assistance of other people to manage their daily lives. Individuals who adopt such compensatory strategies, even if they do not report having difficulty with daily activities, are also included under the disability umbrella to the extent that they are at increased risk for developing limitations.

Public health and aging professionals benefit from the perspectives of many fields as they attempt to understand the intersection between disability and aging. Demographers have focused largely on the population-level trends in disability, their causes, and identifying high-impact opportunities for intervention. Epidemiology has been concerned with identifying risk factors for the onset of activity limitations and functional decline, and more recently with understanding trajectories that individuals follow from onset through end of life. Clinical geriatrics emphasizes prevention of the loss of capacity and, in the face of such loss, the deceleration or mitigation of the effects of such losses on the progression of basic activity limitations—difficulty and dependence in bathing, dressing, eating, toileting, and basic mobility. The rehabilitation and professional therapy fields (occupational, physical, and speech) have focused on regaining and maintaining antecedent skills and making changes to the environment that translate into participation in a much broader range of activities.

The field of public health and aging draws on each of these perspectives but yet maintains a unique focus on implementing programs to create the conditions under which older adults can maintain and maximize physical function well into late life. To some extent, each of these fields speaks a slightly different language, so we begin this chapter with a review of the language and measurement of disability.

THE LANGUAGE OF DISABILITY

Well-trained graduate students know that before formulating a research hypothesis, whether for their thesis, dissertation, or graduate course in Public Health and Aging, they should first review and synthesize the relevant literature on their topic. Now imagine you are interested in designing a public health intervention to prevent the onset of disability among older adults through physical activity. A Medline search of studies using key words "exercise," "prevent," and "disability" with limitation fields set to find only clinical or randomized trials and age group 65 and older, yields 10 articles. After eliminating the five that do not actually examine disability or functioning as an end point in a trial, the remaining five studies define and operationalize disability (or functioning) in at least four different ways: (a) impairments in physical capacity related to mobility including strength, gait, and functional reach; (b) speed of performance of daily tasks and/or walking; (c) self-reports of difficulty with self-maintenance; and (d) self-reports of difficulty or the need for personal assistance with self-maintenance or mobility.

Such a finding—that the term disability is used at least a half a dozen different ways—is not atypical in the study of disability and aging. In some studies, the term may mean having impaired physical functioning; in others, it may mean reporting difficulty with daily activities, needing help with such activities, or receiving help. Policy discussions around public health goals for disability have been hampered by such a lack of a universally accepted and understood terminology. Not only have researchers used the term to connote a variety of concepts about undertaking activities important in daily life, but federal policies also use an equally wide range of definitions. A search of the United States Code found 67 acts or programs that define disability in at least 14 different ways (CESSI, 2003). Whether discussing the size of the population with late-life disabilities or interventions to minimize avoidable dependency, diminished quality of life, and lost productivity of older individuals and family members, the clarity surrounding such conceptual distinctions is critically important.

Recognizing the absence of universally accepted and understood terms and concepts as a major barrier to consolidating knowledge about disability and developing interventions to maximize functioning, the Institute of Medicine's Committee on the Future of Disability in America recommended in its 2007 report the adoption and refinement of the World Health Organization's International Classification of Functioning, Disability and Health (ICF) as the language for disability monitoring and research.

The International Classification of Functioning, Disability and Health (ICF)

The ICF language is presented in Table 5.1. The framework starts with the concept of *health conditions*, which encompasses disease, disorders, injuries, and trauma. Examples of health conditions include cataracts, chronic obstructive pulmonary disease (COPD), or congestive heart failure (CHF). *Impairments* may occur to either body functions (for example, impaired vision, reduced lung function, or reduced cardiac function) or body structures (loss of a lens or narrowing of a heart valve). *Activity limitations* are difficulties an individual may have in executing activities related to learning, communicating, mobility, self-care, or domestic life. *Participation restrictions* are problems an individual may experience in involvement in life situations such as school, work, or community life.

Disability and functioning are used as umbrella terms, rightly reflecting the myriad of uses that currently exist in the research, public health, and policy spheres. In fact, in the pictorial representation of the ICF, the terms do not appear at all (Figure 5.1).

What do appear are the terms "environmental factors" and "personal factors," and these clearly influence and are influenced by all other functioning domains. Environment is defined broadly in the ICF to include products and technologies, the physical environment and human-made changes to it, and attitudes, as well as services, systems, and policies. Personal factors are contextual factors related to the individual, such as age, gender, social status, and life experiences.

Table 5.1

MAJOR CONCEPTS IN THE INTERNATIONAL CLASSIFICATION OF FUNCTIONING DISABILITY AND HEALTH

Health condition: includes disease, disorder, injury, or trauma

Impairment in body function or structure: problems in body function or structures, including physical, mental, and sensory

Activity limitation: difficulties in executing activities related to learning, communicating, mobility, self-care, or domestic life

Participation restriction: problems in involvement in life situations such as school, work, or community life

Disability: umbrella term for impairments, activity limitations, and participation

Functioning: umbrella term for body functions and structures, activities, and participation

Adapted from *The Future of Disability in America* (p. 38, Box 2-1), by Institute of Medicine, 2007, Washington, DC: National Academies Press.

Embedded in the various documents that accompany the classification system, including the introductory guide (World Health Organization [WHO], 2002), is another important distinction between the *capacity* to carry out activities and the actual *performance* of those activities. The former relates to an individual's ability to function without aids or help from another person, whereas performance concerns itself with whether, how often, and with what supports an individual actually carries out particular activities.

Thus, the revised WHO model blends both social and medical models of disability. Disability is not an attribute of the individual, but rather a feature of person-environment relationships (WHO, 2001). In contrast, definitions that frame disability as exclusively caused by a health condition—with treatment of that condition the only focus—are symbiotic with the medicalized model of disability.

The ICF language, which has broad acceptance worldwide, offers several advantages for public health and aging. First, components can be expressed in both "positive and negative terms" (WHO, 2001, p. 10; e.g., functioning and disability), thus changing the dialogue from disability prevention to maximizing functioning. Second, it introduces the notion of participation in activities beyond those necessary for self-care

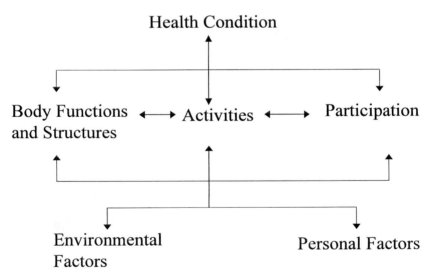

Figure 5.1 International Classification of Functioning, Disability and Health (ICF).

Source: From *International Classification of Functioning, Disability and Health,* by World Health Organization (p. 18), 2001, Geneva, Switzerland: Author.

(so-called ADLs) and domestic life (so-called IADLs). Gerontology and to some extent public health and aging has been almost singularly focused on these outcomes for many years. The ICF facilitates research and policy around additional activities and life situations that may be valued at different points in the life course. Third, in the ICF there is an explicit role for environmental factors of central interest to public health, including services, systems, and policies in filling the gap between capacity and performance.

Despite these advantages, the Institute of Medicine (2007) also pointed out several directions for refining and improving the ICF to better serve research and public policy purposes. The ICF does not currently offer crisp distinctions between activity and participation, an omission that researchers are working to rectify (Jette, Haley, & Kooyoomjian, 2003; Jette, Tao, & Haley, 2007). Current measures available in most surveys and studies of later life have measures that were developed in line with the Nagi disablement model (described below) and, therefore, do not map precisely into the ICF, making it difficult to use with many existing data resources. Nor does the ICF language link directly to quality-of-life measures and paradigms (see Chapter 8 for discussion of quality of life).

Finally, and perhaps most important in the public health and aging context, the ICF is not inherently a dynamic model. Like the International Classification of Diseases (ICD-10), the ICF is inherently a classification system that offers standardized internationally accepted language. For understanding dynamic relationships among factors predicting changes and maintenance of functioning, however, elements of the Nagi model of disablement (described below) remain useful to consider.

The Nagi Model of Disablement

The Nagi disablement model (Verbrugge & Jette, 1994) differs from the WHO approach in asserting a strict four-part temporal and causal sequence shown in Figure 5.2.

In the Nagi model, *pathology* (e.g., sarcopenia) first leads to *impairment* (e.g., lower extremity weakness evident in manual muscle testing). When lower extremity weakness crosses some threshold, *functional limitation* becomes evident, measurable perhaps in gait speeds below age- and gender-appropriate norms. When gait speed in turn drops below the minimum speed required to cross at a signaled intersection, a person is

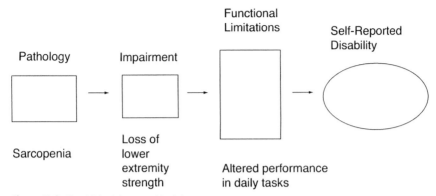

Figure 5.2 Nagi Disablement Model.

likely to report difficulty or a need for help crossing the street, that is, *disability*.

Note that in this framework, unlike in the ICF approach, the term disability more narrowly encompasses only: (a) *self-reported* difficulty or need for assistance, (b) a *need* rather than use or receipt of assistance, and (c) difficulty or need due to impairment, that is, a problem with one's *health*. The first condition construes disability is a matter of subjective evaluation. The second condition, the stress on need rather than on use, is important because it gives due recognition to unmet need (Allen & Mor, 1998). Only some of the elders with a need for assistance receive such assistance, so that restricting disability to the group actually receiving assistance would severely underestimate disability. Indeed, difficulty and dependence define important distinctions (Gill & Kurland, 2003), with the former more prevalent among older adults than the latter. Finally, the third condition requires that self-reports of disability be due to health conditions rather than solely to an environmental restriction, personal motivation, or other nonhealth sources of task restriction. This distinction may be hard to maintain in some cases, because environmental restrictions can also be considered legitimate targets for public health interventions and disease may affect motivation (as in the case of depression).

What of the older adult who uses personal assistance or equipment to complete ADL tasks? Ambiguity exists in the Nagi model, as specified above, as to whether this person would be considered to have a disability. In their elaboration of the model Verbrugge and Jette (1994) have made the additional important distinction between underlying difficulty—the level of difficulty without help or special equipment—and residual difficulty—that is, with whatever assistance is generally used. (The former is similar to the notion of capacity in the ICF.) Agree and Freedman (2003) refer more generally to behavioral compensations for impairments, such as using personal care, update of devices, or altering the demands of the environment, as accommodations. Individuals who make such compensations to complete daily tasks and carry out social roles would be considered to have underlying disability but, depending on the effectiveness the compensation, perhaps not residual disability.

The Nagi model has been used as a framework to identify early signals for the development of disability later in life. One advantage of the Nagi model for such work is the solid tradition of measurement behind it (Guralnik & Ferrucci, 2009). Even in people who do not report mobility problems, for example, weakness in lower extremity strength predicts future mortality and onset of limitations in daily activities (Guralnik et al., 1995). Likewise, people who do not report difficulty in ADL but report they have changed the way they perform these tasks have an increased risk for incident mobility limitations (Fried et al., 1996, 2000). More recently, the Nagi model has been used as the basis for identifying older adults at risk for interventions designed to deter the onset of activity limitations (Pahor et al., 2006).

Yet the Nagi model also has some important limitations. Because the environment is not an explicit domain in the model, for example, the emphasis to date in the literature has been on individually focused rather than population-level levers to reduce activity limitations. Indeed, many public health interventions that might reduce residual difficulty in a population—for example, changing the timing of traffic lights or extending health insurance to cover assistive technologies or motorized wheelchairs that may be used to enhance participation—have been overlooked. The ICF, in contrast, makes clear that environmental factors influence all aspects of functioning.

The Nagi model also makes disability an outcome and uses a fairly narrow definition of disability. This approach has been criticized for neglecting other components of daily life, such as non-ADL activity and general participation in social life, which can be preserved even with severe ADL limitations, and which may be more important to personal identity and self-worth than independence in ADL. Studies focusing, for example, on the ill effects of social isolation (both objective and subjective) among frail older adults (Simonsick, Kasper, & Phillips, 1998) and the beneficial effects of social engagement, in particular, volunteerism (e.g., Fried et al., 2004) might benefit from the more inclusive language that ICF has to offer.

Which approach is superior? The question sets up a false choice and is inappropriate because the ICF is not meant to describe disablement, but rather to inspire more extensive integration of environmental and personal factors into the management of impairing conditions. While the disablement model suggests clinical strategies, the ICF language offers a broader, common framework and language for taking action (Jette, 2009). As the authors state, if "disability is not an attribute of the individual, but rather a complex collection of conditions, many of which are created by the social environment," then "the management of [disability] requires social action, and it is the collective responsibility of society at large to make the environmental modifications necessary for the full participation of people with disabilities in all areas of social life" (WHO, 2001, p. 20). Efforts to bring the ICF language into studies of aging with a dynamic context are in progress (see for example, Freedman, 2009).

THE MEASUREMENT OF DISABILITY

Centrality of the Activities of Daily Living in Measuring Late-Life Disability

summary

Activity limitations have long been a central focus of studies of late-life disability. Indeed, avoiding difficulty and need for help with the tasks of everyday life has been a focal point of chronic disease research. Chronic disease can also cause symptoms or changes in physical, social, affective, and cognitive capacity, an increased risk of hospitalization and death, a need for regular medications and physician visits to monitor indicators of disease progression or therapy, changes in behaviors such as dependency on people or equipment in daily self-maintenance activities, depression and anxiety, and changes in self-image and sense of control. All of these outcomes are appropriate targets for public health inquiry, but activity limitations are central because of their implications for each of these alternative outcomes.

Chronic disease, as described in Chapter 4, may cause difficulty or make it impossible for people to learn, go to school, work, play sports, travel, participate in conversation, drive, or complete the basic tasks required for independent living, such as eating, bathing, dressing, grooming, using the toilet, or moving between a bed and a chair. In short, chronic disease may lead to activity limitations or participation restrictions. The former are often operationalized in later life as the "activities of daily living" (Katz et al., 1963) or "personal self-maintenance activities" (Lawton & Brody, 1969), which over time have picked up the prefix of "basic" or "physical" ADL (hence, BADL and PADL) to distinguish them from more complex, household (or "domestic") tasks usually considered IADLs.

In public health and aging, there has been an almost exclusive focus on the activities of daily living. The reasons for this focus are numerous. Perhaps the most salient reason is that, traditionally in public health ADL competencies were typically considered the primary sphere of activity in old age, on a par with attending school for children and working or running a household for adults (Sullivan, 1966). Whereas older adults do not work or attend school at rates anywhere near those of younger people, an increasing proportion do; and we may want to rethink this rationale for the focus on ADL. (Indeed, the early Sullivan [1966] classification also considered housework the primary sphere of activity for adult women under age 65.)

Second, *ADLs are the basic and universal competencies of adulthood.* The loss of basic ADL competencies—the ability to toilet or bathe oneself—is a severe threat, not just to social participation and safety, but also to adulthood as we understand it, and hence self-worth. (However, note that there is some variability by culture in the degree to which this sort of independence is considered central to adulthood [Albert & Cattell, 1994]) Loss of ADL competency, then, represents a major milestone in the progression of chronic disease. From a public health perspective, providing the services to care for individuals who do not have the basic competencies in place is an enormous intergenerational obligation, one that is projected to grow in the United States as the population ages.

A third reason is *the universality of ADLs: all people need to accomplish ADL tasks; and people perform these tasks on all or most days.* Thus, all older people can be asked whether they have difficulty bathing or dressing or using the toilet. The tasks are not gender-specific, optional, or subject to variation in lifestyle. This is not the case with other competencies, such as the IADLs. The IADLs are household competencies, which typically include managing finances, going shopping, doing housework, doing laundry, using the telephone, and taking medications. The need, desire, and training to perform IADL tasks varies by gender, education, health status, lifestyle, and culture. The same applies to the so-called advanced ADL, such as using a microwave oven, programming a VCR, or using a computer, and to any of the more general lists of activities that have been proposed as indicators of adult competencies.

A fourth reason for the focus on ADLs relates to their measurement properties; that is, the tasks are hierarchical in nature. *ADLs differ in task complexity, and hence in motor and cognitive demand, and as a result appear to be gained and lost in a generally consistent (but not necessarily fixed) order.* Early on, Katz et al. (1963) suggested that the order in which ADL tasks are acquired in childhood development (first, feeding and transfer; later, toileting and dressing; last, bathing) is the reverse of the order in which they are lost in chronic disease (so that the first lost is bathing, the most complex of the tasks), as well as the order in which they are regained in recovery from stroke or brain injury (so that the last competency reacquired is again bathing). For this reason, Katz considered the ADL a measure of "primary sociobiologic function." His early research showed that the disability status of almost all elders in a skilled care setting adhered to this rough hierarchy of preservation and loss of task ability, which formed a Guttman scale. That is, people who were unable to do just one task from this set of tasks almost always had lost the ability to bathe. Likewise, people who could not dress themselves independently were also very likely to have trouble bathing independently. People who could perform only one task independently from the set of ADLs were likely to have retained the ability to feed themselves. In fact, a simulation study has shown that a number of alternative patterns, mostly relating to the order of the most primitive of the ADL tasks, form equally good hierarchical scales (Lazirides, Rudberg, Furner, & Cassel, 1994). However, it is well to remember that Katz and his colleagues (who developed the measure in the late 1950s and early 1960s) did not have access to sophisticated modeling software and that their clinical judgment regarding the scalability of the items was essentially accurate.

It is worth mentioning, as well, that a number of changes in task items have been introduced since Katz first proposed the measure. The original Katz items included bathing, dressing, toileting ("going to the toilet room for bowel and urine elimination; cleaning self after elimination, and arranging clothes"), transferring, continence (ability to control urination and bowel movements), and feeding. These items were initially developed as observations made by clinicians in institutional settings. Over the years these measures have made their way onto national surveys and studies in which older adults, typically in a community setting, are asked to self-report their level of difficulty or need for help or use of help with daily activities. Current measures of ADL competency generally include only one toileting item, and have added indoor mobility and expanded dressing in some cases to include personal grooming. Also, the original Katz scale items had very detailed descriptors for categories of ability. Each item was assessed on a three-point scale, and the scale values were quite detailed. For example, the middle scale point for dressing was "gets clothes and gets dressed without assistance except for assistance in tying shoes." Current versions of the measure typically use a single underlying measure for all ADL tasks: either level of difficulty (none, some, a lot, unable) or need for help (none, sometimes, all the time).

A last point involves the source of information about ADLs. While the ADL items have been selected to minimize "does not apply" or "don't know" responses (since the tasks are both basic and universal), cognitive impairment prevents a small proportion of the young-old (approximately 6% of people under age 75) and a much larger proportion of the old-old (about 20% of people aged 75 and older and perhaps 50% of people residing in nursing homes) from answering the questions. For information about the ADL status of these respondents, researchers and clinicians must rely on proxy reports, that is, information from family or service providers. But for people able to report on ADL status, it is their judgment that defines disability. As in the case of quality-of-life measures (see Chapter 8), this seems appropriate: who other than the person at hand is better able to report on the degree of difficulty he or she faces in performing daily tasks (Gill & Feinstein, 1994)? In fact, studies comparing patient and proxy reports of patient ADL status show moderate levels of agreement, and if patient factors affect accuracy (i.e., denial, loss of insight, wish for a more intense level of services), so do proxy factors (i.e., degree of contact with patient, mental health, perceived burden as caregiver) (Magaziner, Simonsick, Kashner, & Hebel, 1988).

Still, even with these limitations, the ADL hierarchy is highly robust. For example, the Venn diagram shown in Figure 5.3 demonstrates that in a sample of more than 2,000 elders *none* had difficulty with feeding or toileting without also having difficulty in bathing, grooming, or dressing.

Functional Status: WHICAP

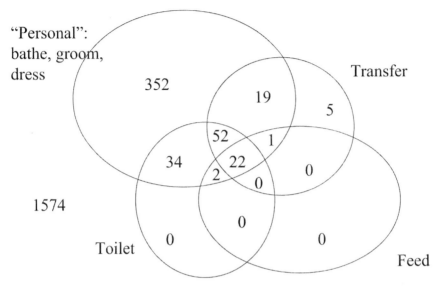

Figure 5.3 Functional status: Washington Heights-Inwood Columbia Aging Project.

Difficulties in Measuring Activity Limitations Among Older Adults

The centrality of BADLs and IADLs as measures of disability is clear, but measuring these most basic tasks is not simple. Kovar and Lawton (1994) describe many issues to be considered in assessing self-reports. These include:

1. Decisions about which activities should be assessed ("the number of possible IADL tasks seems almost limitless");
2. Ceiling effects ("the ADL/IADL scales do best at identifying the most-disabled minority");
3. Problems with the standardization of question formats to control for interpretation of environmental effects ("estimates of functioning reflect an unknown mix of personal disability and contextual constraint");
4. Effect of emphasizing different components in question formats ("dependence" vs. "difficulty" vs. "limitation") or combining them (Gill, Robison, & Tinetti, 1998);

5. Effect of proxy reporting (proxy respondents are more likely to report limitations than self-respondents, but they may be the only source of information for people with severe impairment);
6. Relevance of cultural differences ("socially or culturally assigned roles are obvious conditioners of IADL task performance and, conceivably, capability");
7. Cognitive factors in interpreting questions ("help from another person" can mean ongoing help, occasional help, or indirect help, that is, purchasing an assistive device).

An additional challenge relates to the variation across questions in whether underlying or residual difficulty is being assessed (Freedman, 2000). That is, sometimes questions explicitly ask, "without help or special equipment, do you have difficulty," whereas others ask simply, "do you have difficulty ____." The former are problematic in that respondents may not consider their assistive devices "special" and those who use equipment all the time may be answering about a hypothetical situation; the latter are problematic in their ambiguity, particularly for people who may not always carry out a task the same way every time (e.g., use their cane only some of the time).

These measurement challenges may be responsible for the different prevalence estimates of ADL limitations evident in national surveys. In their now classic study, Wiener, Hanley, Clark, and Van Nostrand (1990) identified substantial variation among the major national probability surveys of disability in the 1980s in the number of ADLs queried, whether "disability" in an ADL required a specified period of duration, and whether distinctions were made between need for assistance and receipt of personal assistance, use of special equipment, and standby help. The prevalence of receiving help with any ADL ranges from 5.0% (Supplement on Aging, 1984) to 7.8% (National Long Term Care Surveys, 1982 and 1984). Given the common definition of "receives help from another person," these differences are impressive. This variability applies to disability in all the ADLs, both those with relatively high prevalence, such as bathing (4.6%–6.3%), and those with low prevalence, such as eating (0.7%–2.5%).

Rodgers and Miller (1997) conducted a similar exercise, analyzing the prevalence of reporting any difficulty and receiving help with six ADLs in the Asset and Health Dynamics of the Oldest Old Study (now the oldest cohorts in the Health and Retirement Study). At the end of their interviews, respondents to the survey were randomly assigned additional ADL questions from existing health and aging surveys. Thus, unlike the comparisons in Weiner et al. (1990), estimates from Rodgers and Miller are generated from the same study sample. A summary of their findings is presented in Table 5.2.

Note the differences in prevalence for the same respondents in the same survey are even greater for different measures of difficulty than they are for measure of help. The difference between the estimate from the Asset and Health Dynamics of the Oldest Old (AHEAD) Study and the National Long Term Care Survey (NLTCS) is especially striking: one survey yields a prevalence of approximately 24% and the other survey yields closer to 11%. Such a large discrepancy is potentially of major public health significance. One only needs to consider the costs of providing support in the community for 24% of the population versus 11%

Table 5.2

PREVALENCE OF ACTIVITY LIMITATIONS AMONG ASSET AND HEALTH DYNAMICS OF THE OLDEST OLD COHORT, NHIS SUPPLEMENT ON AGING, AND NATIONAL LONG TERM CARE SURVEY (AGES 70 AND OLDER AND LIVING IN THE COMMUNITY)

	RECEIVES HELP		HAS DIFFICULTY/ UNDERLYING DIFFICULTY		HAS DIFFICULTY/ PROBLEM	
	AHEAD	SOA	AHEAD	SOA	AHEAD	NLTCS
Waking	3.2	3.9	17.2	24.3**	19.3	6.7**
Dressing	3.8	2.7	8.9	5.0**	10.0	4.6**
Bathing	3.9	3.1	8.0	6.3*	7.9	5.8**
Eating	2.6	0.8**	3.9	2.1**	2.7	1.0**
Transferring	1.3	1.8	6.5	6.9	7.8	3.5**
Using Toilet	0.6	0.6	1.9	3.4**	2.4	1.6*
Any	9.1	6.7+	26.7	24.1+	24.4	10.8+
N (Module)	N = 845 (3)				N = 915 (4)	

* $p < .05$, ** $p < .01$ difference from AHEAD; +, statistical test not reported.
From "A Comparative Analysis of ADL Questions in Surveys of Older People," by W. Rodgers and B. Miller, 1997, *The Journals of Gerontology. Series B, Psychological Sciences and Social Sciences, 52,* Tables 5, 8, 13, and 15.

of the population to begin to appreciate how meaningful these estimates are. And, although significance tests were not reported for this particular contrast, given that all the other contrasts between the AHEAD and NLTCS approach to asking ADL items—including some much smaller differences—reach statistical significance, it is highly likely that this difference also reached statistical significance.

Measuring Capacity: Performance-Based Tests

Elicitation of capacity to perform activities—in Nagi's model, functional limitations—usually involves self-reports of difficulty or need for assistance in a global sense; for example, "By yourself, that is, without help from another person or special equipment, how much difficulty do you have climbing stairs?" As explained previously, these types of questions pose problems of interpretation (Is the handrail or my cane special equipment?) and may even require some individuals to consider a hypothetical situation (Would I have difficulty climbing if I did not use the railing or my cane?).

Fortunately, a growing arsenal of tools is available to the field of public health and aging to measure capacity with performance-based assessments. Physical performance measures involve an individual performing a movement or task according to a standardized protocol and a trained observer rating the performance by use of objective, predetermined criteria. Batteries have been developed to measure the basic components of functioning (strength, balance, coordination, flexibility, endurance) as well as physical movements (e.g., walking speed) and goal-oriented functions (e.g., ADLs and IADLs). For example, the Short Physical Performance Battery (SPPB; Guralnik et al., 1994), assesses the time it takes respondents to walk 4 m and stand up repeatedly from a chair, and asks participants to hold progressively more complicated stances. Quartiles established within each of the three tests are then used to establish a "physical performance" score with a range of 0 (poorest performance on all three measures) to 12 (top quartiles of performance on all three measures). Such tests have been administered by interviewers in the home environment in population-based studies such as the Established Populations for Epidemiologic Study of the Elderly (EPESE) and the Women's Health and Aging Study (WHAS), and are now incorporated into the designs of population-based studies such as the large, national studies, the Health and Retirement Study and the English Longitudinal Study of Ageing (ELSA). Evaluations of the SPPB suggest that it is a strong predictor of incident activity limitations (Guralnik, Fried, Simonsick, Kasper, & Lafferty,1995b; Guralnik et al., 2000) and is particularly useful for detecting change within individuals (Guralnik et al., 1999; Onder et al., 2002).

Other tools from the occupational therapy field may also be useful, because they tap the antecedent skills necessary to perform a range of activities. In the Assessment of Motor and Process Skills (AMPS) test mentioned earlier, occupational therapists obtain *performance-based ratings of specific motor and cognitive skills* used in completing two tasks from a pre-specified list of 54 IADL/BADL tasks (Fisher, 2006a, 2006b). An occupational therapist, having undergone a 5-day training program in the AMPS, makes the ratings. Each of the motor and cognitive or "process" skills, drawn from extensive experience in occupational therapy with a variety of patient populations, is rated on a 4-point scale (competent, questionable, ineffective, deficit). The skills (and domains) are shown in Table 5.3.

An important advantage of the AMPS is its use of a many-faceted Rasch measurement model. The Rasch model has been used to (a) calibrate difficulty levels for the 54 tasks, (b) establish difficulty levels for ratings of each skill item, and (c) combine these skill ratings and task difficulty ratings to establish a single score for respondents on separate motor and cognitive/process skill dimensions. The equating of AMPS

Table 5.3

ASSESSMENT OF MOTOR AND PROCESS SKILLS

AMPS Motor Skills:

Posture: stabilizes, aligns, positions.

Mobility: walks, reaches, bends.

Coordination: coordinates, manipulates, flows.

Strength and Effort: moves, transports, lifts, calibrates, grips.

Energy: endures.

AMPS Cognitive/Process Skills:

Energy: paces, attends.

Using Knowledge: chooses, uses, handles, heeds, inquires.

Temporal Organization: initiates, continues, sequences, terminates.

Space and Objects: searches/locates, gathers, organizes, restores, navigates.

Adaptation: notices/responds, accommodates, adjusts, benefits.

tasks, linked by common skill items, makes it possible to compare the ability of respondents who perform *different* sets of tasks.

An advantage of this approach is its explicit focus on the skill elements elders use *to get tasks done*, as observed in home settings by using prespecified but ecologically valid tasks. In this way it differs from existing IADL or BADL performance tests (e.g., Karagiozis, Gray, Sacco, Shapiro, & Kawas, 1998; Lowenstein et al., 1992; Muharin, DeBettignies, & Pirozzolo, 1991; Myers et al., 1996), which are limited to only a few tasks, require subjects to perform tasks they may not do in normal activity, and do not yield measures of ability or skill that are involved in all IADL/BADL tasks.

Measuring the Environment

The emergence of the ICF highlights the need to improve measures of the environments in which older adults conduct their daily activities. Indeed, the expansion of measures of assistive technology and the physical environment would allow analysts to more fully understand the reasons for population-level changes in disability prevalence, and could further understanding at the individual level of the accommodation process and interventions to enhance independence and participation.

Keysor (2006) summarizes three general approaches to environmental measurement. The first approach involves assessment of an individual's perceptions of how the environment influences his or her participation. For example, the CHIEF (Whiteneck et al., 2004) is a 24-item self-report instrument that asks how often various barriers in the environment have been a problem in the past 12 months (and, if so, whether it has been a big problem or a small problem). The CHIEF focuses on barriers related to attitudes and support, services and assistance, physical and architectural features, policies, work, and school. A second approach is to literally observe study subjects and characterize avoidance and/or encounters with various features in the physical environment. Shumway-Cook and colleagues (2003), for example, used this approach to assess eight dimensions of the physical environment that may influence mobility: temporal, physical load, terrain, postural transitions, distance, density, attentional demands, and ambient conditions. A third approach is to ask research participants to characterize the presence or absence of various features in the environment (rather than perceptions about their roles as barriers). Keysor, Jette, and Haley's (2005) 36-item Home and Community Environment Instrument and the Pilot

Study of Aging and Technology (PSAT) instrument (Freedman, Agree, & Cornman, 2005) are examples of the latter strategy.

Such measures are beginning to make their way into clinical studies and national surveys. An example of the latter, the items from the PSAT were incorporated into an experimental module in the Health and Retirement Study in 2006, to assess the existence, acquisition, and use of assistive home features and devices by adults ages 52 and older (Freedman & Agree, 2008). Findings suggest that assistive home features are common: 78% of this age group have one or more features, 37% have added them, and 53% used them in the past 30 days. Of particular concern for public health and aging, one in four near-elderly and older adults were found to be at risk for a home modification, that is, had a mobility limitation and an unmodified barrier at the entry to their home, inside their home, or in the bathroom (either shower/bath area or toilet area). Adults receiving Medicare through the Disability Insurance program were identified as having elevated chances of being at risk for a home modification, suggesting a possible programmatic opportunity for reaching such a population.

TRENDS IN DISABILITY PREVALENCE AND ACTIVE LIFE EXPECTANCY

A central question for demographers interested in population aging is, "what are the implications for lengthening life for the health of the older population?" Simply put, the question is, are these additional years spent in good health and function or in a state of dependence?

Trends in Prevalence

Early studies on this question suggested that longer life implied worsening health, as measured by increases in self-reported activity limitations and chronic disease. Some researchers have questioned whether these increases were due to changing social forces during the period that made reports of disability more acceptable. The evidence for the 1980s and early 1990s was much more mixed, with Manton and colleagues first noting large declines in activity limitations (Manton, Corder, & Stallard, 1993) and Crimmins and colleagues concluding that there was no clear ongoing trend (Crimmins, Saito, & Reynolds, 1997b). A review of these inconsistencies by the Committee on National Statistics of the National

Research Council (Freedman & Soldo, 1994), concluded that there had been modest declines in the proportion of older people with limitations in IADLs, but inconsistencies across surveys in trends in ADLs.

In the 15 years since that workshop more than a dozen studies have focused on late-life disability trends. A review by Freedman, Martin, and Schoeni (2002b) highlighted methodological considerations in the comparison of trends in prevalence across surveys and reported findings for a range of outcomes, including physical, cognitive, and sensory limitations, as well as ADL and IADL limitations. Of the 16 studies identified, the authors analyzed 8 unique surveys: for the purposes of trend analysis, 2 were rated as good, 4 were rated as fair, 1 was rated as poor, and 1 was rated as mixed (fair or poor, depending on the outcome). Studies rated fair or good consistently showed substantial declines in IADL limitations. For example, evidence from the National Health Interview Survey (NHIS) suggests that between 1982 and 2004 there was a 6% decline in the population ages 70 years and older needing help with only routine care (but not personal care) activities, such as shopping, preparing meals, and managing money, sometimes called IADLs. Subsequent analysis of data from the NLTCS suggested that declines in limitations in three IADL activities—managing money, shopping for groceries, and doing laundry—were notably large from 1984 to 1999; however, among those reporting a limitation in ADL or an IADL, the severity of disability increased over time (Spillman, 2004).

At the time that the review was published, disagreement remained about whether there had been a decline in the proportion of older Americans having difficulty with self-care activities, such as bathing, dressing, toileting, and walking around inside, sometimes called ADLs. The answer was sorted out by a technical working group that analyzed five national surveys conducted from the early 1980s through 2001 (Freedman et al., 2004). The 12-person panel prepared estimates by use of identical methodologies and investigated sources of the inconsistencies among the population age 70 years and older. They found that during the middle and late 1990s consistent declines on the order of 1%–2.5% per year for two commonly used measures in the disability literature: difficulty with daily activities and help with daily activities. Mixed evidence was found for a third measure: use of help or equipment with daily activities. In comparing findings across surveys, the panel found that the time period, definition of disability, treatment of the institutional population, and standardization of results by age were important considerations.

More recently, the NLTCS suggested that declines continued from 1999 to 2004 (Manton, Gu, & Lamb, 2006), but other surveys, such as the Medicare Current Beneficiary Survey (Federal Interagency Forum on Aging-Related Statistics, 2008), suggested a possible leveling off of "any limitation." Disagreement also exists about trends among the generations approaching late life (see Martin et al., 2009; Seeman, Merkin, Crimmins, & Karlamangla, in press; Soldo, Mitchell, Tfaily, & McCabe, 2007; Weir, 2007) and some have warned that trends in obesity and other potentially disabling conditions among working-age adults could offset future improvements in late-life functioning (Bhattacharya, Choudhry, & Lakdawalla, 2006; Sturm, Ringel, & Andreyeva, 2004). Hence, reconciling disparate findings remains an important focus among demographers.

Trends in Active Life Expectancy

Prevalence measures are helpful policy and planning tools but do not yield information on whether increasing years of life are active. Measures of active life expectancy are needed to ask whether, on average, older adults spend more of their lives living free from limitations. Active life expectancy is a summary measure that combines information on age-specific mortality with age-specific activity limitations. Some researchers use cross-sectional activity limitation information ("Sullivan method") and others have drawn on transition probabilities in making these calculations, but in either case the concept is similar: how many years on average could an individual be expected to live without activity limitations if age-specific rates of such limitations and mortality held over a hypothetical cohort's lifetime. Comparisons of active life expectancy estimates over time are subject to many of the same threats to validity as are prevalence trends.

What have the studies shown? Several studies of the 1970s suggested that increases in active life expectancy were being accompanied by an increase in the number of years lived with a limitation, but this trend appeared to reverse during the 1980s and more recently. Three studies using different measures, methods, and dates (Cai & Lubitz, 2007; Crimmins et al., 1997b; Manton et al., 2006) suggest surprisingly similar results: all three show an increase in the expected number of years of active life and in the percentage of life expectancy expected to be spent without activity limitations. A fourth study (Crimmins, Hayward, Hagedorn, Saito, & Brouard, 2009) suggests stable levels of active life expectancy between the 1980s and 1990s that are the result of several underlying processes: declines in the onset of limitations, increases in the chances of recovery, and reductions in mortality among those living with an activity limitation at age 70.

Disparities in Trends and Causes

Adopting a public health focus, we may ask, have all groups benefited equally from these trends or are some groups being left behind? Although the evidence is thin, and with few exceptions, statistical tests have not been performed to determine whether these differences are due to chance, the answer appears to be no, at least when the population is sliced by major racial and socioeconomic groups. In one of the few studies including such tests, Schoeni, Martin, Andreski, and Freedman (2005), found persistent gaps in activity limitations between Blacks and other groups and widening gaps between socioeconomic groups from 1982 to 2002. Educational disparities in both the prevalence of activity limitations and in the extent of expansion in active life are also evident. For instance, older adults with less than a high school education as a group have experienced increases in the prevalence of basic activity limitations, while other groups have experienced declines (Schoeni et al., 2005). Similarly, a study by Crimmins and colleagues found a compression of morbidity—that is, an increase in the percentage of life expectancy to be lived in an active state—for highly educated groups but an expansion of morbidity for less educated groups (Crimmins & Saito, 2001).

In searching for ways to promote further declines in late-life disability prevalence, we might ask, what are the causes of trends to date and are those forces expected to continue as the Baby Boom generations reach late life? Four distinct realms of explanation have been explored to date: demographic and socioeconomic shifts; changes in chronic disease and related treatments; trends in underlying physical, cognitive, and sensory functioning; and environmental changes, in particular, growth in the use of assistive devices.

Research to date suggests that the decline is likely the result of a combination of factors and not any single underlying trend (Schoeni, Freedman, & Martin, 2008). For example, the improvement has been attributed in part to the greater educational attainment of older adults today compared with cohorts who were in late life in the mid-1980s. Yet such changes account for only a portion—and not all—of the decline in limitations. One analysis suggests that impending increases in education levels will continue to contribute to improvements in late-life functioning, albeit at a reduced rate (Freedman & Martin, 1999).

Other evidence also suggests that the extent to which some chronic conditions are expressed in terms of disability may have been ameliorated in recent decades. In particular, arthritis, vision-related conditions such as cataracts, and cardiovascular diseases appear to be less debilitating even as the prevalence of these and related conditions has increased in the older population (Schoeni et al., 2008). It could be that earlier diagnosis and better management of such conditions has led to lower reported rates of disabilities. Evidence supporting this possibility is lacking, however.

A third area of focus has been on trends in underlying physical, cognitive, and sensory functioning. Self-reported measures of capacity (using Nagi's functional limitations—difficulty with body movements such as reaching, bending, and lifting) have shown consistently large declines (Freedman, Martin, & Schoeni, 2002b), but no study of trends in performance measures has been conducted to date because of data limitations. Evidence regarding trends in cognitive function among the elderly population is not as well developed, although there may be some positive movement in that regard (Langa et al., 2008). Vision impairments appear to be less debilitating than they were 10 years ago, possibly because of the increases in cataract surgery over the past decade (Schoeni et al., 2008).

A final avenue of inquiry has focused on the role of assistive technology in disability trends. Well-known shifts have been occurring in the forms of assistance available to help people cope with disability in later life, and the use of technology without personal care has increased markedly among those reporting reduced functional capacity (Freedman, Agree, Martin, & Cornman, 2006a). Some researchers have also attributed declines in IADL disabilities to the increased availability of modern conveniences, such as no longer having to go to the store to shop or to the bank to manage money, and having microwave ovens to facilitate cooking (Spillman, 2004). Moreover, many more seniors are living in supportive living environments that provide assistance with these tasks, such as continuing-care retirement communities, assisted living facilities, and other retirement communities. The role of these pervasive technologies and specialized living environments has not been quantified.

THE EPIDEMIOLOGY OF DISABILITY: RISK FACTORS
FOR FUNCTIONAL DECLINE

Prospective cohort studies have proven very productive in helping to identify factors that increase the risk of developing an activity limitation in later life. In these studies, a group of people without difficulty in daily activities at baseline is monitored during some defined interval. Onset of disability is recorded, typically at 1- or 2-year intervals, sometimes more frequently. We are thus able to identify incident (new) cases and go back to baseline assessments to see how these people differ from people who never reached the end point of interest. Typically, we examine a series of baseline risk factors and calculate the risk associated with a factor, independent of other risk factors that make up a person's profile. Features associated with the disability outcome are "risk factors"; features that reduce likelihood of incidence are called "protective factors." We often calculate these risks by use of logistic regression models, or proportional hazards models if we wish to incorporate a time dimension into analyses (i.e., time to onset rather than simply onset).

In a comprehensive review, Stuck and colleagues (1999) summarized findings across a large number of such studies, with a focus on potentially modifiable risk factors for functional loss. Findings varied somewhat between studies, according to the demographic composition of the cohort, the length of follow-up, how attrition was handled, how risk factors were categorized, and how competing risks (for death and disability) were handled. Nevertheless, the review identified some consistent findings across studies. Consistent predictors of functional loss included, for example, cognitive, vision, and lower body impairments; depression; comorbidity; high/low body mass index; few social contacts; low physical activity; and smoking as consistent predictors of functional loss. Stuck also identified several areas that required further investigation, including the role of biological factors (earlier in the disablement pathway) and the environment.

Since Stuck's review, progress has been made on both fronts. On the biological front, potential biomarkers for disability have been identified. For example, serum albumin level (g/liter) is a risk factor for both incident activity limitations and mortality. Within the EPESE cohort, serum albumin concentration and activity limitations were strongly related at baseline. Moreover, at follow-up, greater serum albumin concentration was associated with a greater risk of mortality within categories of baseline functioning. A new set of biomarkers for function is currently under investigation, including C-reactive protein, interleukin-6 (IL-6), and other cytokines.

In addition, strides have been made in understanding the relationship among inflammation, frailty, and loss of physical capacity that precedes limitations and frank limitations. Chronic inflammation, visible in elevations in IL-6, fibrinogin, C-reactive protein, and tumor necrosis factor-alpha, and decreases in serum albumin, are associated with loss of lean muscle mass (shrinking), low energy, decreased appetite, and the other symptoms of frailty. For instance, in the Women's Health and Aging Study, high levels of IL-6 and C-reactive protein were shown to predict incident difficulty with daily activities independent of other risk factors (Ferrucci et al., 1999). The mechanism for this effect is the catabolic effect of IL-6 on muscle, which leads to sarcopenia and, hence, loss of muscle strength in the lower extremities. This, in turn, leads to limitations in mobility and ultimately ADLs. Examination of changes in knee extensor strength and walking speed suggest that IL-6 affects muscle mass, and that this effect is responsible for the increased risk of disability. That is, the effect of IL-6 on risk of disability was attenuated when changes in muscle mass were introduced into regression equations. This attenuation in risk suggests that "change in muscle strength is intrinsic to the causal pathway leading from high IL-6 to the development of new disability" (Ferrucci et al., 2002). This is an indirect demonstration of the causal mechanism, but it is consistent with other research showing an association between high levels of IL-6 and lower muscle mass and strength (Visser et al., 2002a), as well as lower muscle mass and poorer lower extremity function (Visser et al., 2002b). A stronger demonstration would show an increased risk of disability among people whose IL-6 serum levels have increased (or a lower risk of disability in a group whose IL-6 levels have declined, perhaps as a result of a therapeutic intervention). This growing body of work suggests that intervention strategies that might prevent IL-6 and other cytokines from affecting muscle may be ready for investigation.

With respect to environmental influences, the role of neighborhoods in facilitating or impeding late-life function has been a recent focus (e.g., Balfour & Kaplan, 2002; Clarke & George, 2005; Freedman, Grafova, Schoeni, & Rogowski, 2008; Schootman et al., 2006). Balfour and Kaplan (2002), for example, found that functional loss among persons 55 and older in Alameda County, California, was related to self-reported problems with neighborhoods, including excessive noise, inadequate lighting at night, heavy traffic, and limited public transportation. Clarke and George (2005) found that among adults age 65 and older living in North Carolina, greater independence in IADLs (e.g., shopping, managing money, household chores) was reported among those living in environments with more land-use diversity, and that among those with functional limitations, housing density was inversely related to self-care disability. Schootman and colleagues (2006) found that among middle-aged African Americans around St. Louis, Missouri, adults living in areas with 4–5 versus 0–1 fair/poor conditions were more than 3 times as likely to develop a lower body limitation. And, Freedman et al. (2008) have found by using tract- and county-level data linked to the nationally representative Health and Retirement Study that neighborhood economic advantage is associated with a reduced risk of lower body limitations for both men and women, and that high connectivity of the built environment is associated with reduced risk of limitations in instrumental activities for men.

While of interest to public health, such studies stop short of providing communities with the information they need to create environments that support functioning and well-being of older adults. Fortunately, progress has been made on this front through the Visiting Nurse Service of New York's AdvantAge Initiative (Feldman, Oberlink, Simantov, & Gursen, 2004). Based on the premise that communities matter in the daily lives of older adults, AdvantAge began by exploring what makes a neighborhood "elder friendly." By talking with people in four communities, they identified four domains of the elder-friendly community: (a) addressing basic needs, (b) optimizing physical health and well being, (c) maximizing independence for older adults who are frail or have disabilities, and (d) promoting social and civic engagement. They then developed a 33-item instrument for communities to rate their elder-friendliness (Feldman & Oberlink, 2003). In addition, they surveyed older adults in 10 communities to understand older adults' perceptions of the 33 indicators. Information was reported back to communities in chart book form. National survey results (Feldman et al., 2004) based on 1,500 older adults made norms available to communities so that they had a basis of comparison for each indicator. The national survey underscored the disparate experience of two groups of older adults—the vibrant, successfully aging seniors dubbed the "fortunate majority" and a smaller group referred to as the "frail fraction." The latter are living in ill health, with inadequate resources, and in nonsupportive and sometimes dangerous communities.

In an equally important companion project, the AdvantAge initiative identified and profiled best practices to promote health and independence among older adults. The resulting report highlighted several key "ingredients" to the success of community-based programs (Feldman & Oberlink, 2003). These ingredients are so fundamental to successful community-based interventions—whether related to elder friendliness or any other public health and aging topic—that we provide a summary here:

1. Broad stakeholder support throughout the planning, implementation, and life of the program
2. Knowledge of the community and how to tailor programs to that community
3. Leadership—both in terms of lead agency and lead person
4. The "right" lead agency and person
5. Building and sustaining relationships with all those involved in the effort
6. Marketing with tailored messages
7. Flexibility to change and grow with community needs

The information provided to participating AdvantAge Initiative communities has been used to help give a voice to the older adults of the community, as well as to identify barriers and solutions to promoting elder friendliness.

A CLINICAL PERSPECTIVE: IDENTIFYING DISABLEMENT PATHWAYS

For prevention of disability progression and frailty in older adults, a good target is the older adult with reduced capacity to carry out the building blocks of activities—those with mobility limitations, upper and lower body limitations, sensory limitations, and mild cognitive impairments. In ICF-language, by focusing on capacity in the domains upon which activities are built, it is possible to identify persons at risk for activity limitations and participation restrictions. (Put in terms of the Nagi formulation, it is important to measure *functional limitation* antecedent to *disability*.) The aim is to identify factors associated with reports of disability among individuals who demonstrate a range of limitation in the abilities or skills needed to undertake daily activities. Such "skill elements"—for example, sequencing steps in a task, organizing a work-space, or maintaining bodily alignment—have been well-examined in occupational therapy research and have been defined, with clear scoring criteria, as in AMPS (Fisher, 2006a, 2006b).

The Link Between Capacity and Performance

What is the relationship between the motor and cognitive skills used in performing daily activities (functional limitation) and IADL/BADL limitations? A first investigation in this area involved the relationship be-tween leg strength and gait speed. Buchner et al. (1996) found that the relationship between leg strength, measured in an exercise ma-chine test, and gait speed was nonlinear. In such a nonlinear relation-ship (or flattened S-shaped curve), three regions are defined, as shown hypothetically in Figure 5.4. The figure relates gait speed, a measure of mobility capacity, to difficulty or needing help in bathing, a measure of activity limitation. However, this type of nonlinear relationship be-tween capacity and activity limitations has been established for other indicators, including balance and gait speed, and between gait speed and IADL/BADL measures (Jette, Assmann, Rooks, Harris, & Craw-ford, 1998).

When mobility speed is extremely low, people are essentially un-able to walk or stand, and disability in bathing is complete. The curve is flat (region A), indicating that until gait speed exceeds a certain mini-mum (despite some minor improvements), limitation in bathing will not change. In other words, there is a threshold of leg strength or gait speed required for bathing. Once this threshold is crossed, gait speed and in-dependence in bathing are directly related, as shown in region B, so that each additional unit of leg strength or gait speed is associated with a proportional gain in independence or efficiency (or ease) in bathing. Once leg strength or gait speed exceeds a certain level again, a second threshold is crossed, defining the beginning of region C. At this point, additional gait speed or leg strength does not translate into greater bath-ing efficiency. Given the biomechanical and ergonomic properties of the task, individuals are already performing as efficiently as possible and any additional leg strength contributes to physiological reserve but does not affect the speed or efficiency of bathing. Above this threshold, incre-ments in strength or skill are not associated with reduction in disability but only with increased reserve (Buchner et al., 1996; Sonn, Frandin, & Grimby, 1995).

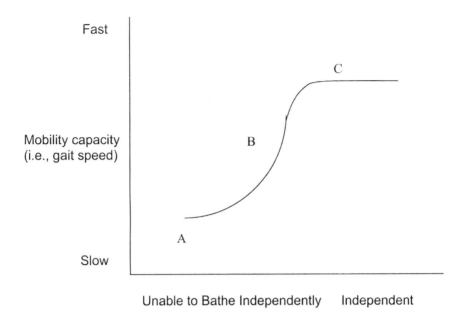

Figure 5.4 Hypothetical relationship between mobility capacity and bathing disability.

Identification of these thresholds may be clinically important, because these indicate the point on a continuum of ability, physical or cognitive, when capacity has implications for limitations. The thresholds also help set goals for intervention and rehabilitation. For example, a clinical trial seeking to prevent or reduce activity limitations by improving strength would not show benefit if targeted to individuals in region C of the curve. These individuals are already beyond the threshold where improvements in strength will affect performance of daily tasks. Similarly, only with large improvement in capacity could we expect to see reduction in limitations in region A. By contrast, people along region B of the curve might be the best target for such a trial. In this group, even small changes in underlying capacity can be expected to translate into increases in independence and efficiency.

Buchner et al. (1997) have shown the relevance of these considerations in a clinical trial of exercise to reduce the incidence of falls. The trial was part of the FICSIT initiative, "Frailty and Injuries: Cooperative Studies of Intervention Techniques." The study recruited elders with extensive functional limitation; all were unable to do an eight-step tandem gait test without errors, and all were below the 50th percentile in knee extensor strength based on norms for weight and height. A program of endurance and strength training led to increases in isokinetic strength and aerobic capacity, but no improvements in gait speed or balance. This lack of consistent benefit (reduction in measures of impairment, no benefit in measures of functional limitation) already suggests that selection criteria for the study were too stringent. People recruited for the study were likely near or within region A of the curve shown in Figure 5.4, so that improvement in underlying capacity might not lead to reduction in limitations. Indeed, in this study 1-year fall rates in the intervention group were 42%, better than the control group rate of 60%, but no different than the risk of falls typical of older people living in the community (Tinetti, Speechley, & Ginter, 1988). Buchner concludes that "the eligibility criteria selected a sample on the verge of substantial decline, and exercise prevented this decline." A more efficient design would have selected a less impaired sample.

The nonlinear relationship between underlying capacity and activity limitations also appears to hold for cognitive capacity. Figure 5.5 is a scatterplot of limitations (reported by caregivers) by number of errors by care recipient on a cognitive screening measure, derived from a sample of caregivers to elders with a diagnosis of Alzheimer's disease. Scores ranged from 24 (best score: independent all the time in 12 tasks) to 0 (worst score: dependent all the time in all 12 tasks assessed). Elders completed a 15-item cognitive screening test, which included items from a series of brief cognitive status tests (CARE-Diagnostic Screen; Gurland et al., 1995). These items assess a person's orientation, short-term memory, attention, and language ability. The scatterplot stratifies by number of comorbid conditions to better isolate the effect of cognitive capacity on dependence in daily activities.

The least-squares regression lines shown in Figure 5.5 were derived using a curvilinear regression model. The R^2 for the model in subjects without other comorbid conditions (thick line, $n = 78$) increased from 0.41 to 0.52 with introduction of a quadratic term, suggesting that the nonlinear curvilinear model offers a better fit. By contrast, in the two groups with other concurrent disease, linear models provided an adequate fit. Subjects with cognitive impairment in the absence of other comorbid disease are not likely to have reported limitations until they made five or more errors on the cognitive screen. This relationship should be compared with that of subjects with cognitive deficit and one or two or more comorbid conditions. They report greater dependency at every

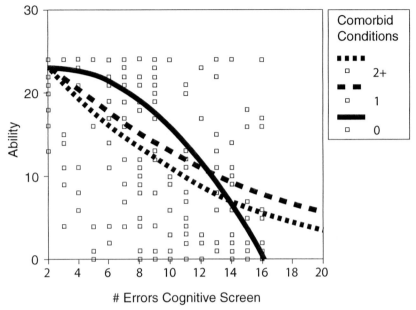

Figure 5.5 Relationship between disability and cognitive status.

level of cognitive ability. We conclude that the relationship between cognitive impairment and activity limitations may follow that demonstrated for physical indicators and disability.

The Role of Accommodations

Both the ICF language and the Nagi disablement model support questions about the compensatory processes and environmental modifications that prevent reduced capacity from resulting in activity limitations or participation restrictions. Four major types of accommodations exist: change in how the activity is performed (e.g., frequency, duration, or positioning), uptake of assistive technology, changes to the environment to support performing the activity, and reliance on help from another person. Although much attention has focused on the latter, in particular, caregiving to older adults, these other types of accommodations that may facilitate independent performance of activities have only recently come into focus.

Perhaps the most common—yet least studied—accommodation is simply altering the frequency of a task or changing the way a task is performed (Weiss, Hoenig, & Fried, 2007). This is the first and most basic adaptation. If a shoulder range-of-motion limitation makes it difficult for someone to wash his or her hair, the first response probably will be a reduction in the frequency of hair washing or a change in bathing routine, such as washing hair only when someone is available to help. These are effective modifications for mild-to-moderately severe functional limitation. With progression of functional limitation, completing ADL tasks may become impossible without further modifications, either alteration of the physical environment (washing hair in the sink rather than shower, use of a grab bar or bath stool, use of walk-in shower stall), or recourse to personal assistance (regular help getting into the tub, balance support, and personal assistance with the application of shampoo).

More subtle forms of behavioral adaptation involve drawing on other faculties to compensate for reduced capacity in another area. For example, older persons with severe balance deficit (impairment) who still perform well in daily tasks, such as vacuuming or cooking, have presumably relied more on other faculties to prevent the balance disorder from disabling them in these daily tasks. We know very little about these processes, although efforts from kinesiology and neuroscience are underway to specify this effect. A simpler example is seen in the elder with mild cognitive impairment who uses other brain regions, visualized in functional magnetic resonance imaging, to perform better than expected in certain memory tasks. This elder probably uses mnemonics or other strategies to perform the memory task and, hence, draws on other relatively spared domains of brain function. Such subtle changes may suggest that a person's capacities might be increased through recruitment of remaining, relatively spared abilities. This process is less well explored than any of the other behavioral accommodations described here, but may be at least as important. It suggests far more extensive use of rehabilitative technologies to teach older people (and, indeed, anyone facing reductions in capacity) how to reorganize the way they do tasks by drawing on other remaining abilities.

One challenge for defining the population with activity limitations, already mentioned, is that people who have made successful adaptations of this sort may not report difficulty with the task. After all, they are successfully performing the task and have, to a great extent, overcome the change in capacity that might have otherwise caused this difficulty. Behavioral changes that individuals make to compensate for changes in underlying capacity may then be an important clue for clinicians to look for in predicting who will develop limitations—or who might benefit from an intervention to prevent this process from unfolding. For example, people reporting no difficulty with ADL, but who also say they have reduced the frequency of these ADL tasks, have lower grip strength, gait speed, dexterity, and balance scores, and a higher risk of developing ADL limitations (Fried et al., 1996).

Also widespread is the use of assistive technologies and environmental modifications. Cornman and colleagues (2005) have found, for example, that estimates of assistive device use across several national surveys range from 14% to 18% for the population of adults aged 65 and older, and range from 39% to 44% for the 85 and older population. Devices are used most often for mobility and bathing, and less often for toileting and transferring. However, questions about such devices are often restricted to individuals who report difficulty with daily activities and, therefore, omit a potentially sizeable group—those who use assistive devices but report no difficulty with daily activities. If this group is included the prevalence of both device use—and of those at risk for developing limitations because of reductions in capacity—are significantly higher.

The fact that assistive technology may in many cases bridge the gap between capacity and the environment is not surprising. Using the 1994–1995 Disability Supplement to the NHIS, for example, Verbrugge and Sevak (2002) show that equipment only or equipment with personal assistance is more likely to reduce difficulty than personal assistance alone. To explain this result, they point out "First, equipment is designed for the task, can be modified to suit the individual, and is generally on hand when needed. . . . Second, equipment maintains an individual's self-sufficiency. This can foster pride and keen perception of task improvements." This is an important result and suggests the need for further development of assistive devices. However, it is also worth recognizing the limits of equipment use in the case of cognitive disability, a major source of disability in late life (see Chapter 6).

An Example of Accommodations: Bathing

We can tie these insights on disability and efforts to mitigate the effects of reduced capacity with a closer look at a particular activity. A good candidate is bathing. As we have seen, it is the most prevalent ADL limitation and one that lends itself to a variety of accommodations and the use of compensatory processes.

In a study of nearly 200 older adults, all aged 70 and older, with mild to moderate activity limitations (reported difficulty in one to three domains of upper extremity, lower extremity, IADL, and ADL function, but not all four), 9.5% reported they had difficulty with bathing (Albert, Bear-Lehman, Burkhardt, Merete-Roa, & Noboa-Lemonier, 2006). These self-reports were quite stable. In the whole sample, less than 2% changed their self-report between a telephone interview and an in-home assessment. Respondents reported a variety of sources for their difficulty bathing, including fear of falling and concern about balance, pain, weakness, swollen legs (edema), and shortness of breath. People who reported difficulty bathing were more likely to report they had changed the frequency of bathing and the way they bathed. For example, of those reporting difficulty bathing, 87.5% said they had changed the way they bathe during the past 12 months. In people who did not report difficulty bathing, only 24.8% reported a change in the way they bathe. Thus, reports of difficulty and attempts to modify environments to mitigate difficulty go hand in hand.

If we look only at people who said they had no difficulty bathing, we find further evidence that environmental modification is a response to changes in underlying capacity. People who reported they had changed the way they bathe showed lower grip strength, slower gait speed, and less efficient performance on the AMPS assessment (the occupational therapy assessment described above) than people who reported no change. We find this pattern even when we restrict the sample further to people who report they have not changed the frequency with which they bathe. People who have changed the way they bathe score more poorly on the measures. Thus, changes in behavior, indicated by changes in frequency and mode of performing the ADL, are clearly related to degree of capacity.

In the same sample, we also investigated one facet of compensation in the face of reduced capacity. We established the poorest balance group by examining the distribution of scores on a series of progressively more difficult static stances. Those in the lowest tertile (or third) showed a great range of motor performance in the AMPS assessment. In fact, nearly half scored above the cutting score on the motor dimension, indicating an ability to live independently despite poor balance. Of those with poor balance but good motor performance, 13.3% reported difficulty bathing. By contrast, nearly 40% of people with poor balance and poor motor performance reported difficulty bathing. Thus, some elders in the poor balance group were able to draw on other abilities to achieve reasonable motor performance despite balance deficit. These elders were also less likely to report bathing difficulties. We need to know more about this process.

PUBLIC HEALTH INTERVENTIONS TO MAXIMIZE LATE-LIFE FUNCTIONING

To this point we have considered disability and aging from three vantage points. The demography literature teaches us that, although activity limitations may be declining, not all groups have benefited equally, and continued declines in prevalence will be important to achieve as the large Baby Boom cohorts begin to retire this decade. Epidemiology has pointed to a list of important risk factors—from biological, to medical, to social and behavioral to environmental—that increase individuals' chances of developing activity limitations. Clinicians have added important insights about how accommodations and compensatory strategies may be individualized to bridge gaps between an individual's capacity to perform activities and their desire to perform both essential and valued activities. The public health and aging professional's interest cross cuts these disciplines as it seeks to establish public programs to ensure maximization of functioning among older adults. Here, we illustrate this sprawling literature by reviewing one especially important and promising avenue—fall prevention programs, and follow this with a discussion of how to compare the likely effects of interventions at the population level.

Preventing Falls → Online Article

Falling is a common event among older people. Approximately 30% of people aged 65 and older residing in communities and 40% of people aged 80 and older fall each year (Tinetti et al., 1988). According to the Web-based Injury Statistics Query and Reporting System, available at http://www.cdc.gov/injury/wisqars/index.html and shown here in Table 5.4, in 2006, nearly 17,000 people aged 65 years or older died because of falls, up from 10,000 in 1999.

The number of reported injuries because of falls in this population exceeded 1.8 million. Approximately one in four older people who fall experience either a severe injury (e.g., fracture, trauma to the head, serious lacerations, joint dislocation) or limitation. Among those who sustain hip fractures, recuperation from depressive symptoms, cognitive loss,

Table 5.4

FALL-RELATED DEATHS AND INJURIES, 2001–2006, 65+ AND 85+ POPULATION

YEAR	# DEATHS	CRUDE DEATH RATE	# INJURIES	CRUDE INJURY RATE	POPULATION
65 and Older Population:					
2001	11746	33.25	1,642,533	4649.12515	35,329,945
2002	12961	36.42	1,640,080	4608.48203	35,588,294
2003	13820	38.44	1,822,590	5069.980707	35,948,651
2004	15028	41.4	1,851,602	5101.258967	36,296,965
2005	15917	43.32	1,802,172	4904.367212	36,746,273
2006	16747	44.95	1,840,564	4940.703674	37,253,065
85 and Older Population:					
2001	5366	121.47	504,704	11425.32486	4,417,415
2002	6020	132.41	503,708	11079.13089	4,546,457
2003	6436	136.5	554,978	11770.56146	4,714,967
2004	6993	144.26	555,070	11450.80042	4,847,434
2005	7561	149.57	545,958	10800.07957	5,055,128
2006	8052	152.33	573,804	10855.21849	5,285,976

From Web-based Injury Statistics Query and Reporting System (WISQARSTM).

and upper-body limitations generally occurs within a few months; however, lower body functioning takes on average a year or so to regain pre-fall status (Magaziner et al., 2000). Some older adults who fall also curtail activities because of a fear of falling again. As a result, individuals who experience falls have two or three times the relative risk of developing activity limitations as those who do not fall.

There are many known risk factors for falling. Tinetti et al. (1998), for example, found in a cohort of community-dwelling adults age 70 and older that sedative use, cognitive impairment, functional limitation in the lower extremities, poor reflexes, abnormalities of balance and gait, and foot problems were all risk factors for falling. An important finding from this study was the important role of environmental and ergonomic factors in falls. While 77% of the falls occurred at home, in a familiar environment, 44% of the falls involved modifiable home hazards. In these falls, people tripped over objects or slipped on stairs. Also, most falls involved particular kinds of activities, mainly those that displaced a person's center of gravity. These activities included getting up or sitting down, bending over or reaching, or stepping up or down. These particular environmental and ergonomic factors, along with medical risk factors identified in this effort, suggest a number of interventions to reduce the risk of falling.

Over the past two decades, a series of randomized clinical trials have shown that the risk for falls can be reduced. In a review of 40 such fall prevention trials, the most effective interventions were multifactorial falls risk assessments with management programs (Chang et al., 2004). Exercise programs alone were also effective in reducing the risk of falling, but not as effective as multifactor approaches. For example, one of the early, yet most notable, intervention studies linked reduction in the risk of falling to modification of particular risk factors. In the trial conducted by Tinetti and colleagues (1994), the Yale FICSIT trial, 35% of the intervention group fell, compared with 47% of controls, over a 1-year period. In this trial, one inclusion criterion was use of four prescription medications, a risk factor for falling, and a target of this multifactorial intervention. As part of the intervention, medication use for people in the intervention group was evaluated and adjusted, as needed. Sixty-three percent of the intervention group continued to take four or more medications, compared with 86% of controls. The trial also showed that many other risk factors for falling were modifiable, including balance impairment, difficulty with toilet transfer, and gait impairment. Each was modified through a combination of behavioral training, exercise program, or environmental change. The prevalence of impairments in the intervention group declined relative to controls; and this reduction appears to have been responsible for the reduction of falls.

A reanalysis of the data (Tinetti, McAvay, & Claus, 1996) showed that improvements in balance and reduction in blood pressure (to lower fall risk associated with orthostatic hypotension) were associated with lower rates of falling. Also, the reanalysis showed that fall risk declined in both treatment and control groups according to degree of reduction in a composite measure of fall risk. In the treatment group, the average number of risk factors declined by about one (of seven different risks), but this degree of risk factor reduction was enough to reduce falls by approximately 35% (Buchner, 1999). Together, these findings suggest that altering or eliminating specific risk factors for falls can reduce fall risk.

In other developed countries these types of tailored programs have been packaged with community-focused interventions, with reasonable success (McClure et al., 2005). Specific interventions varied but generally involved a combination of community-wide education, reduction in risks in homes and communities, training of health care personnel, and/or visits to the homes of high-risk individuals. A review of five prospective community trials with matched control communities suggested that, despite methodological limitations, fall-related fractures potentially could be reduced by 6%–33%.

In the United States, public health efforts to prevent falls have greatly expanded since the FICSIT trials. The AoA, for example, has been providing grants to states to mobilize the aging, public health, and nonprofit networks at the state and local level (see Chapter 3). Four evidence-based fall prevention programs have been included in these grants in more than a dozen states: Matter of Balance, Stepping On, Tai Chi, and Step by Step. In partnership with AoA, the CDC has funded evaluations of these fall prevention packages, and has also independently funded projects to translate this research into practice and to disseminate findings to communities. With respect to the latter, CDC has compiled a compendium of successful interventions for public health practitioners and community-based organizations, which covers exercise programs, home modification programs, and multifactor fall prevention programs (Stevens & Sogolo, 2008).

A companion guide for community-based organizations offers practical advice for planning, development, implementation, and evaluation of fall prevention programs (Stevens & Sogolo, 2008). In addition to providing essential program components (e.g., education, exercise, medication management, vision assessment, and home hazard identification), the guide also provides tips to communities on building and maintaining partnerships that will foster sustained prevention programs. Like the AdvantAge Initiative described earlier, critical ingredients for a successful and sustained fall prevention program involve community building, leadership and resources, and flexibility.

Comparing Potentially High-Impact Interventions

How does one go about comparing potentially high-impact interventions at the population level? That is, if one were to attempt to maximize the population's functioning, what approaches would be most effective? An interdisciplinary team recently tackled this question (Freedman et al., 2006) and identified critical information needed to compare the effects of interventions at the population level. Their framework drew on the notion of illness trajectories, that is, that individuals follow one of several prototypical experiences in terms of declines in function at the end of life, and that interventions might alter these trajectories or the demands placed on individuals by the environment. Their exercise started with the simple goal of reviewing the literature to identify the interventions with the greatest potential to reduce disability prevalence in the older population.

Their plan to compare interventions was complicated by several factors. First, most randomized studies evaluate interventions in terms of their influence on one or more proximate risk factors for disability, rather than on disability itself. Thus, to assess short-run effects, they considered three pieces of information—the prevalence of the risk factor of interest, the effect of the intervention on the targeted risk factor, and the relationship between the risk factor and the disablement process. Second, a variety of measures of functioning were found in the literature, and many studies evaluating interventions omitted measures of functioning altogether and instead focused on more proximate outcomes (e.g., leg strength or balance). Thus, the effects of interventions on the progression of activity limitations in many cases cannot be calculated precisely. Third, because interventions may influence not only disability, but also length of life, their short- and long-term effects may differ. Despite these complications, however, the investigators were able to assess the *relative* magnitude of effects on the prevalence of activity limitations by comparing interventions according to the following dimensions: the size and selectivity of the intervention's target population, the risk of disability associated with the risk factor addressed by the intervention, the effect of the intervention on the targeted risk factor, and the influence of the intervention on length of life and competing risks.

The team implemented this strategy for three potentially high-impact strategies: physical activity, depression screening and treatment, and fall prevention. Because of the large population at risk for falling, the demonstrated efficacy of multicomponent interventions in preventing falls, and the strong links between falls and activity limitations, they concluded that in the short run, multicomponent fall-prevention efforts would likely have a higher impact than either physical activity or depression screening and treatment. However, they stressed that "longer-term comparisons [could] not be made based on the current literature and may differ from short-run conclusions, since increases in longevity may temper the influences of these interventions on prevalence" (p. 493).

More generally, although there are a number of promising approaches to facilitating functioning in later life, there are real challenges to widespread implementation of high-impact interventions. Here, we outline five such challenges:

1. Disablement and functioning are complex processes with multiple risk factors at work. In general, multifactor interventions that are tailored to individual needs seem to work better than single interventions, but public health and aging programs are not always equipped to individualize services.
2. Ideally, public health and aging interventions need to be developed at multiple levels—not just aimed at the individual, but also at the families and communities in which people live. As we have seen, some examples of fall prevention interventions combine individual- and community-based approaches, but on the whole these have not been adopted in the United States.
3. Identifying the appropriate target population and window of time for targeting an intervention is critical to its success. The curvilinear relationship between underlying capacity and activity limitations complicates this targeting effort.
4. Attention throughout the process to the issue of sustainability and/or adherence is critical for long-term success.
5. Finally, the complex interactions between functioning and length of life complicate the equation. Interventions can influence both but will only reduce the prevalence of activity limitations and/or participation restrictions if the intervention lengthens active life at least as much as it lengthens life expectancy. These relationships are very difficult to predict and more research is needed to link interventions to disability and mortality outcomes.

SUMMARY

Language of Disability. The internationally accepted World Health Organization's International Classification of Functioning, Disability and Health (ICF) provides a useful language for disability research and public health interventions. Key terms include activity limitation, participation, the environment, and distinctions between capacity and performance. Unlike the Nagi model of disablement, the ICF language is not a dynamic model. To blend the benefits of the ICF language with those of the Nagi model is an important next step for disability and aging research.

Measuring Disability. Difficulty and need for help with activities of daily living have been central measures of interest in the study of public health and aging. New measures capturing the capacity to perform daily activities, the environment, and behavioral accommodations that individuals make to bridge the gap between capacity and the environment are gaining importance in the field.

Disability Trends. The prevalence of activity limitations declined during the 1980s and 1990s and active life expectancy increased. Declines were larger for instrumental activities of daily living than for the more severe activities of daily living, and more advantaged groups experienced larger declines. The reasons for these trends are complex and include shifts in socioeconomic status of the older population, in the distribution of underlying conditions and limitations in capacity that may be related to use of medical treatments, and in the uptake of assistive and other convenience technologies. In recent years this trend may have leveled off, and there are some signs that, in the future, this course may even reverse. Reconciling disparate findings remains an important focus among demographers.

Risk Factors for Functional Loss. Consistent predictors of functional loss included cognitive, vision, and lower body impairments; depression; comorbidity; high/low body mass index; few social contacts; low physical activity; and smoking as consistent predictors of functional loss. In addition, in recent years, our understanding of the biology of disability and the role of inflammation has increased. Studies of environmental factors, especially those focused on neighborhood characteristics that influence late-life disablement, suggest a role for the economic and built environments as well. These latter findings have not yet been translated into multilevel interventions.

Disablement Pathways. Clinicians have documented nonlinear relationships between measures of physical and cognitive capacity and activity limitations. Such findings indicate that there may be zones of opportunity for maintenance or improvement in functioning and other subgroups for whom intervention around underlying capacity may be less productive. Three distinct types of behavioral accommodations were also discussed in detail: changes in how the activity is performed (e.g., frequency, duration, or positioning), uptake of assistive technology, and changes to the environment to support performing the activity. The latter two are highly prevalent, but less is known about behavioral accommodations. One promising, but poorly understood, type of behavioral adaptation involves drawing on other faculties to compensate for reduced capacity in another area.

Public Health Interventions to Maximize Physical Functioning. Research to date is incomplete in guiding public health practitioners as to which interventions will maximize the functioning of the population in the long run. However, it appears that fall prevention efforts may be a useful place to start for short-term results. One especially promising avenue includes combining individually and community-focused efforts. The design and implementation of interventions to maximize physical functioning holds many challenges. Such challenges include the need to design multifactor, multilevel interventions that are targeted at the appropriate population, that are sustainable, and that lengthen active life expectancy at least as much as life expectancy.

6 Cognitive Function: Dementia

Alzheimer's disease and the other dementias are a major source of morbidity and disability in older people. The medical and supportive care needs of people who have dementia are a major challenge to families, medical care, and every component of long-term care services, not to mention to older people themselves, who perceive declining memory. More and more, they are given a diagnosis of "mild cognitive impairment," often without being told what the diagnosis means for risk of Alzheimer's (Albert, Dienstag, Tabert, Pelton, & Devanand, 2002a). Because the risk of dementia is highly related to age, with diagnosis of dementia occurring in the vast majority of people at the oldest ages, dementia is a central problem in geriatric care. The strong association between age and risk of dementia also makes the study of cognitive deficit and its consequences a key element in the epidemiology of aging.

The Alzheimer's Association reports a prevalence of 5.1 million Americans with Alzheimer's disease (AD) in 2009, with a projected increase to 7.7 million in 2030 (Alzheimer's Association, 2009). About 5%–10% of people aged 65 and older and between one-third and one-half those aged 85 and older meet criteria for the disease. Survival with the disease from the point of diagnosis averages about 8 years, but evidence suggests a very long latency, with progressive cognitive decline over a period of 20 or more years before people come to medical attention and receive the diagnosis. In fact, many older people in the community meet criteria for AD but have not received a diagnosis (Ross et al., 1997) and may not receive the diagnosis until quite late in the course of the disease (or may even die without ever receiving the diagnosis).

Families confronting the disease face the very difficult problem of deciding when driving should cease, when supervision is required for safety, when older people can no longer live alone, and when parents or spouses are no longer competent to handle money, take medications, or manage their lives independently. They will likely have to contend with the personality changes, psychiatric symptoms, and challenging behaviors typical of the more advanced stages of the disease. They may have to perform ADL care or manage supportive care staff hired to assist the elder, or more likely both sets of tasks, possibly at a distance. They may face the difficult decision to admit the Alzheimer's patient to a nursing home. Or, as is increasingly common, older people themselves may choose residences (such as assisted living or continuing care retirement communities) that can accommodate Alzheimer's or nursing-home levels of care, should they need such services.

A central question for public health with respect to Alzheimer's disease is to ask whether early diagnosis would make lives better for patients and families. A new array of technologies, including magnetic resonance imaging (MRI), that allows quantification of amyloid load and impaired hippocampal blood flow, now offer increasingly early detection. Does early detection do any good? Does it translate into better use of existing therapies, more effective planning for the future, and reduction in the excess morbidity associated with the disease, such as falls, depression, car accidents, weight loss and dehydration, or self-neglect? At this point, cognitive assessments, with notification of families and physicians, are not standard elements in primary care, and research is only now underway to determine whether such testing leads to changes in clinical management or family planning for long-term care needs.

The explosion of research in Alzheimer's and other dementing diseases makes this realm difficult to summarize. We address the following topics in this chapter: definitions of dementia, the question of normal memory decline and pathological changes, including the significance of awareness of declining cognitive ability and early effects of cognitive decline on daily activities; estimates of the incidence and prevalence of AD; risk factors for AD (genetic and environmental risk factors, as well as concurrent medical status predictors); and outcomes for people with dementia.

WHAT IS DEMENTIA?

DSM-IV (*Diagnostic and Statistical Manual of Mental Disorders*, 2000) has established criteria for a dementia diagnosis. A person meets criteria for dementia if he or she has:

Definitions

- *Memory impairment,* defined as an impaired ability to learn new information or recall previously learned information; and
- One or more of the following additional impairments in cognition:
  - *Aphasia,* difficulty in language comprehension or production manifested in difficulty finding the right words, and marked by the presence of frequent word substitutions, breaking off in midsentence, and repetition;
  - *Apraxia,* difficulty performing movements in response to verbal commands despite intact motor function;
  - *Agnosia,* difficulty recognizing familiar faces, objects, and places despite intact sensory function; or
  - *Executive function deficits,* difficulty in planning or sequencing activity, or difficulty completing a task in the presence of interference from another task.

In addition, these cognitive deficits must be severe enough to cause significant impairment in social or occupational function and must represent a significant decline from a previous level of functioning. For Alzheimer's disease to be diagnosed, the course of this general cognitive disorder must, in addition, be characterized by gradual onset and continuing, progressive decline. The defect in cognition should not be attributable to other central nervous system conditions that cause progressive deficits in memory and cognition, such as cerebrovascular disease, Parkinson's disease, Huntington's disease, subdural hematoma, normal-pressure hydrocephalus, or brain tumor. Nor should the cognitive disorder be caused by systemic conditions that are known to cause dementia, such as hypothyroidism, vitamin B12 or folic acid deficiency, niacin deficiency, hypercalcemia, neurosyphilis, or HIV infection. Substance-induced conditions should also be excluded. Finally, the cognitive deficits should not occur exclusively during the course of delirium, an acute and temporary confusional state. Delirium, unlike dementia, is usually the result of a general medical condition, a medication reaction, or substance use, and resolves with treatment.

The distinction between dementia and delirium is important. Delirium is characterized by fluctuating disturbances in cognition, mood, attention, arousal, and self-awareness. This clouding of consciousness and disorientation is acute, and will resolve with appropriate medical treatment. It is highly prevalent in some settings: 10%–30% of hospitalized medical patients, and up to 80% of terminally ill patients in the last weeks of life, have been reported to have episodes of delirium (Inouye et al., 1999). It is also common in nursing homes. Delirium can affect a patient with dementia, and, in these cases, distinguishing between the two may be difficult.

The Alzheimer's Disease and Related Disorders Association (ADRDA) (McKhann et al., 1984) has developed additional criteria for diagnosing dementia of the Alzheimer's type. A definitive AD diagnosis requires that clinical criteria for probable AD be met and, in addition, that histopathological evidence from biopsy or autopsy be available. "Probable AD" is defined by the criteria listed above, but a diagnosis of "possible AD" can also be made based on the dementia syndrome described above in "the presence of variations in the onset, presentation and clinical course" or in "the presence of a second systemic or brain disorder sufficient to cause the dementia but not considered to be the cause of the dementia." These are the criteria for diagnosis of the National Institute of Neurological Disorders and Stroke-Alzheimer's Disease and Related Disorders Association (NINCDS-ADRDA).

The "possible AD" distinction is important because dementia can also be a feature of other neurodegenerative diseases, such as Parkinson's or vascular disease, and can also accompany stroke or trauma. In other adults, these diseases or effects from disease can co-occur. In such cases, the diagnosis of AD may depend on which came first; for example, if dementia precedes Parkinson's disease, it is reasonable to call this person an incident case of AD, with a further complication from Parkinson's. In other cases, the temporal sequence is less clear and a diagnosis of "possible AD" may be warranted.

Lack of diagnostic specificity in the NINCDS-ADRDA criteria and the discovery of a series of biomarkers for Alzheimer's disease have led to a new set of proposed criteria. These biomarkers include imaging technologies (structural MRI to identify characteristic brain signatures), molecular neuroimaging (positron emission tomography [PET] scanning with use of new ligands to quantify amyloid), cerebrospinal fluid analyses (that identify amyloid and tau proteins), and familial genetic mutations that cause AD. The newly proposed diagnostic criteria for Alzheimer's disease include memory impairment along with a positive finding in one of the biomarkers (Dubois et al., 2007). The new criteria are designed to reflect the activity of drug therapies ("disease modifying agents") that affect these basic processes (such as amyloid clearance). Indeed, changes in the biomarkers are now viewed as indicators of successful therapy.

This shift to a biological rather than purely clinical phenotype is notable. Apart from the absence of clear definitions (for example, the amount of brain atrophy or combination of cerebrospinal fluid markers required for diagnosis), the newly proposed criteria shift attention from clinical problems, such as memory loss or IADL limitations, to the neurodegenerative process assumed to underlie Alzheimer's. This approach is reasonable if these are indeed the primary neurodegenerative processes and if therapies can successfully modify them. But without clear specification of the level of biomarker required for diagnosis, the new criteria introduce uncertainty in the meaning of the diagnosis and may allow a vast expansion of the prevalence of the disease based on the presence of risk factors alone.

A comparison with osteoporosis may be instructive. Based on norms available for people at much younger ages, we define osteoporosis as bone mineral densities less than a certain T score (bone mineral densities in the lowest 2.5% or 5% of a population distribution of 35-year-old women, for example). We consider women with this level of bone loss to have the disease and prescribe therapies, such as bisphosphonates, that help with bone remodeling and turnover and can be said to modify the disease. This is precisely what is missing in the revised criteria for Alzheimer's. We lack norms and distributions for the proposed biomarkers. Moreover, we cannot be sure that these biomarkers are the critical ones. Finally, we still have only equivocal evidence that current therapies modify these measures of underlying neurodegeneration.

MAKING AND RECEIVING THE DIAGNOSIS OF ALZHEIMER'S DISEASE

When an elder is brought to medical attention because of memory disorders or progressive inability to manage independently in a household, the treating physician is likely to assess cognitive status with the Folstein Mini-Mental State Examination (MMSE), a 30-point assessment of orientation, memory, attention, language, calculation, and visuospatial construction skills, typically used as a screening test. The MMSE is shown in Table 6.1. Current recommendations suggest that a score greater than 24 is considered normal, a score of 15–24 shows mild-to-moderate impairment, and a score less than 15 shows definite impairment. Nevertheless, the test is not a diagnostic tool and should be considered only a first-line glimpse at cognitive function.

Properties of the MMSE have been investigated intensively. Performance on the measure is related to age and education, apart from dementia status, suggesting that these influences must be considered when interpreting scores on the test. In one effort, the MMSE was administered to over 18,000 adult participants selected in a probability sample within census tracts and households (Crum, Anthony, Bassett, & Folstein, 1993). Median MMSE scores ranged from 29 in people 18–24 years of age, to 27 in people aged 70–74, and to 25 in people aged 80 and older. The median MMSE score was 29 in people with 9 or more years

Table 6.1

EXCERPT FROM MINI-MENTAL STATE EXAMINATION (MMSE)

Orientation to Time

"What is the date?"

Registration

"Listen carefully. I am going to say three words. You say them back to me after I stop. Ready? Here they are . . .

APPLE (pause), PENNY (pause), TABLE (pause). Now repeat those words back to me."

[Repeat up to 5 times, but score only the first trial.]

Naming

"What is this?" [Point to a pencil or pen]

Reading

"Please read this and do what it says." [Show examinee the words on the stimulus form]

CLOSE YOUR EYES

of school, 26 for people with 5–8 years, and 22 for people with 0–4 years. Because a score of less than 24 is often taken as an indicator of possible dementia, education obviously needs to be taken into account in interpreting performance. The need for caution in applying cutoff scores in the MMSE is even clearer when we examine older people with low education. For people with 0–4 years of school, the median MMSE score for people under age 65 ranges from 22 to 25, but it is 21–22 in people aged 70–79 and 19–20 in people aged 80 and older. Research suggests that literacy may be as important as years of school for MMSE performance (Albert & Teresi, 1999), and that quality of education should also be considered when interpreting education-referenced scores, especially among minorities (Manly, Jacobs, Touradji, Small, & Stern, 2002).

One way to grade the severity of dementia is through instruments such as the Clinical Dementia Rating, or CDR (Hughes, Berg, Danziger, Cohen, & Martin, 1982). The original scoring categories and criteria are shown in Table 6.2. The CDR involves six dimensions: three cognitive (memory, orientation, and judgment and problem-solving) and three functional (home and hobbies, community affairs, and self-care). The original system allows a diagnosis of normal, "questionable," "mild," "moderate," and "severe" dementia. The CDR has also been expanded to include a "profound" and "terminal" level of severity (Dooneief, Marder, Tang, & Stern, 1996).

Scoring of the CDR requires a semistructured interview with both the caregiver and patient. In particular, caregivers provide information that the clinician can use in his or her discussion with the patient to check a patient's level of insight on the extent of memory deficit. Washington University has prepared a series of training videotapes that illustrate effectively the variation in the severity of dementia. The tapes are good teaching tools not only for rating severity, but also for showing features of dementia, such as lack of insight, difficulty with verbal production and comprehension, retardation of motor activity, depression, and confabulation to mask memory difficulty. Students unfamiliar with dementia who view the tapes report how difficult, even excruciating, it is to see someone struggle with language and the simplest comprehension tasks.

Scoring of the CDR can take a number of forms. Clinicians can use it to formulate a global impression, or they can more formally assign severity according to the sum of box scores or some other algorithm for weighting dimensions in making an assignment.

The CDR score offers an important end point for studies of dementia progression or treatment efficacy. What proportion of patients with mild

Table 6.2

CLINICAL DEMENTIA RATING (CDR)

	IMPAIRMENT LEVEL AND CDR SCORE (0, 0.5, 1, 2, 3)				
	NONE 0	QUESTIONABLE 0.5	MILD 1	MODERATE 2	SEVERE 3
Memory	No memory loss or slight inconsistent forgetfulness	Consistent slight forgetfulness; partial recollection of events; "benign" forgetfulness	Moderate memory loss; more marked for recent events; defect interferes with everyday activities	Severe memory loss; only highly learned material retained; new material rapidly lost	Severe memory loss; only fragments remain
Orientation	Fully oriented	Fully oriented except for slight difficulty with time relationships	Moderate difficulty with time relationships; oriented for place at examination; may have geographic disorientation elsewhere	Severe difficulty with time relationships; usually disoriented to time, often to place	Oriented to person only
Judgment & Problem Solving	Solves everyday problems & handles business & financial affairs well; judgment good in relation to past performance	Slight impairment in solving problems, similarities, and differences	Moderate difficulty in handling problems, similarities, and differences; social judgment usually maintained	Severely impaired in handling problems, similarities, and differences; social judgment usually impaired	Unable to make judgments or solve problems

Community Affairs	Independent function at usual level in job, shopping, volunteer and social groups	Slight impairment in these activities	Unable to function independently at these activities although may still be engaged in some; appears normal to casual inspection	No pretense of independent function outside home; appears well enough to be taken to functions outside a family home	No pretense of independent function outside home; appears too ill to be taken to functions outside a family home
Home and Hobbies	Life at home, hobbies, and intellectual interests well maintained	Life at home, hobbies, and intellectual interests slightly impaired	Mild but definite impairment of function at home; more difficult chores abandoned; more complicated hobbies and interests abandoned	Only simple chores preserved; very restricted interests, poorly maintained	No significant function in home
Personal Care	Fully capable of self-care		Needs prompting	Requires assistance in dressing, hygiene, keeping of personal effects	Requires much help with personal care; frequent incontinence

From http://www.adrc.wustl.edu/adrc/cdrGrid.html.

dementia (CDR 1), for example, progress to moderate or more severe dementia (CDR 2+) over a defined interval? Natural history studies of incident cohorts provide information of this sort, which is important for assessing the efficacy of a therapy in delaying progression. The risk of progression from mild to more advanced dementia in an incident AD cohort is approximately 6%–10% per year (see below); thus, a reasonable goal for delay of disease progression would be a rate significantly lower than this.

Measures that tap cognition alone (as opposed to cognition and function, like the CDR) are also valuable tools. Neuropsychological assessment allows fairly fine differentiation of strengths and weaknesses in a variety of cognitive domains. Age- and education-based norms, in different languages, are now available for an increasingly wide range of tests (which now offer multiple forms, an advantage for longitudinal studies that must consider "practice effects"). With so many tests, scored in so many different ways, however, it is often difficult to decide how best to use the measures. Should tests be aggregated according to the cognitive domain they have been designed to assess (such as memory, visuospatial skill, language, or executive function), or according to data reduction techniques (such as factor analysis)? Assuming we combine tests, should we count the number of tests 1 or 2 standard deviations below norms to compute a "deficit score," or should we standardize scores and compute a sum of z scores? After we have computed a composite measure, should we be concerned with mean performance or variation in the test scores over time (Holtzer, Verghese, Wang, Hall, & Lipton, 2008)?

One factor-analytic study of neuropsychological test performance offers some reassurance for these questions. Mayeux and colleagues reported a stable and plausible factor structure for test performance in a sample of elders without dementia (Mayeux, Small, Tang, Tycko, & Stern, 2001). In this effort, three factors emerged:

Memory: Total recall, long-term recall, delayed recall, long-term storage, cued long-term recall, and total recall over six trials of the Selective Reminding Test (Buschke & Fuld, 1974);
Visuospatial/Cognitive Skill: Matching and recognition components of the Benton Visual Retention Test (Benton, 1955), Rosen Drawing Test (Rosen, 1981), and Identities and Oddities of the Mattis Dementia Rating Scale (Mattis, 1976);
Language: Boston Naming Test (Kaplan, Goodglass, & Weintraub, 1983), Controlled Oral Word Association Test (Benton, 1967), and WAIS-R Similarities (Wechsler, 1981).

In this study, composite scores for each factor were computed and used to examine decline in cognitive performance over follow-up in a community-dwelling cohort of elders without dementia drawn from Medicare enrollee files. The authors used the scores without reference to norms because the purpose of the study was not to establish impaired performance, but rather to track change in different cognitive domains.

Change in cognitive test scores may be an unreliable indicator of drug efficacy in clinical trials if these changes are small. The clinical significance of such small changes is not clear. For example, if participants in the active arm of a trial retain baseline scores and participants in the placebo group decline by a mean of 1.2 words on a 15-word memory test, is the difference meaningful? Can we say the therapy has blunted the memory decline typical of AD? Does this difference in short-term memory performance matter for daily performance of ADL or IADL tasks? Research to establish the clinical significance of such often subtle change is difficult. In the absence of such research, the gold standard for clinical trials is to insist on an additional favorable global impression of clinical change as a criterion (Leber, 1991; Schneider & Olin, 1996). Thus, the Food and Drug Administration (FDA) considers therapies efficacious only if they demonstrate improvement in cognitive performance along with a global impression of relative improvement. The latter establishes the clinical significance of otherwise small changes in performance.

COGNITIVE DECLINE WITH AGE: DISTINCT FROM ALZHEIMER'S DISEASE?

Earlier, in Chapter 1, we showed that people enter late life with different cognitive and health resources, along with differences in wealth and family support. Differences in the case of cognitive resources, or "cognitive reserve," are especially important. By age 65 or 70 any sample of older adults without dementia will show a wide range of performance on tests of memory and other cognitive domains. But older people scoring more poorly on measures of memory, for example, can be expected to reach the dementia end point, or "convert" to AD, sooner (adjusting for other differences) than older adults with better memory performance. This difference in cognitive resources at the beginning of old age means some people are closer to the threshold of detectable dementia even when they are not very old, as shown schematically in Figure 6.1.

The figure shows that we must consider the decline in memory performance typical of aging and also ask whether the pathological process of AD is something separate from this decline. Figure 6.1 shows two groups of older persons, one entering old age (for convenience, age 65) with high cognitive reserve (a score of 1.5 on a hypothetical cognitive score), the other entering old age with low reserve (cognitive score of 0.5). The two groups can have different trajectories according to whether memory changes in ways typical of "normal aging," or whether memory declines much more quickly as the result of a potentially distinct Alzheimer's pathological process. The figure also includes an "Alzheimer's threshold," a cognitive score (for convenience, set at zero) that is associated with disability and clinical diagnosis.

If we look only at the decline in memory associated with normal memory (see below), we see that the high-reserve group does not reach the Alzheimer's threshold even as late as age 85. The low-threshold group, by contrast, crosses the dementia threshold shortly after age 75. Note that this difference would occur even if the slope of memory decline in the two groups were equivalent, shown by parallel or nearly parallel lines. If we look instead at the declines in memory associated with the pathological process, we see that the high-reserve group now crosses the Alzheimer's threshold at approximately age 80 and the low-reserve group crosses at age 75 or so. Again, the slope of decline in the two groups could be equivalent, represented by parallel lines, or we might hypothesize an important interaction, in which low reserve and the pathological process together result in a steeper slope of decline.

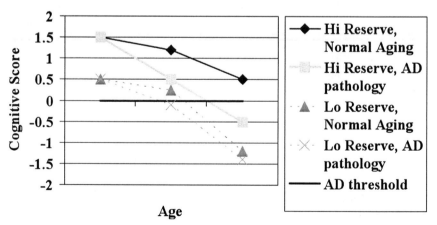

Figure 6.1 Schematic presentation of cognitive resources/reserve as risk factor for dementia.

The big question in this kind of inquiry is whether distinct slopes for normal and pathological memory change in aging exist at all. Within the high- or low-reserve groups, we will find variation in rates of change. Do the changes in memory at either end of this range represent different underlying brain processes, or is a single process enough to account for this variation? More simply, are the declines typical of Alzheimer's just one end of the continuum of changes typical of aging?

Research suggests that memory declines typical of Alzheimer's disease may be distinct from normal aging. Mayeux et al. (2001) first identified a cohort of nearly 600 older people who never met criteria for dementia over 7 years, who were evaluated, on average, every 20 months. The mean age of the cohort was 75.9 at baseline, and 14.2% had one or more *APOE*-e4 alleles. The *APOE* gene is the only gene identified so far for Alzheimer's risk in older adults (as opposed to *PS1, APP, SORL,* and other genes associated with familial disease and much younger onset). The increased risk of AD associated with the e4 allele has been confirmed repeatedly in large prospective cohort studies (Maestre et al., 1995). Mayeux and colleagues (2001) monitored their cohort to investigate the relationship between declines in cognitive performance and *APOE* status. Declines in cognitive domains in people without the e4 allele could plausibly identify normal age-related changes in cognition. People with the e4 allele, who have a higher risk of AD, could plausibly represent early AD and should show steeper declines in memory performance.

In this cohort, memory performance mostly declined over time; two-thirds had a negative slope on the composite memory measure described earlier. Older age and lower education were each associated with poorer memory scores at baseline and at follow-up assessments. Individuals with an *APOE*-e4 allele had steeper declines in memory performance, suggesting early changes typical of Alzheimer's disease. This steeper slope was evident only in people with low education, or low cognitive reserve, suggesting an interaction between low reserve and the Alzheimer's pathological process.

It is noteworthy that memory was the only cognitive domain that declined in this cohort of people who never met criteria for dementia. Visuospatial and language performance were stable across the 7 years of follow-up. Scores in the visuospatial and language domains were stable even in people with an *APOE*-e4 allele.

These findings suggest that memory decline typical of aging can be separated from the pathological aging typical of AD. They also suggest the sensitivity of the memory domain for identifying age-related changes and the risk of AD. In a second set of analyses, Mayeux et al. (2001)

also examined changes in the three domains in a separate group of 228 people who did not meet criteria for AD at baseline but progressed to AD over the follow-up period. These people showed significant declines with time in all three domains, showing a more generalized decline of cognition in people closer to the Alzheimer's threshold.

Mayeux's study is valuable for showing that memory decline is common in a group of older people who do not develop AD over a long period, but also more pronounced (steeper, in terms of Figure 6.1) in a group with an AD risk factor who are still, however, far from the AD threshold. These elders showed declines in memory only. It stands to reason, then, that areas of the brain involved in memory, such as the entorhinal cortex of the hippocampus, should be different in younger people and older people without AD. Differences in anatomy would not be expected, because the older people in this case do not have AD and would not be expected to show the pathological lesions (amyloid plaques, neuritic tangles) typical of the disease. However, differences in physiology might be expected, because poorer memory presumably must reflect differences in cellular processes. In fact, recent research suggests just such a difference, with older people selectively showing less MRI signal than younger people only in this region of the hippocampal formation (Small, Tsai, De La Paz, Mayeux, & Stern, 2002).

These kinds of differences have been confirmed in studies using Pittsburgh Compound B (PiB), an amyloid ligand, in PET imaging (Klunk et al., 2004). Amyloid deposition correlates with AD severity, presence of *APOE*-e4 alleles, and therapeutic activity. In addition, PiB studies have shown that seniors without AD or with mild cognitive impairment short of frank AD have more amyloids than elders who perform at normal levels on cognitive assessments (Aizenstein et al., 2008).

COGNITIVE DECLINE PRIOR TO FRANK DEMENTIA

Mild cognitive impairment (MCI) is typically defined by the following criteria: subjective complaints of memory problems and memory performance below age- and education-referenced norms, with normal performance in other cognitive domains and absence of impairment in the instrumental and basic activities of daily living (Peterson et al., 1997; Peterson, 2000). Another definition of mild cognitive impairment is "questionable dementia," which involves both mild deficits in cognitive status and mild deficits in functional status. This state is recognized in the 0.5 category of the CDR (Hughes et al., 1982). Still other alternative nosologies include "age-associated memory impairment," which involves poor memory performance relative to people under age 50 (Crook et al., 1986; Feher, Larrabee, Sudilovsky, & Crook, 1994) and "aging-associated cognitive decline," which involves defective performance in any cognitive domain, relative to age-matched elders (Levy, 1994; Richards, Touchon, Ledesert, & Ritchie, 1999). The different definitions all strive to establish an intermediate cognitive status: people with MCI do not meet criteria for dementia but show deficits in memory or other domains of cognition. These deficits are evident to elders and distressing enough to lead them and their families to seek medical attention. They may presage advancing Alzheimer's disease.

Even within the domain of "questionable dementia" it is possible to make distinctions based on prognosis. Morris and colleagues assigned MCI patients ascertained in a clinic setting into three groups: CDR 0.5 but likely demented, CDR 0.5 with likely progressive dementia ("incipient AD"), and CDR 0.5 with uncertain dementia (Morris et al., 2001). All three groups faced a high risk of developing Alzheimer's disease (CDR 1.0 or greater) over a 5-year follow-up period: 60.5% for the likely dementia group, 35.7% for the likely progressive dementia group, and 19.9% for the uncertain dementia group. These rates should be compared with a control group (CDR 0, no cognitive or functional impairment) over the same time period, in which the incidence of Alzheimer's disease was 6.8%. Given these results Morris and colleagues conclude, "individuals currently characterized as having MCI progress steadily to greater stages of dementia severity at rates dependent on the level of cognitive impairment at entry." People in the three groups who died and came to autopsy had neuropathogical evidence of AD, again suggesting that MCI, at least when defined by CDR 0.5 criteria, is a dementia prodrome rather than a benign variant of aging.

The situation is less clear for patients who do not meet CDR 0.5 criteria but whose cognitive performance is lower than expected. Ritchie and colleagues assessed mild cognitive impairment in a population-based, rather than a clinic-based, sample (Ritchie, Artero, & Touchon, 2001). Only 11.1% of patients progressed to dementia. Moreover, these people moved back and forth across the dementia threshold, changing diagnostic category at different assessments. With more restrictive definitions identifying greater cognitive impairment, 28.6% met the dementia end point over 3 years.

In general, studies suggest that dementia incidence in elders who report cognitive complaints and demonstrate mild deficits in cognitive assessment is much higher than that for elders as a whole, 18% over 3 years, compared with perhaps 3%–6% in the population of older adults as a whole (Ritchie et al., 2001). Consequently, mild cognitive impairment cannot be considered benign or a normal feature of healthy aging, and elders with mild cognitive impairment in this sense (i.e., complaints of memory impairment supported by neuropsychological performance >1 SD below age norms) are indeed at risk for developing Alzheimer's over a 3- to 5-year period.

Of course, the annual risk of transition to AD among people with mild cognitive impairment will depend heavily on the definition of MCI, and even limiting definitions to a single type of MCI shows substantial variation. The "isolated amnestic" variant, that is, memory performance below age- and education-adjusted norms without involvement of other cognitive domains, ranges from 3% to 12.5% in community-based samples (Manly et al., 2005). The annual risk of progression to Alzheimer's disease was 5% in a New York City sample (Manly et al., 2008). If we examine this risk among people who already demonstrate some kind of cognitive impairment, but one short of dementia, the annual risk of transition to AD is 10%–12% (Plassman et al., 2008).

Insight on Declining Cognitive Ability

Older adults with MCI describe their difficulties with memory in this way:

> I do feel the difference. I can't retrieve words easily. I lose words. It will take me a few minutes . . . and it takes me a while to retrieve it. Sometimes I can't, and that's disturbing. And to think of walking into a room and forgetting why you walked in is a killer. It's strange. Or getting a list in my head, and not writing it down . . . and then forgetting what I want to do. That kind of thing. I'm sure it happened before, but not as frequently as now. It's happening more.

The woman reporting these memory problems met criteria for MCI. She had a Global Deterioration Score (GDS) of 3, as indicated by a score below age- and education-adjusted norms on the Logical Memory II subscale of the Weschler Memory Scale; she did not meet criteria for dementia, as indicated by a Mini-Mental State Examination (MMSE) score greater than or equal to 24; and she did not report difficulty in daily occupational, self-care, home management, or community activities, as indicated by a Clinical Dementia Rating of 0.5.

Still, she was concerned that her memory problems might presage Alzheimer's disease. Mainly, she was concerned that she might be denying the extent of her problems, which she recognized as a feature of memory impairment and incipient Alzheimer's disease. She was also concerned that she was not pushing herself as hard as she might and that this circumscription of daily activities and interests might be the result of her memory deficit. Was she actually avoiding situations that would reveal her difficulty with memory?

Her assessment and the new label of "MCI" did not help. She reported great frustration with the clinical label: "They said there was some memory loss, that it might not mean anything, and that they would like to re-evaluate me in a couple of years to see if it's progressing. [But] the significance of it is what I'm interested in, and [that] they didn't tell me" (Albert et al., 2002). *online → Insight on Dementia*

Mild Cognitive Impairment and Disability *Summary*

Aside from "questionable dementia," the other definitions of mild cognitive impairment, reviewed earlier, assume no impairments in instrumental (household management) or basic (personal self-maintenance) activities of daily living, but leave open the possibility of deficits in higher level functions, such as the ability to work, travel, participate in community affairs, or manage complex activities (such as driving to a new place, appearing in front of an audience, planning an event, participating in competitive games, or taking part in activities that involve some degree of risk from slow reaction times or poor judgment). As Ritchie et al. (2001) point out, "No guidelines have been given as to what constitutes activities of daily living restriction in MCI." Recent studies show that people with MCI who ultimately progress to Alzheimer's disease do show mild functional deficits (such as occasional need for help or need for cuing and supervision in activity) and reductions in physical activity before AD diagnosis (Friedland et al., 2001; Touchon & Ritchie, 1999).

Estimates of the proportion of seniors with cognitive impairment short of dementia vary, but are surprisingly high. The Aging, Memory, and Demographics Study (ADAMS) surveyed a national probability of Americans in 2002. It used a fairly liberal definition of "cognitive impairment without dementia." People were considered to fall into this category if (a) they did not meet criteria for dementia, and (b) participants or their proxies reported cognitive or functional impairment, *or* participants performed 1.5 *SD* below published norms for neuropsychological tests. By this standard, 22.2% of older people demonstrated cognitive impairment without dementia, of which 8.2% were considered to demonstrate prodromal AD.

Cognitive impairment short of dementia is clinically meaningful. In prior research, Albert and colleagues (1999) found that quite mild cognitive impairment is associated with less frequency and diversity of advanced functions, as indexed by the Pfeffer Functional Activities Questionnaire (Pfeffer, Kurosaki, Chance, & Filos, 1982). The Pfeffer scale records perceived difficulty with writing checks, assembling tax or business records, shopping alone, playing games of skill, making coffee or tea, preparing a balanced meal, keeping track of current events, paying attention and understanding while reading or watching a TV show, remembering to take medications and attend family occasions, and traveling out of the neighborhood. Close informants to people with "minimal cognitive impairment" reported that these elders had more difficulty in these tasks than a group with no cognitive impairment. In this study we considered someone to have mild cognitive impairment if they were not demented (score of 23 or greater on the MMSE), but had performance >1 SD below norms on one or more of a series of neuropsychological tests (recall of 2 of 3 objects at 5 minutes, delayed recall in the six-trial Selective Reminding Test (SRT), or a Wechsler Adult Intelligence Scale [WAIS] performance IQ score of >15 points below the WAIS verbal IQ score).

We have also shown that a discrepancy measure indicating lack of awareness of functional deficits (i.e., greater informant- than self-reported functional deficits) predicted risk of Alzheimer's disease more efficiently than self- or informant reports alone (Tabert et al., 2002). In these models, which controlled for sociodemographic differences and cognitive status, self-reports of functional status at baseline were not associated with the risk for diagnosis of Alzheimer's disease. By contrast, informant reports of deficits at baseline were a significant predictor of dementia over follow-up. A discrepancy of $1+$ deficit in the Pfeffer scale, relative to those with no discrepancy, was associated with a fourfold increase in the risk of a future AD diagnosis. These findings support research by Tierney et al. (1996), who showed that informant- but not self-reported cognitive deficits (i.e., memory for lists, events, and names, finding one's way around home and neighborhood, and financial management) also predicted risk of AD.

Other research suggests that older adults meeting criteria for MCI performed worse than older adults performing within age- and education-based norms on tasks involving fine and complex motor skills (mainly tests of manual dexterity) (Kluger et al., 1997). These findings suggest a gradient of motor and cognitive performance in which people with MCI again fall between people with no cognitive impairment and people who meet criteria for Alzheimer's disease.

Finally, occupational therapist ratings of efficiency and safety in IADL tasks, such as cooking and cleaning, were lower in people with MCI compared with older adults without cognitive impairment. The therapists use the Assessment of Motor and Process Skills, a standardized measure of motor and process skills (Fisher, 2001), to rate older adults as they performed daily tasks. Therapists were blinded to the cognitive status of these seniors (Albert, Bear-Lehman, & Burkhardt, 2006).

The upshot of this research is that MCI affects high-level function, not basic self-care, that people with MCI are not fully aware of the extent of their functional impairment, and that families recognize functional deficits in people with MCI. Furthermore, functional deficit, as reported by families and *not* reported by elders, may be useful for identifying MCI patients with a high likelihood of rapid progression to Alzheimer's disease (Albert et al., 2002).

PREVALENCE AND INCIDENCE OF ALZHEIMER'S DISEASE

Surprisingly little information about the national prevalence and incidence of Alzheimer's disease has been available in the United States. Early estimates of the number of people with AD in this country ranged from 1.09 to 4.58 million (Brookmeyer, Gray, & Kawas, 1998). Such estimates were based on studies in four communities: Rochester, Baltimore, Framingham, and East Boston. Each study measured AD in a different way; for instance, the Rochester study included only cases coming to medical attention, whereas the East Boston study (which had higher rates) included both mild and moderate cases.

U.S. General Accounting Office (GAO) estimates from the 1990s fall in the middle of this range. In a synthesis of 18 prevalence surveys, the GAO estimated that 1.9 million people aged 65 and older were identified as meeting criteria for Alzheimer's disease in 1995. Prevalence rises to 2.1 million if we include possible or mixed cases, that is, cases marked by AD and some other source of dementia. If we restrict cases to moderate or more severe AD, the prevalence is 1.0 million with the narrow definition and 1.4 million if we include possible and mixed cases. All told, in the mid-1990s, 5.7% of Americans aged 65 and older had AD, with 3.3% meeting criteria for moderate or more severe AD (GAO, 1998).

In 2002 estimates became available from one of the first studies designed explicitly to produce national estimates of AD and other dementias. ADAMS, an add-on to the Health and Retirement Study, examined a nationally representative sample of people age 71 and older with cognitive assessments (Plassman et al., 2007). Of Americans over age 71, 13.9% met criteria for dementia, and 9.7% met criteria for AD. The absolute number of older adults with dementia was 3.4 million (with a 95% confidence interval [CI] of 2.8–4.0 million). The absolute number with AD was estimated to be 2.4 million (95% CI 1.8–2.9 million). Including people aged 60–70 yields a prevalence of 4.7 million Americans with dementia and 3.3 million with AD (Plassman et al., 2008). These prevalence estimates are considerably higher than the median reported for a recent synthesis of published studies, which suggested an AD prevalence of 2.5 million (Hirtz et al., 2007).

Table 6.3 reports the GAO prevalence by age and gender for the U.S population aged 65 and older in 1995. The table shows that prevalence doubles every 5 years, both for men and women, reaching approximately 40% for people aged 95 and older. The proportion with moderate or more severe AD in the oldest age group reaches approximately 25%. The prevalence of AD is higher in women than in men in every age group, with the gap widening at successively older ages. This gender disparity most likely reflects greater risk of AD for women, but this finding is controversial. Some prospective cohort studies have found a greater risk of AD for women (Launer et al., 1999); others have not (Tang et al., 2001). Results from ADAMS do not suggest differences by gender or race in the prevalence of AD. In addition, in ADAMS the prevalence of AD in people over age 80 was 18.1% and in people over 90, it was 29.7%.

If prevalence doubles every 5 years, then delaying the disease by 5 years would reduce prevalence by half. This is an important public health goal. With this delay, dementia-free life expectancy would increase, a greater number of older adults would live their last years without the need for costly supportive care, and older people at these late ages would die of other causes. Such a delay would obviously have a major impact on disability in late life and caregiving demands. In simulation studies using available data on population growth, Brookmeyer, Gray, and Kawas (1998) suggests that a delay of even 1 year in the incidence of the disease would result in nearly 800,000 fewer prevalent

Table 6.3

PREVALENCE OF ALZHEIMER'S DISEASE, UNITED STATES, 1995

| | ALZHEIMER'S DISEASE | | | |
| AGE | ALL | | MODERATE+ | |
	MEN	WOMEN	MEN	WOMEN
65–69	0.6	0.8	0.3	0.6
70–74	1.3	1.7	0.6	1.1
75–79	2.7	3.5	1.1	2.3
80–84	5.6	7.1	2.3	4.4
85–89	11.1	13.8	4.4	8.6
90–94	20.8	25.2	8.5	15.8
95+	35.6	41.5	15.8	27.4

Table entries are percentages meeting criteria for Alzheimer's disease, CDR 2+.
From "Alzheimer's Disease: Estimates of Prevalence in the U.S.," by GAO, 1998.
Retrieved from http://www.gao.gov/archive/1998/he98016.pdf.

cases over the next 50 years. A delay of 2 years would cut prevalence by 2 million cases.

A number of prospective cohort studies have examined the incidence of Alzheimer's disease. These studies are superior to retrospective studies that ask family proxies to date disease onset (i.e., "when did _____ first report memory problems or first go to the doctor because of difficulty with memory?" [Wolfson et al., 2001]). Retrospective studies do not allow formal diagnosis and are always subject to recall bias. Prospective studies begin with a dementia-free cohort and monitor the cohort over multiple assessments to track onset of disease.

However, prospective cohort studies of AD are complicated not just by differences in the definition of the disease, but also by different approaches to establishing the date of onset. Even with a regular schedule of follow-up assessments, it is not possible to establish the date when a person first met criteria for the disease. Further, most studies do not have long follow-up or closely spaced assessment intervals. The result has been imprecision in the true date of diagnosis, which affects calculation of person-years of dementia-free follow-up. In the face of this problem, the European Community Concerted Action on the Epidemiology and Prevention of Dementia Group (EURODEM) carried out a pooled analysis of AD incidence, which used a statistical adjustment: "To account for the fact that reliable data regarding when the dementia started is difficult to obtain, we used an iterative procedure that provides a best estimate for time of onset based on the patient's age and age-specific dementia rates" (Launer et al., 1999). A simpler approach, if multiple follow-up assessments are available, is to call the incidence date the date of the assessment when the respondent first met criteria for the diagnosis (Tang et al., 2001).

The incidence of AD is closely related to age. For people aged 65–74, the annual incidence ranges from <0.5% to 1.3%. For people aged 75–84, the range is 1.5%–4.0%, and for people aged 85 and older the range is 4.7%–7.9% per year (Launer et al., 1999; Tang et al., 2001). Thus, for someone aged 85 and older, the risk of meeting criteria for AD for the first time is approximately 5%–10% per year, a very high rate.

Even within age strata, the incidence of AD varies considerably among groups defined by race and ethnicity. In New York City, for example, incidence was considerably lower among Whites than among African Americans and Hispanics. African Americans and Hispanics were 2–3 times as likely to develop AD; thus, for example, the risk among Whites aged 75–84 was 2.6% per year and among African Americans and Hispanics it was 4.4% (Tang et al., 2001). This difference persisted even with adjustment for socioeconomic (education, literacy status, gender) and disease (hypertension, diabetes) factors. It also persisted when analyses were limited to people with the *APOE*-e3 allele (Tang et al., 1998) to control for the effects of this genetic risk factor (see below). Thus, minority status is among the most important risk factors for AD. Given the increasing number of older adults in the United States who belong to minority racial and ethnic goups, this disparity has great public health significance.

These rates for AD incidence apply to the entire population at risk in any given year. If we restrict risk estimates to the group of older people who report memory complaints or demonstrate mild cognitive impairment, annual AD incidence is, of course, much higher. The risk of AD in these older adults is between 10% and 25% per year, depending on ascertainment site (community versus clinic) and the stringency of the definition of mild impairment (Peterson et al., 2001).

How many older adults in the United States will have AD in the future? As the number of adults reaching old age increases, so will the number of Americans living with AD. Projections by Hebert suggest the number may reach 7 million in 2030. This estimate is based on incidence rates reported in several neighborhoods in Chicago. Projections based on Brookmeyer's study, which relies on rates from four community-based studies, put the figure closer to 5 million in 2030. To our knowledge, projections have not been undertaken that take into account both shifts in age and education level using national estimates of either prevalence or incidence.

RISK FACTORS FOR ALZHEIMER'S DISEASE

Genetic Risk Factors

The role of genetic factors in the development of AD is an active research area but at this point is still underdeveloped. Only approximately 7% of early-onset AD (younger than age 65) and less than 1% of late-onset AD has been linked to mutations on particular genes (Whalley & Deary, 2001; Whalley et al., 2000). Early-onset Alzheimer's disease has been linked to mutations on a number of genes (located on chromosomes 1, 14, and 21). Risk of late-onset AD is associated with the e4 allele of the *APOE* gene on chromosome 19. The mechanism for the APOE-AD relationship is not completely understood.

Although mutations for early-onset AD have been identified, their relevance for late-onset AD, which represents the vast majority of cases, is unclear. For public health purposes, attention is centered on *APOE*, the apolipoprotein E gene, which produces a plasma protein involved in the transport of cholesterol and other hydrophobic molecules (Farrer et al., 1995). Whereas some forms of apolipoprotein E have been linked to disorders of cholesterol metabolism and coronary heart disease (Saunders et al., 1993), this protein product has also been shown to raise the risk of AD. A number of studies have shown overrepresentation of the *APOE*-e4 allele in people with AD. Of individuals with AD 34%–65% carry the *APOE*-e4 allele, compared with only 24%–31% of people without AD of the same age (Jarvik et al., 1995; Myers et al., 1996; Roses et al., 1994). The number of *APOE*-e4 alleles is associated with earlier age of onset (Corder et al., 1993). The *APOE*-e2 allele, by contrast, may be protective against AD, but this finding has been challenged (Corder et al., 1994; Talbot et al., 1994; van Duijn et al., 1995).

Despite the association between *APOE* and AD, *APOE* testing is currently not recommended as a screening tool. A number of reasons have been advanced. First, the presence of an e4 allele is not necessary for the development of AD (35%–50% of persons with AD do not carry

an e4 allele) (Roses et al., 1994). Second, the AD diagnosis is not difficult to make, and the extra predictive power provided by genetic testing
would not add a great deal to clinical tools. Third, no treatment beyond
tertiary symptomatic therapies is available in any case, so that awareness
of AD risk before disease onset would not have practical benefit. And,
finally, discrimination or other untoward effects are possible with such
information, reducing the possible gain further.

A task force investigating the issue concluded:

> Because most patients presenting to physicians with dementia have AD,
> the additional information gained by genotyping would be useful only if it
> reduced the necessity for other more expensive or invasive tests. Individu-
> als homozygous for epsilon-4 are the most likely candidates for disease, but
> they comprise only 2% to 3% of the general population; [and] even among
> AD patients, only 15% to 20% have this genotype. Most symptomatic epsi-
> lon-4 homozygotes will in fact have AD, but any uncertainty will oblige the
> physician to exclude other forms of dementia.

They go on to conclude: "Thus, although *APOE* genotype may be a
risk factor for AD, it cannot yet be considered a useful predictive genetic
test" (Farrer et al., 1995). The 2008 U.S. Task Force on Preventive Services concurred with this recommendation.

Socioeconomic Factors And Cognitive Reserve

Earlier we discussed lifelong cognitive resources as a predictor of Alzheimer's risk. The significance of cognitive resources early in the life
span for this late-life outcome has become increasingly clear in studies that have linked risk of AD in late life to childhood IQ (Whalley &
Deary, 2001; Whalley et al., 2000), educational accomplishments and
leisure activities (Helzner, Scarmeas, Cosentino, Portet, & Stern, 2007;
Scarmeas, Albert, Manly, & Stern, 2006; Wilson et al., 2004, 2009), occupational attainment and job demands (Stern et al., 1994), language skills
in early adulthood (Snowdon et al., 1996), diversity of physical and cognitive engagement over the life span (Friedland et al., 2001), parental
socioeconomic status, and literacy (Albert & Teresi, 1999; Manly, Jacobs,
Touradji, Small, & Stern, 2002).

The case of childhood cognitive ability and AD risk is revealing. In a
Scottish case-control study involving a match-back to childhood IQ tests,
Whalley and Deary (2001) found that people who developed AD after

age 65 had lower scores on this early measure of cognitive ability compared with people who did not develop AD. Differences in Alzheimer's risk, then, were already apparent at age 11. It is noteworthy that people who developed *early-onset* AD did not differ from other elders on the childhood IQ measure, suggesting an important difference in mechanism between early and late-onset AD.

What do these findings mean? One interpretation is that cognitive ability is similar to grip strength: differences (in muscle fiber density, in neuronal integrity or number) already apparent at birth or in the perinatal period (and which develop or set limits on development over the life span) provide variable reserves against depletions that occur with aging. These resources put one closer or further away from the threshold of disability associated with the loss of physical and cognitive function that occurs over the life span. In this view, development of AD is not so much a disease as one kind of aging, and some kind of early strengthening of cognition to build up reserve would be an appropriate intervention. The association between a cognitive resource and AD risk, then, is not evidence of an independent risk factor (as it is usually portrayed); instead, it is the identification of an early phase of the process that will ultimately result in AD.

Medical Morbidity: Hypertension and Vascular Disease, Diabetes, Bone Mineral Density Loss, Estrogen Deficiency, Depression

An increasing number of medical conditions have been shown to increase the risk of Alzheimer's disease. For the most part, these are considered secondary risks, in that they do not represent the primary mechanism for development of AD, but recent research suggests that the insulin pathway may have direct effects on the hippocampus. In any case, treatment of these secondary conditions may offer avenues for reducing Alzheimer's risk and may indicate points in the pathway of Alzheimer's neurodegeneration that may be amenable to intervention. The findings for these morbid conditions in some cases remain controversial.

Hypertension, Stroke, Diabetes, Cholesterol

Hypertension has been associated with cognitive performance, so it stands to reason that this condition might be associated with later risk of AD. However, one large prospective study failed to confirm this association (Posner et al., 2002). In this cohort, 731 of 1,259 subjects (58.1%), all free of AD at baseline, had a history of hypertension associated with diabetes, stroke, or heart disease. A history of hypertension was not associated with an increased risk for AD, but it did raise the risk for vascular dementia. The increased risk of vascular disease was evident only in respondents who had multiple morbidities. Respondents with hypertension and heart disease had a threefold increase in risk for vascular dementia, whereas respondents with hypertension and diabetes faced a sixfold increase.

These results stand in contrast to results from the double-blind, placebo-controlled Systolic Hypertension in Europe (Syst-Eur) Trial, in which randomly selected patients with hypertension were offered active study medication after the end of the trial for a further period of observation (Forette et al., 2002). In this add-on component, long-term antihypertensive therapy reduced the risk of dementia by 55%, from 7.4 to 3.3 cases per 1,000 patient-years, a finding that remained after adjustment for sex, age, education, and entry blood pressure. In a "number needed to treat analysis," the trial showed that treatment of 1,000 patients with hypertension for 5 years would prevent 20 cases of dementia.

Whether through an AD or vascular dementia process, diabetes is now increasingly recognized as a risk factor for cognitive decline. In the Study of Osteoporotic Fractures, women with diabetes (n = 682) had lower baseline scores than women without diabetes on a variety of cognitive measures (Digit Symbol, Trials B, MMSE). These women also faced greater likelihood of cognitive decline in models that adjusted for age, education, depression, stroke, visual impairment, heart disease, hypertension, physical activity, estrogen use, and smoking (Gregg et al., 2000). But, again, other research has shown only a modest association between diabetes and risk of AD (Luchsinger, Tang, Stern, Shea, & Mayeux, 2001).

Vascular risk factors may offer insight on mechanisms of AD. Wu and colleagues (2008) were able to show that diabetes and brain infarcts are each associated with hippocampal dysfunction, a key site for Alzheimer's pathology, but affect separate subregions and therefore may indicate distinct underlying mechanisms (Wu et al., 2008). "The hippocampal subregion linked to diabetes implicated blood glucose as a pathogenic mechanism, [while] the hippocampal subregion linked to infarcts suggested transient hypoperfusion as a pathogenic mechanism." This analysis suggests that elevations in blood glucose and hypoperfusion due to infarcts are separate sources of hippocampal degeneration. The implication is that Alzheimer's dementia may have different sources. We await studies that definitively establish the value of aggressive control of hypertension (a risk factor for strokes and brain infarcts) and glycemia for prevention of Alzheimer's.

Cholesterol may also be a risk factor for cognitive decline. Among people with Alzheimer's disease, higher prediagnosis low-density lipoprotein cholesterol and a history of diabetes was associated with faster cognitive decline (Helzner et al., 2009). This again points to the role of vascular factors in the course of AD and also as risk factors for the disease. This line of investigation is confirmed in other research showing associations between obesity earlier in life and risk of AD (Fitzpatrick et al., 2009) and the protective effects of the Mediterranean diet (Scarmeas et al., 2006).

Bone Mineral Density Loss and Estrogen Deficiency

Animal models and preclinical studies suggest that estrogen use may promote the growth and survival of cholinergic neurons and may also decrease cerebral amyloid deposition. Given the reduction in estrogen production that follows menopause, estrogen supplementation in women is a plausible strategy for delaying the onset of Alzheimer's disease. Hope for this approach was strengthened by prospective studies that showed a lower incidence of AD in postmenopausal women taking estrogen compared with women who did not. In a group of 1,124 older women who initially did not have Alzheimer's disease, Parkinson's disease, and stroke, the age at onset of Alzheimer's disease was significantly later in women who had taken estrogen. Alzheimer's disease was diagnosed in 5.8% of the estrogen users compared with 16.3% of nonusers, even after adjustment for such differences as education, ethnic origin, and *APOE* genotype (Tang et al., 1996).

Even a well-planned prospective study with statistical adjustment cannot rule out selection factors that are confounded with estrogen use (such as better education, income, and more proactive health behaviors). For this effort, randomized controlled trials are required. Confidence in estrogen replacement as a *treatment* strategy has been shaken by a series of negative clinical trials. A Cochrane Review (2002, and updated in 2009) assessed high-quality trials of estrogen use (selected from a review of all double-blind, randomized controlled trials on the effect of estrogen, alone or in combination with progestrin, for cognitive function in postmenopausal women with AD or other types of dementia). Meta-analyses showed no significant benefit and actually suggested that such treatment may be associated with worse outcomes in a number of cognitive domains.

The negative result for these treatment trials does not rule out a protective effect for estrogen as a *preventive* agent if given earlier to women who have not yet developed AD. A number of long-term prevention trials have been conducted or are underway to examine this potential benefit. However, expectations of success have been dampened by findings from the Heart and Estrogen/Progestin Replacement Study (HERS), a randomized, placebo-controlled trial involving 2,763 women with coronary disease. Participants at 10 of the 20 HERS centers (n = 517 estrogen, n = 546 placebo) completed a cognitive function substudy. At approximately 4 years of follow-up, the groups did not significantly differ on a variety of cognitive tests (modified MMSE, Verbal Fluency, Boston Naming, Word List Memory, Word List Recall, and Trials B) (Grady et al., 2002). This trial had only a single cognitive assessment at the end of the trial and did not examine incident Alzheimer's disease, so the question of the efficacy of estrogen replacement as a prevention strategy remains open. Still, these negative results are not reassuring. Combined with reports from the Women's Health Initiative of an increased risk of some cancers and stroke in women using estrogen replacement therapy (leading to early termination of the unopposed estrogen arm of the trial; Shumaker et al., 2003), estrogen replacement so far has not turned out to be useful as an anti-dementia agent. Meta-analyses suggest that "benefits of HRT include prevention of osteoporotic fractures and colorectal cancer, while prevention of dementia is uncertain. Harms include CHD, stroke, thromboembolic events, breast cancer with 5 or more years of use, and cholecystitis" (Nelson, Humphrey, Nygren, Teutsch, & Allan, 2002a). The Women's Health Initiative Memory Study and Women's Health Initiative Study of Cognitive Aging did not show clear benefit for hormone therapy (Asthana et al., 2009). The value of estrogen supplementation early in life remains an open question (Henderson, 2009).

Other evidence suggests that estrogen may turn out to be critical for cognitive health and risk of AD after all. For example, bone mineral density (BMD) is a marker of cumulative estrogen exposure and has been associated with cognitive function in older women without dementia (Yaffe, Browner, Cauley, Launer, & Harris, 1999b). In the Study of Osteoporotic Fractures (n = 8,333 older community-dwelling women not taking estrogen), women with low-baseline BMD had up to 8% worse baseline cognitive scores and up to 6% worse repeat cognitive scores.

For women who declined 1 *SD* in hip or calcaneal BMD, the risk of cognitive deterioration (defined as the most extreme 10% of those who declined) increased by about a third, compared with women with stable BMD. The same was true for women who had vertebral fractures. These women had lower cognitive test scores at baseline and greater odds of cognitive deterioration similar to those who declined 1 *SD* in BMD.

Thus, the relationship between estrogen and risk of AD remains unclear, but the preponderance of evidence suggests that it is not an appropriate therapy in old age. The effect of earlier use at or around menopause is still under investigation.

Depression

Depressed mood may be an early sign of AD or a risk factor in its own right. Prospective studies cannot settle the issue but do suggest that older people without dementia who have a depressed mood face an increased risk of AD. In one cohort study (*n* = 478 without dementia at baseline, mean of 2.5 years follow-up), depressed mood at baseline increased the risk of incident dementia nearly threefold. The effect persisted after adjustment for age, gender, education, language of assessment, and functional status (Devanand et al., 1996). The role of depression in subsequent cognitive decline has been confirmed (Yaffe et al., 1999a). However, a definitive treatment trial, in which depression would be treated to see if treatment response improves cognition or delays AD, remains to be completed.

Depression may also increase the risk of poor cognitive performance short of frank dementia. In one longitudinal cohort, depressive symptoms at baseline predicted declines in a number of memory domains (Panza et al., 2009).

OUTCOMES ASSOCIATED WITH ALZHEIMER'S DISEASE

Mortality

Table 6.4 presents U.S. mortality from AD by age and race strata in 1998. Approximately 50,000 deaths per year are attributed to AD, making AD the eighth most common cause of death in the United States. Mortality from AD is exceedingly rare in people under age 65: less than 1:100,000 per year. But AD very quickly becomes a prominent cause of

Table 6.4

MORTALITY AND ALZHEIMER'S DISEASE, UNITED STATES, 1998

AGE	TOTAL	WHITE		AFRICAN AMERICAN	
		MEN	WOMEN	MEN	WOMEN
45–54	0.1				
55–64	1.1	1.2	1.2		
65–74	10.4	10.6	11.1	7.4	8.1
75–84	70.0	69.3	74.8	50.2	59.2
85+	299.5	257.9	336.2	142.5	202.5

Table entries are deaths per 100,000.
From http://www.cdc.gov/nchs/datawh/statab/unpubd/mortabs/gmwk51.htm.

death at later ages. It is noted on death certificates in 10 (ages 65–74), 70 (aged 75–84), and 300 (aged 85 and older) of every 100,000 deaths. This is almost certainly an underestimate, because AD may be a contributory cause and not appear on the death certificate, especially if the certificate is prepared by a funeral home director, coroner, or doctor unfamiliar with the patient. The lower attribution of mortality to AD among African Americans may represent greater likelihood of death certificates completed in this way.

Alzheimer's disease increases the risk of mortality. Compared with older adults without dementia matched for age, drawn from the same community, and similar in socioeconomic features, these elders face a mortality risk 2–3 times higher. Figure 6.2 presents Kaplan-Meier plots of time to death in three groups first assessed in 1989–1992 and monitored for up to 10 years. These elders were recruited from a Medicare enrollee sample and AD registry, both in the Washington-Heights Inwood community, northern Manhattan, New York City.

In 1989–1992, people met criteria for AD when they were first seen (*prevalent AD*), or developed AD sometime in this period (no dementia at baseline visit, dementia at later visit over the follow-up period: *incident AD*), or never met criteria for AD over the entire follow-up period (*without dementia*). A convenient measure of mortality risk is

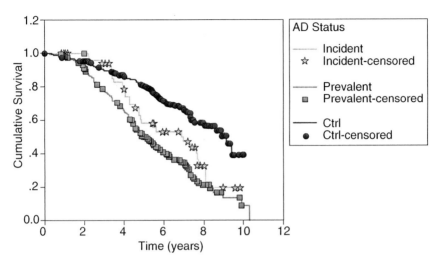

Figure 6.2 Survival in AD: prevalent, incident, and elders without dementia, New York City, 1989–1999.

to note the point in follow-up time when 50% of people in each of the three groups have died. As the figure shows, this point was reached in 5.2 years in the prevalent AD group, 7.0 years in the incident AD group, and 9.2 years in the without dementia group. Although an impressive difference, this approach does not adjust for differences in age or other factors, an important limitation, since age is related to AD risk, as we have already seen. To control for this confounding, proportional hazards models can be used to separate the effects of age and AD, as well as the influence of other factors. In such a model, we found that prevalent AD was associated with a twofold increase in mortality risk and incident AD was associated with a 1.7-fold increase, both highly significant effects.

It is not surprising that survival with AD depends heavily on the age at diagnosis. Results from the Baltimore Longitudinal Study of Aging show that median survival after diagnosis ranged from 8.3 years in people aged 65 to 3.4 years for people aged 90. Comparing this survival with elders without dementia showed that AD reduces life span by approximately two-thirds for people in whom AD is diagnosed at age 65 and by approximately 39% for people in whom AD is diagnosed at age 90 (Brookmeyer, Corrada, Curriero, & Kawas, 2002). These differences reflect the effect of competing risks of mortality, which increase at later ages.

Survival after a diagnosis of AD may in fact be shorter than these early estimates. A number of studies now suggest that AD is associated with a median survival of 4–5 years; (Helzner et al., 2008; Larson et al., 2004; Wolfson et al., 2001).

Nursing Home Care

Alzheimer's disease is a major risk factor for nursing home placement. In the Washington Heights-Inwood, New York City sample, described above, we tracked nursing home admission in up to 10 years of follow-up. This sample has the advantage of long follow-up and careful diagnostic assessment for AD, but it is probably atypical for estimating the absolute rate of nursing home use, because New York City offers an extensive alternative Medicaid-funded home care benefit. In addition, this study enrolled a largely minority sample, and research has shown that minorities are less likely to use skilled nursing home care than Whites.

In the Washington Heights cohort, 8.8% of prevalent cases entered nursing homes, compared with 3.5% of people who never met criteria for AD. Incident cases were intermediate, with 5% entering nursing homes. With this background of relatively low rates of nursing home placement, it is still impressive to see that incident AD was associated with a large increase in the risk of nursing home admission. Using a time-dependent approach, in which the date of AD diagnosis is used as a predictor of time to nursing home placement, we found that incident AD was associated with an eightfold increase in risk in models that controlled for age, race-ethnicity, and education.

In other settings, nursing home placement is more frequent. Among participants in a clinical trial of selegiline and tocopherol, all with moderate dementia and living in the community, two-thirds of the 341 patients followed up entered nursing homes over 2 years (Knopman et al., 1999). Dementia progression was the strongest predictor of placement, such that people progressing to severe dementia (CDR 3) were eight times as likely to enter nursing homes as people who had moderate dementia. Despite sociomedical determinants of nursing home placement (such as features of caregivers, e.g., caregiver burden, perceived skill or efficacy, presence of family support, and system-level features, such as availability of beds or alternative home-based services), nursing home placement remains an important outcome for assessing disease progression and treatment. To take these sociomedical factors into account, Stern and colleagues have developed a measure of "dependency" and "equivalent institutional care" that tracks need for services provided in institutional settings (Stern et al., 1994).

Nursing home placement is driven by exhaustion or depletion of caregiver resources, as well as by the progression of disease (Gaugler, Yu, Krichbaum, & Wyman, 2009). New research in this area has focused on assessment of risk domains that predict caregiver inability to manage Alzheimer's care at home. One promising approach involves screening of "caregiver risk" to identify domains amenable to support or intervention. The Resources for Enhancing Alzheimer's Caregiver Health (REACH II) Study has developed such a risk appraisal measure, which involves assessment of caregiver depression, burden, self-care and health behaviors, social support, safety, and patient problem behaviors (Czaja et al., 2009). We examine caregiver interventions in more detail below.

Hospitalization and Primary Care

Do people with Alzheimer's disease face an increased risk of hospitalization? This simple question is actually quite hard to answer. People with AD may enter the hospital for other reasons, and AD may not be recorded on the discharge diagnosis. Moreover, risk of hospitalization may be elevated in early stages of disease, when patients are likely to fall, fail to take medications, or have a psychiatric admission, and decline with more severe stages of dementia. Patients with the most severe dementia may reside in nursing homes, which provide medical care for many conditions, or may simply not be brought in for hospital care as part of a general strategy of less aggressive treatment. In addition, whereas the use of Medicare billing records, which include ICD-10 diagnoses of AD, can be used to establish hospital episodes and volume of costs, these sorts of analysis are prone to an observation bias, in which the most severe cases are overrepresented (Newcomer et al., 1999). Because AD is a terminal disease, it is hard to distinguish end-of-life care from AD care. Finally, the proper test would be a comparison between people with similar medical conditions and health status except for AD, but this comparison is difficult because AD may itself be associated with medical conditions, such as falls or injuries, wasting and dehydration, or pneumonia and infectious disease.

With these caveats, it is not surprising to see considerable variation in yearly rates of hospitalization in people with AD. The Consortium to Establish a Registry for Alzheimer's Disease (CERAD) reported a rate of 370 hospitalizations per 1,000 AD patients per year in a clinical cohort (Fillenbaum, Heyman, Peterson, Pieper, & Weiman, 2000). In a community cohort in New York City, the rate was 100 per 1,000 AD cases per year (Albert et al., 1999). In any case, what seems clear is the elevation of this risk relative to matched elders without AD. In the New York sample, 10% of AD cases had a hospitalization in a year, compared with 6.8% among elders without dementia. In logistic regression models that control for differences in age, gender, education, number of comorbid conditions, and death in the follow-up period, severe AD (CDR 3+) was associated with an elevated risk of 2.3. This study had the advantage of a large population-based cohort in which hospitalizations were tracked with an innovative electronic medical record. This risk was comparable with the added risk associated with the presence of two comorbid conditions.

The association between dementia and hospitalization has been confirmed in population-based studies. A large record-linked Australian study found that older people with dementia spent an average of 30 days in the hospital in the last year of life (Zilkens, Spilsbury, Bruce, & Semmens, in press). Among older people, in general, the length of stay in U.S. hospitals in the last year of life is 10–17 days (Fonkych, O'Leary, Melnick, & Keeler, 2008). However, variations across different health care systems make these comparisons difficult (Van den Block et al., 2007).

Primary care use and associated costs also seem to be elevated in AD. In the New York City cohort, people with recent diagnoses of AD were more likely to have more medical care encounters than people without AD, even 1–2 years before diagnosis (Albert, Glied, Andrews, Stern, & Mayeux, 2002b). Other studies have not found excess primary care costs in the prodromal period (Liebson et al., 1999).

Disability and Psychiatric Morbidity

The hallmark of progressive dementia is increasing dependency in ADLs and an increase in both "negative" (apathy, withdrawal) and "positive" (agitation, aggression, delusions, hallucinations, wandering) psychopathological symptoms. In the most severe stages of dementia, the prevalence of some symptoms declines (such as delusions), presumably because caregivers can no longer recognize these symptoms as patients become increasingly vegetative.

Cognitive performance in patients and ADL ratings from proxies (or from clinicians) are highly correlated in people with AD. For example, in one series of people with AD, correlations between the Blessed Memory-Concentration-Information Test, a mental status measure similar to the MMSE, and IADL and ADL (personal self-maintenance scale, PSMS) ratings were 0.83 and 0.78, respectively (Green, Mohs, Schmeidler, Aryan, & Davis, 1993). In this sample of 104 clinic patients with probable AD, PSMS scores were collected every 6 months and tracked for change. The PSMS items include toileting, feeding, dressing, grooming, indoor mobility, and bathing. These were scored on a scale of 1 (no difficulty) to 5 (maximum difficulty), so that total scores ranged from 6 to 30. In this sample, PSMS scores declined, on average, 2.44 points over 12 months, with a standard deviation of 3.87.

These numbers are important for gauging the clinical significance of changes in functional scales used in clinical trials in AD. A recent meta-analysis of the effect of cholinesterase inhibitors, the primary approved therapy for treatment of AD, showed a significant but small effect size of 0.1 *SD* favoring treatment. Using the standard deviation of 3.87, cited above, 0.1 *SD* is equivalent to 0.387, or about a 0.4-point change on the PSMS scale. Because the mean PSMS change over 12 months was 2.44, the 0.4 change is roughly equivalent to the decline patients can expect over a 2-month period (Trinh, Hoblyn, Mohanty, & Yaffe, 2003). Delaying decline by 2 months per year is a small but important benefit to patients and family caregivers.

A large trial of donepezil (Aricept) to assess preservation of ADL function in AD confirmed this benefit in an alternative way (Mohs et al., 2001). The trial sought to assess whether this cholinesterase inhibitor delayed "clinically evident decline in function," which was defined as progression to moderate or more severe levels of difficulty with particular ADL, or loss of 20% of instrumental ADL function, or onset of more advanced dementia, as assessed by the CDR. Fifty-six percent of patients receiving the placebo met the end point, compared with 41% of patients receiving donepezil. The median time at which patients met this end point was 208 days among patients receiving placebo and 357 days in patients receiving donepezil. The therapy, then, slowed progression by approximately 5 months in a 1-year period.

Cholinesterase inhibitors also showed benefit for the reduction in frequency of AD psychopathology. A meta-analysis showed that this class of therapies reduced Neuropsychiatric Inventory scores (NPI scores; Cummings, 1997), on average, by nearly 2 points, an improvement in the frequency or severity of one psychiatric symptom (Trinh et al., 2003). Because the presence of psychiatric symptoms is an important predictor of nursing home placement, not to mention caregiver distress and burn-out, these therapies offer an important benefit, at least in the short run.

Thus, at this point, AD cannot be prevented and disease progression remains relentless. Available therapies offer benefit mostly as a holding action, delaying time to severe disability and nursing home placement. Schneider and colleagues have shown that when adverse events from antipsychotic medications are factored into assessments of benefit, differences between treatments and placebo are minimal and may actually favor placebo (Schneider et al., 2006).

Family Caregiving

Families provide the vast majority of Alzheimer's care. Although patients with Alzheimer's are common in nursing homes, accounting for perhaps half of the residents, these residents represent a minority of the population with Alzheimer's disease. As we discuss in Chapter 9, nursing home use has declined among older adults over the past decade in the United States as alternative residential care settings have expanded. Nursing home residence in people aged 65 and older declined from 54 per 1,000 in 1985 to 46.4 per 1,000 in 1995, and to 34.8 per 1,000 in 2004 (Federal Interagency Forum on Aging-Related Statistics, 2008). Most people with AD are cared for at home, use a variety of in-home (home attendant, allied health) and out-of-home services (adult day care, acute rehabilitation), and will enter nursing homes very late in the course of the disease, if at all.

In fact, people residing in nursing homes now are likely to be older and frailer than prior nursing home cohorts. They are also less likely to spend long periods of time in these institutions. The nursing home is becoming more of a short-stay rehabilitative or palliative care unit, funded by Medicare, than a long-term care residence (traditionally funded by Medicaid). The commonly cited estimate of a lifetime prevalence of 40% for nursing home residence (Kemper & Murtaugh, 1991), then, must be interpreted in this light.

How many people with Alzheimer's disease are cared for in the community? If we consider older people with three or more ADL limitations, we have an imperfect but reasonable indicator of dementia in the community. About half of these people relied exclusively on family and friends for assistance in 1994, a decline from two-thirds in the 1980s (Feder, Komisar, & Niefeld, 2001). This change reflects an expansion in financing for long-term care that occurred in the 1990s. Medicare spending for home health care grew from approximately $4 to $18 billion in the first half of the 1990s. Home care for Alzheimer's disease has benefited from this change. More recently, however, cost controls have been introduced into this health sector (Balanced Budget Act of 1997) that have reduced growth in Medicare-funded home care.

Estimates of the absolute number of family caregivers providing supportive care for older people, and also older people with Alzheimer's disease, are available in the 1996 panel of the Survey of Income and Program Participation (SIPP). In 1998, 6.7 million family members were providing help to some 4.5 million older adults with disabilities (Alecxih, Zeruld, & Olearczyk, 2000). This estimate is slightly lower than the estimate of 7.1 million derived from the National Long-Term Care Survey. The SIPP allows estimates of particular features of Alzheimer's caregiving. In 1998, approximately 473,000 family members or friends were serving as primary caregivers to people with diagnoses of Alzheimer's disease. These people were providing most of the nonpaid support received by people with dementia living in the community and were nominated as the person most involved in such care. They spent an average of 48 hours per week providing care and had been providing such care for a mean of 7 years. This compares with a mean of 24 hours per week and a mean duration of 5 years for all nonpaid caregivers in the community (Alecxih et al., 2000). Thus, Alzheimer's care is more demanding than standard care by this measure of caregiving intensity.

One investigation by Albert and colleagues (1998) tracked hours of care provided to people with Alzheimer's disease according to severity of dementia and also over a period of nearly 2 years. Family caregivers reported that more than half of the time they spent with these elders involved direct hands-on care, defined as help with ADL. Caregivers reported a mean of 7.2 hours per day of ADL care, or 50.4 hours per week. This report is quite close to the SIPP results. These informal, or nonpaid hours must be interpreted in light of the total hours of supportive care provided for these elders, which in this New York City sample were extensive. Total weekly hours were 56.7 for people with mild dementia, 81.2 for people with moderate dementia, and 112.0 for people with severe or greater dementia. Family contributions were 30.8 for people with mild dementia, 57.5 for people with moderate dementia, and 29.4 for people with severe dementia, suggesting substitution of formal for informal care in the most severe levels of dementia.

However, these cross-sectional findings can be deceiving. In longitudinal analyses, Albert and colleagues (1998) found that caregivers did not, in fact, reduce the number of hours they provided as elders progressed to more advanced dementia. Rather, formal hours increased, suggesting that these caregivers were already providing the maximum of hours they could provide.

What are the tasks of families who provide care for elders with dementia? Family caregivers certainly provide help with ADL, but providing ADL support at home to a family member is not well described by ADL measures. Although the ADL/IADL measures tell us that someone has a particular care need, satisfying that need takes place in a complex environment. Take bathing, for example. The ADL measure tells us that someone is dependent in bathing. It does not tell us the reason why the person cannot bathe independently, which may involve impairments in mobility and balance, or limb weakness, or cognitive incapacity, or psychiatric disorder, or some combination of these deficits. As a result, the ADL measure does not tell us if the person is cooperative during bathing, whether he or she helps wash parts of his/her body once in the tub, or whether he/she needs supervision throughout the entire course of bathing or only when getting in and out of the tub. Yet, these are the features that make caregiving for someone with bathing disability more or less difficult for families (Albert, 2004).

Thus, although a count of ADL/IADL needs will certainly be correlated with indicators of caregiving challenge (how many hours daily, reported burden and fatigue, risk of nursing home placement), these correlations will be low. Indeed, ADL status explains only a modest amount of the variance in caregiver reports of burden (Poulshock & Diemling, 1984).

The ADL/IADL measures also fail to capture the full context in which families provide care. What kinds of home modifications have family members made to facilitate caregiving? To return to our bathing example, providing bathing care will be easier if families have installed grab bars, or have a home with a walk-in shower or a flexible shower head. Similarly, what kinds of care arrangements have families put in place to ensure such care if they work, or wish to travel, or are themselves weak or ill? These too will determine how challenging ADL/IADL care may be. These sorts of care management tasks are a critical part of the work of caregiving, but are not considered in traditional ADL/IADL measures.

Thus, providing care is not simply the mirror image of the need for care, as expressed in ADL/IADL status (Albert, 2004). We have argued that ADL/IADL care should be subsumed within a wider, multidomain formulation that gives adequate scope to *how* people need ADL care and *how caregivers develop environments for providing it*. This is an especially salient issue in the care of people who have cognitive disorders, such as AD.

Even if we limit ourselves to traditional ADL tasks, we quickly see that caregivers who provide such care mention many additional factors that make ADL care easy or difficult, manageable or unbearable. One is *timing:* whether care is required rarely, frequently but in predictable ways, or frequently in unpredictable, unexpected ways (Hooyman, Gonyea, & Montgomery, 1985). AD care is characterized by great unpredictability in the timing of ADL care because of poor sleep hygiene, psychiatric complications, incontinence, inability to communicate care preferences, and noncooperation.

A glaring example of the central role of timing is nighttime care. People who routinely need to be taken to the toilet at night, disrupting a caregiver's sleep, are clearly more challenging than people who can be taken to the toilet during the day and sleep through the night, even though both equally need assistance in toileting (McCluskey, 2000). More generally, caregivers forced to adopt care receivers' schedules are likely to be the most burdened, because they are the most captive to caregiving.

A second dimension is *caregiver proximity* in the ADL task. Is it enough that a caregiver is in the house while someone eats a meal or bathes, or does the caregiver need to be in the same room standing by, or does the caregiver need to provide hands-on help? Stand-by help can be quite burdensome in that it limits caregivers to the home even if they do not have to provide hands-on help at all times. In fact, stand-by help, in some cases, may be more burdensome, because family members need to be available (and, hence, are prevented from doing other tasks) without a sense that they are providing care. This is a typical feature of caregiving to the elder with mild dementia.

A third dimension is the kind of *effort* caregivers need to exert to see that the ADL need is met. Someone with a need for help in bathing may only require supervision, or coaxing and support, or complete guidance and direction. It is possible that coaxing and support, in some cases, may be more challenging than complete guidance and control. For example, taking someone to the toilet every 2 hours may be more burdensome than complete continence care involving disposable diapers (Albert et al., 1999).

Finally, it obviously matters whether care receivers participate, actively resist, or are passive as receivers of ADL care (Feinstein, Josephy, &

Wells, 1986). Helping a person who is cooperative is far different from helping a person who is resisting assistance in bathing or eating (Reinhard, 2004). Unfortunately, care offered to people with severe dementia is often met with resistance.

The effects of providing care to a person with AD have been studied intensively. Marital discord and divorce, depression and anxiety, loss of employment, restriction of social life, invasion of privacy, impoverishment, and substance abuse have all been linked to caregiving stress. Buffering factors that mitigate these negative effects include support from family, religiosity, strong personal mastery and self-efficacy, satisfaction with caregiving, and adopting strategies to reduce the burden of care.

Caregiving strain has also been linked to mortality risk, as suggested in the Caregiver Health Effects Study, a study of the bereavement experience of people who cared for spouses who died during follow-up (Schulz & Beach, 1999). Spouses who provided care and reported burden from caregiving were more likely to die than noncaregivers, but caregiving spouses who did not experience burden did not face an elevated risk. Schulz concluded that mental or emotional strain is an independent risk factor for mortality among older spousal caregivers.

Caregiving is also associated with poorer work performance. In a study of a large employer database, employees reporting elder care responsibilities were more likely to report certain chronic conditions (such as diabetes), poorer attention to their own health (as evidenced in lower use of clinical preventive health services, less opportunity for physical activity), and greater overall medical care costs, in addition to greater absenteeism and poorer perceived productivity on the job (National Caregiver Alliance and MetLife Mature Market Institute, in press). We examine caregiving in more detail below, when we consider interventions to support families.

Quality of Life in AD

One central problem for people with AD is their inability, with later stages of the disease, to report on subjective states: their perceptions of pain, satisfaction, comfort, enjoyment, contentment, anxiety, or well-being. Because quality-of-life assessment is unthinkable without a patient's reports of such states (see Chapter 8), it would seem that assessment of quality of life in people with AD would be impossible. Severely affected patients (patients with MMSE scores below 12 or patients with more than moderate cognitive impairment) cannot reliably complete self-report questionnaires. Yet it is clear, even to the casual observer, that people with AD have good and bad days, that facial expressions and body posture reliably communicate information about internal states, and that these perhaps primitive indicators of mood or well-being are associated with changes in environment (Albert & Logsdon, 2001). If we can perceive mood changes and illness behaviors in animals, we can certainly recognize such changes in people with dementia. Thus, the challenge in advanced AD is to identify indicators of internal states that reliably convey information about mood and well-being.

What domains or aspects of daily life are important to patients in the presence of severely compromised cognition and function? The domains included in current measures vary considerably. Among other domains, Rabins includes "awareness of self" and "response to surroundings" (Rabins, Kasper, Kleinman, Black, & Patrick, 2001), and Brod includes "aesthetic sense" and "feelings of belonging" (Brod, Stewart, & Sands, 2001). Logsdon's QOL-AD measure includes items assessing "energy level" and "ability to do things for fun" (Logsdon, Gibbons, McCurry, & Teri, 2001). These are patient or proxy reports and face a variety of limitations. Proxy reports about patient quality of life are correlated with a caregiver's own mood or perceived caregiver burden. People impute moods or symptoms based on their own status. Patients' self-reports will be reliable only up to a point, although some patients are evidently able to complete questionnaires with MMSE scores as low as 10 (Logsdon et al., 2001).

Behavioral observation measures avoid these limitations. The Apparent Affect Rating Scale (APS) (Lawton, Van Haitsma, Perkinson, & Ruckdeschel, 2001), Multidimensional Observational Scale (MOSES) (Helmes, Csapo, & Short, 1987), Discomfort Scale (Hurley, Volicer, Hanrahan, Houde, & Volicer, 1992), and other observer ratings capture negative and positive behaviors in real time (Albert, 1997). "Behavior stream" technologies now allow clocking of the duration of mood or behavior states and the context in which patients express these states, such as "agitation during morning ADL care." Behavior stream measures are complicated by the need for extensive training of raters and limitation to institutional home settings.

One intermediate approach is to adapt behavior stream-like measures to proxy reporting. Albert and colleagues (1996, 1999a, 2001) asked proxies to report on affective states by use of APS items (i.e., facial expressions of the so-called "hot" affects: anger, anxiety, interest, pleasure) and patient activity over the prior 2 weeks (frequency of a series of in-home and out-of-home activities that could be completed with caregiving cueing and supervision). The measures were significantly correlated with dementia severity in both clinic and community samples (Albert et al., 1999a). This is important confirmation of the validity of the quality-of-life measures. Such measures should be correlated with stage of dementia (because dementia severity affects mood and opportunities for engagement) but should also show variance within stage (suggesting that there are other sources of pleasure or engagement relevant to dementia care).

This approach is also useful for specifying time to important quality-of-life milestones in the progression of AD. For example, in a group of people with moderate dementia at the start of follow-up, 50% no longer were leaving their homes at 20 months. In a group with mild dementia, this milestone was not reached until 30 months (Albert & Logsdon, 2001). This study was also able to show a hierarchy of quality-of-life (QOL) outcomes. Onset of home confinement preceded onset of null activity, which in turn preceded onset of null positive affect. Finally, this study showed that proxies identified states of pleasure even among patients with psychopathological behaviors. This finding reminds us that we must pay attention both to positive and negative behaviors if we are to understand dementia adequately.

One promising approach to assessing quality of life in people with AD involves more extensive "care mapping," in which detailed assessment of behavior streams is used for quality assurance purposes (Edelman, Fulton, Kuhn, & Chang, 2005). The premise of this approach is to supply supportive care personnel with real-time reports of environment-affect relationships. The hope is that personnel in skilled nursing facilities or adult day care settings can individualize the way care is provided and use this information to promote greater involvement of patients in activities or social interaction. A similar approach has been used by Schnelle and colleagues for training certified nursing assistants to deliver self-maintenance care and to improve other kinds of daily interactions, as well as to recognize resident pain or discomfort (Schnelle et al., 2009)

Dementia and the End of Life

Family caregivers face difficult decisions related to end-of-life care of relatives in the last stages of the disease (Meier, 1999). Should patients with pneumonia be treated aggressively with intravenous antibiotics, transferred to hospital, and intubated; or should they be treated symptomatically with analgesics, antipyretics, and oxygen? Should a patient with dementia who refuses food or who has trouble swallowing be tube fed? Little is known about the ways families make these decisions.

Persons with advanced dementia suffer serious medical problems, such as pneumonia, urinary tract infections, and fever (Fabiszewski, Volicer, & Volicer, 1990; van der Steen, Ooms, van der Wal, & Ribbe, 2002). Research suggests a high prevalence of intravenous antibiotic use and invasive procedures (Ahronheim, Morrison, Baskin, Morris, & Meier, 1996; Morrison & Siu, 2000). For example, despite the futility associated with aggressive care in end-stage dementia, Evers and colleagues (2002) found that more than 50% of the patients with dementia were treated with systemic antibiotics. Our own clinic series suggests similar trends. In a group of people with probable AD, 31% used intravenous antibiotics and 16% had feeding tubes placed in the 6 months before death. A series of studies have shown that feeding tube placement for people with AD in skilled nursing facilities is not associated with improved outcomes (Casarett et al., 2005; Morrison et al., 2005).

It is still unclear why some families opt for use of life-sustaining technologies in the case of older people with profound or terminal AD. It may be that family caregivers who score high on measures of distress (depression, caregiver burden, lack of social support) are less likely to develop medical care goals that limit aggressive end-of-life care. These families may also be at greater risk for emergency room use of life-sustaining technologies. To our knowledge, no research has investigated this issue. By contrast, AD patients may be less likely to be considered for life-sustaining technologies than other people with terminal conditions. The loss of cognitive ability and, hence, the loss of personhood associated with disease may allow families to "let go" of people who are in the last stages of life.

NON-ALZHEIMER'S DEMENTIAS

Vascular cognitive impairment (VCI), as opposed to Alzheimer's disease, is cognitive impairment related to cerebrovascular disease, such as stroke. VCI is mainly defined by neuroimaging, which allows further differentiation into subgroups that show cortical infarction, white matter changes, or some combination of the two. In cohort studies of incident dementia, such as the Cardiovascular Disease Study, approximately 70% of people meeting criteria for dementia can be classified as AD, another 10% as VCI, 15% as mixed AD and VCI, and the remaining 5% as some other etiology (such as hydrocephalus, metabolic disorders, or Korsakoff's syndrome) (Lopez et al., 2003).

VCI is a risk factor for mortality. In a Mayo Clinic record linkage study, patients with vascular dementia had a greater risk of mortality than matched controls without dementia. Among VCI patients, dementia related to stroke was associated with the highest mortality risk. Patients without stroke, but with imaging evidence of bilateral infarctions in gray matter structures, had a lower mortality risk (Knopman, Rocca, Cha, Edland, & Kokmen, 2003).

Another source of dementia in the older adults is Parkinson's disease (PD). The Parkinson's Foundation has reviewed a series of prevalence and incidence studies of dementia in PD and found that about a quarter of all patients with Parkinson's disease meet criteria for dementia. PD patients with dementia are older but do not differ in the duration of the disease (Lieberman, 2002). The annual incidence of dementia in patients with Parkinson's ranges from 2.7% (ages 55–64) to 13.7% (ages 70–79). Dementia risk in PD may vary according to whether patients have Lewy body inclusions in the brainstem or brain, or have Lewy bodies with Alzheimer's changes as well.

Mortality risk in PD is related to the presence of dementia. Incident dementia in PD increases mortality risk even when the motor effects of PD are controlled (Levy et al., 2002).

INTERVENTIONS TO PREVENT COGNITIVE DECLINE

If physical "prehabilitation" can retard disablement (Gill et al., 2002), could a program of preventive cognitive training have the same effect in the realm of cognitive decline? The Advanced Cognitive Training for Independent and Vital Elderly (ACTIVE) Trial investigated this question in the setting of a randomized clinical trial (Ball et al., 2002). A volunteer sample of nearly 3,000 older adults without cognitive or physical impairment was randomly assigned to one of three intervention groups or a no-contact control group. The three intervention arms involved 10 sessions devoted to training in memory skill (verbal episodic memory), reasoning (problem-solving strategies), or speed of processing (visual search and identification). The intervention program was delivered in small-group settings, with a focus on teaching strategies designed to improve memory, speed, or problem solving. Intervention groups were given exercises to practice and retain skills. In the memory-training arm, for example, participants "were instructed how to organize word lists into meaningful categories and to form visual images and mental associations to recall words and text." In this 2-year study, a subset of participants received booster training just before the 1-year evaluation.

Outcomes in the trial included ability on cognitive tests of these remediated skills, such as episodic memory, identification of patterns, and speed of processing. The trial also examined performance-based and self-reported everyday skills related to these cognitive domains. These included "everyday problem-solving" (for example, the ability to handle medication information), "everyday speed" (for example, the speed with which one looks up a telephone number), driving habits, and ADL and IADL limitations.

The trial showed that these cognitive interventions helped healthy older adults perform better on the specific cognitive skills for which they were trained. These benefits suggest that the slow cognitive declines reported for elders without dementia can be remediated. For example, ACTIVE participants receiving memory training improved by approximately 0.25 SD over 2 years, whereas the cognitive skills of older adults without dementia typically decline at about this rate over a 7-year period. However, these proximal cognitive benefits did not translate into improvements in everyday performance. The authors suggest that the absence of transfer to real-world outcomes is best explained by a ceiling effect in the everyday performance measures. Most subjects were not impaired in driving, in looking up telephone numbers, or in reasoning about medications. The pronounced ceiling effect may have obscured true benefit in this area. In fact, the control group did not decline on many of the everyday performance measures. The authors conclude, "it is not yet clear whether differential functional decline across treatment groups will be observed in the future as this select cohort enters more fully into an age of functional loss" (Ball et al., 2002).

More recent reports from the same trial indicate some generalization of benefit to self-reported quality of life (Wolinsky et al., 2006) and risk of depression (Wolinsky et al., 2009). However, the benefit in functional status has proven more elusive (Willis et al., 2006).

INTERVENTIONS TO SUPPORT FAMILY CAREGIVERS

Family caregiving, as we have mentioned earlier, is a major challenge in care of the elder with dementia. Families overwhelmed by the stresses of caregiving may resort to nursing home placement even when this is not a preferred choice. They may simply feel they have no other option once the stresses of caregiving and lack of respite have undermined coping resources and family function. A program of psychosocial support might strengthen caregiver resources and help them manage the stresses of care better. Would such a program, if effectively delivered, also reduce rates of nursing home placement? This difference in outcome would be a powerful demonstration of the effects of psychosocial support on vulnerable families, and in the case of spouse caregivers, highly vulnerable elders.

Mittelman and colleagues designed such a program for caregiving spouses of people with Alzheimer's disease and tested it in a randomized controlled trial of nursing home placement (Mittelman, Ferris, Shulman, Steinberg, & Levin, 1996). The intervention was designed to guide and support caregivers through the challenging period when spouses progressed to increasingly severe dementia. In the first 4 months of the study, spouses received two individual counseling sessions and four family sessions. "Counseling sessions were task oriented, promoting communication among family members, teaching techniques for problem solving and management of troublesome patient behavior, and improving both emotional and instrumental support for the primary caregiver." This phase was followed by participation in a support group and finally by continuing availability of contact with counselors. The control group received the usual follow-up and information and referral. Thus, "if control subjects asked about obtaining paid help at home, they were given the names of service providers, whereas treatment subjects were given as much help as they needed to find and appropriately use such services" (Mittelman et al., 1996).

After 3.5 years, 58.7% of patients in this sample of 206 families had entered nursing homes and 26.2% had died at home. In addition, not all caregivers in the intervention group agreed to support group participation; only 72% joined support groups. However, 42% of controls joined such support groups. Despite this combined drop-out and "drop-in" dilution of the experiment, patients in the treatment group remained at home significantly longer than patients in the control group. Treatment group patients entered nursing homes about a year later than controls. This difference was obtained in survival models that controlled for age and gender of caregivers, socioeconomic resources, caregiver mental health, and severity of dementia.

Mittelman and colleagues (1996) conclude that "continuously available support and information can enable spouse caregivers of AD patients to withstand the difficulties of caregiving and avoid or defer institution-alization of the patients." This conclusion is supported by the design of the experiment but also by the absence of differences in patient care between intervention and control groups. For example, patients in the two groups were equally likely to receive psychotropic medications and medical care. Thus, the intervention appears to have affected caregivers rather than patients. Patients were equally likely to develop urinary incontinence and equally likely to receive medical care for the condition, but intervention group caregivers, through support from training and counseling, were better able to manage the demands of care related to incontinence.

This finding is reassuring, given the absence or unclear benefit for a variety of other interventions involving patient and caregiver outcomes, including respite programs (Lawton, Brody, & Pruchno, 1991) and home attendant care (Weissert, Chernow, & Hirth, 2003). On the other hand, benefit has been reported for caregiver mental health, as in the Medicare Alzheimer's Disease Demonstration (Newcomer et al., 1999). As the United States moves toward increasing incentives for family caregivers (mostly in the form of tax breaks) and a greater diversity of services that can be provided in homes, it will become increasingly important to determine what kinds of resources families need to be effective caregiving units.

Results from REACH-II, Resources for Enhancing Alzheimer's Caregiver Health, show that training and low-intensity support can have a dramatic effect on caregiver health and well-being as well. This randomized controlled trial assessed the effects of a multicomponent psychosocial behavioral intervention designed to reduce burden and depression among family caregivers. The primary quality-of-life outcome comprised measures of caregiver depression, burden, self-care, and social support and care recipient problem behaviors at 6 months. The intervention group showed clinically significant benefit, which, however, was more pronounced among White and Hispanic caregivers than among African Americans (Belle et al., 2006). Institutional placement of care recipients did not differ over the 6 months. This linkage of targeted training and support to specific problem areas offers great potential for Alzheimer's caregiver support.

Finally, collaborative models to link family caregivers to dementia care consultants based in primary care practices show benefit for supporting caregivers and reducing the risk of nursing home placement (Fortinsky, Kulldorff, Kleppinger, & Kenyon-Pesce, 2009).

SUMMARY

Families confronting dementing disease face the very difficult problem of deciding when driving should cease, when supervision is required for safety, when elders can no longer live alone, and when parents or spouses are no longer competent to handle money, take medications, or manage their lives independently. They will likely have to contend with personality changes, psychiatric symptoms, and challenging behaviors as people reach more advanced stages of disease. Caregivers may have to perform ADL care, manage supportive care staff hired to assist the elder, or more likely both sets of tasks, possibly at a distance. They may face the difficult decision to admit the Alzheimer's patient to a nursing home. Or, as is increasingly common, older people themselves may choose residences (such as assisted living or continuing care retirement communities) that can accommodate Alzheimer's or nursing-home levels of care, should they need such services.

Definition of Dementia. A person meets criteria for dementia if he or she has memory impairment and one or more additional impairments in cognition, such as aphasia, apraxia, agnosia, or executive function deficits. These cognitive deficits must be severe enough to cause significant impairment in social or occupational function and represent a significant decline from a previous level of functioning. For Alzheimer's disease to be diagnosed, the course of this general cognitive disorder must, in addition, be characterized by gradual onset and continuing, progressive decline that is not attributable to other central nervous system conditions.

AD and Memory Decline in Aging. Research suggests that memory declines typical of Alzheimer's disease may be distinct from normal aging. In a cohort without dementia, declines in cognitive domains in people without the e4 allele, representing normal aging, were less pronounced than declines in people with the e4 allele, representing a likely early prodrome of AD.

Mild Cognitive Impairment. MCI is typically defined by subjective complaints of memory problems and memory performance below age- and education-referenced norms, with normal performance in other cognitive domains and absence of impairment in the instrumental and basic activities of daily living. Estimates of the proportion of older adults with cognitive impairment short of dementia range from 5% to as high as 22%. Dementia incidence in elders who report cognitive complaints and demonstrate mild deficits in cognitive assessment is much higher than that for elders as a whole, 5%–12% per year, compared with perhaps 1%–2% in the population of older adults as a whole. Consequently, mild cognitive impairment cannot be considered benign or a normal feature of healthy aging.

Prevalence and Incidence of Alzheimer's Disease. In a nationally representative sample of seniors aged 60 and older, the best estimate of AD prevalence is 3.3 million in 2002. Among elder aged 71 and older, 13.9% of Americans meet criteria for dementia. By 2015, we can expect 4.6 million cases of AD using a narrow definition and 5.3 million if we include mixed cases. About a third of these cases will have moderate or more severe forms of AD.

The incidence of AD is closely related to age. For people aged 65–74, annual incidence ranges from <0.5% to 1.3%. For people aged 75–84, the range is 1.5%–4.0%, and for people aged 85 and older the incidence is 4.7%–7.9% per year. Minority status is among the most important risk factors for AD. Given the increasing number of older adults in the minorities in the United States, this disparity has great public health significance.

Risk Factors for Alzheimer's Disease. Only approximately 7% of early-onset AD (< age 65) and less than 1% of late-onset AD have been linked to mutations on particular genes. For late-onset AD, attention centers on the *APOE* gene. A number of studies have shown overrepresentation of the *APOE*-e4 allele in people with AD. Despite this finding, the current recommendation is against use of *APOE* as a screening tool: "although *APOE* genotype may be a risk factor for AD, it cannot yet be considered a useful predictive genetic test."

The significance of cognitive resources early in the life span for dementia in late life has become increasingly clear in studies that have linked risk of AD to childhood IQ, educational accomplishment and leisure activities, occupational attainment and job demands, language skills in early adulthood, diversity of physical and cognitive engagement over the life span, parental socioeconomic status, and literacy. These findings suggest that cognitive ability is similar to grip strength: differences (in muscle fiber density, in neuronal integrity or number) already apparent at birth or in the perinatal period (and which develop or set limits on development over the life span) provide variable reserve against depletions that occur with aging. These resources put one closer or further away from the threshold of disability associated with the loss of physical and cognitive function that occurs over the life span.

A variety of medical conditions have been shown to increase the risk of AD, including hypertension and vascular disease, diabetes, loss in bone mineral density, estrogen deficiency, depression.

Outcomes Associated With Alzheimer's Disease. Compared to older adults without dementia matched for age and comorbid disease, drawn from the same community, and similar in socioeconomic features, elders with AD face a mortality risk 2–3 times higher than elders with normal cognition. AD is a key risk factor for nursing home admission. AD is also associated with greater risk of acute medical care in the hospital, as well as general medical care in the community.

Families provide the vast majority of Alzheimer's care. Although patients with Alzheimer's disease are common in nursing homes, accounting for perhaps half of the residents, these residents represent a minority of the Alzheimer's population. Most people with AD are cared for at home, use a variety of in-home (home attendant, allied health) and out-of-home services (adult day care, acute rehab), and will enter nursing homes very late in the disease, if at all.

The effects of providing care to a person with AD have been studied intensively. Marital discord and divorce, depression and anxiety, loss of employment, restriction of social life, invasion of privacy, impoverishment, substance abuse, and mortality have all been linked to caregiving stress. Buffering factors that mitigate these negative effects include support from family, religiosity, strong personal mastery and self-efficacy, satisfaction with caregiving, and strategies to reduce the burden of providing care.

Family caregivers and clinicians face difficult decisions related to end-of-life care of relatives in the last stages of AD. Should patients with pneumonia be treated aggressively with intravenous antibiotics, transferred to hospital, and intubated; or should they be treated symptomatically with analgesics, antipyretics, and oxygen? Should a patient with dementia who refuses food or has difficulty swallowing be tube fed? Little is known about the ways families make these decisions, but evidence suggests that use of life-sustaining technologies is common in this terminal population.

Investigation of quality of life in people with AD requires a judicious mix of patient, proxy, and observational measures. A useful QOL measure should be correlated with the stage of dementia (because dementia severity affects mood and opportunities for engagement), and it should show variance within stage (suggesting that there are other sources of pleasure or engagement relevant to dementia care). In this way, QOL investigation may be useful as a guide to clinical care and environmental modifications that will benefit patients and their families.

Interventions to Prevent Cognitive Decline. The ACTIVE trial showed that older adults can be successfully trained in specific cognitive skills. Whether such training reduces the risk of decline is at this point unclear, although some evidence suggests benefit.

Interventions to Support Family Caregivers. Randomized trials of targeted support show that both outcomes for elders (nursing home placement) and caregiver psychosocial status (burden, fatigue, depression) can be improved to mitigate the severe challenges of Alzheimer's care.

7 Affective and Social Function: Suffering, Neglect, Isolation

Symptoms of poor mental health may be different in older people than in younger people (Blazer, 2002). As we will see, older people are less likely to meet standard criteria for syndromal depression or anxiety disorders. Affective disorders are more likely to take the form of "subthreshold syndromes," symptom intensities and frequencies short of standard criteria for diagnoses of clinical disorders. Does this mean that older people are less depressed? Or should we draw the conclusion that depression needs to be redefined in this case because it is a different kind of clinical entity? The disability and excess morbidity associated with subthreshold disorders suggest the latter, as we will see below. These questions also suggest that we consider mental health in older adults within the broader context of emotional and social experience in old age.

Despite these difficulties in diagnosis and definition, late-life mood disorders, and in particular, depression, are highly prevalent and debilitating. Among the almost 35 million Americans age 65 and older in 2008, approximately 2 million experience depression (Reynolds, 2008). Seniors with depression, who often contend with other diseases and disability as well, are less likely to take medications reliably, seek appropriate medical care, or practice optimal disease self-management. Thus, psychiatric conditions which may result in increased risk of suicide, poorer function, and social isolation, carry with them more general threats to well-being. In addition, many seniors with subthreshold disorders also experience disability and are at high risk for developing syndromal clinical depression. Seniors with very mildly elevated depressive symptoms are more likely to have mild cognitive impairment as well (Bhalla et al., 2009). In addition, recognition and treatment of depression may be challenging in primary care settings because of lack of geriatric expertise, time pressure, and pressing concerns to handle more obvious physical illness.

Increasing recognition of these challenges has led to a new concern for bringing depression screening and treatment to community settings. These efforts include developing ways to link social service agencies and mental health care, training aging services staff to recognize and refer cases of depression, and training agency staff to deliver mental health interventions.

BURDEN OF MENTAL ILLNESS

The first Surgeon General's Report on Mental Health (1999) begins by recognizing the immense burden of disability associated with mental illness throughout the world. In more developed countries ("established market economies"), for example, mental health disorders account for approximately 15% of all disease burden, more, in fact, than the burden associated with cancer (Murray & Lopez, 1996). The rank of these diseases in terms of the burden they produce is shown in Table 7.1. Mental illness is exceeded only by cardiovascular disease in years lost to disability and early mortality. Cancer follows, showing that diseases of mental health, because they begin early in life and persist over the life span, produce a greater volume of morbidity and disability. Clearly, treatment and prevention of mental disorders would go a long way toward the reduction of disease burden.

The burden of particular diseases involving mental health relative to total disease burden is shown in Table 7.2. The table shows that the equivalent of 98.7 million person-years was lost to disability or early mortality in the more developed countries in 1990. Unipolar depression, the most prevalent mental illness, accounted for 6.8% of this total burden. Burden associated with depressive disorders exceeded burden associated with cardiovascular disease (more narrowly defined than above), alcohol use, and road traffic accidents.

Table 7.1

DISEASE BURDEN BY SELECTED ILLNESS CATEGORIES IN ESTABLISHED MARKET ECONOMIES, 1990

	TOTAL DALYs,[a] %
All cardiovascular conditions	18.6
All mental illness[b]	15.4
All malignant diseases (cancer)	15.0
All respiratory conditions	4.8
All alcohol use	4.7<
All infectious and parasitic diseases	2.8
All drug use	1.5

[a]Disability-adjusted life year (DALY) is a measure that expresses years of life lost to premature death and years lived with a disability of specified severity and duration (Murray & Lopez, 1996).
[b]Disease burden associated with "mental illness" includes suicide.
From "Evidence-Based Health Policy—Lessons From the Global Burden of Disease Study," by C. J. Murray & A. D. Lopez, 1996, *Science, 274(5288)*, 740–743.

Table 7.2

LEADING SOURCES OF DISEASE BURDEN IN ESTABLISHED MARKET ECONOMIES, 1990

		TOTAL DALYs (MILLIONS)	TOTAL, %
	All causes	98.7	
1	Ischemic heart disease	8.9	9.0
2	Unipolar major depression	6.7	6.8
3	Cardiovascular disease	5.0	5.0
4	Alcohol use	4.7	4.7
5	Road traffic accidents	4.3	4.4

From "Evidence-Based Health Policy—Lessons From the Global Burden of Disease Study," by C. J. Murray & A. D. Lopez, 1996, *Science, 274*(5288), 740–743.

The measure of burden in these comparisons is the DALY, or disability-adjusted life year. This is a summation of years of healthy life lost to disability and early mortality. Whereas the DALY is similar in principle to other measures of health expectancy, discussed in Chapter 10, its calculation differs in an important way. It assigns weights to age, where these weights "reflect the relative importance of healthy life at different ages" (World Bank, 1995). These weights increase up to age 25 and then decline. They have also been designed to reflect the dependence of the young and older people on working age adults. One effect that this age-weighting factor in DALY calculations has is to decrease in the contribution of old age disability to the total years lost to disability. Be that as it may, the DALY approach to burden is useful for highlighting the greater morbidity and disability associated with mental illness.

An alternative indicator of the severe burden of mental illness, especially depression, is visible in self-reports of disability from people with different chronic health conditions. The Medical Outcomes Study examined adult outpatients with a series of sentinel conditions (hypertension, myocardial infarction, arthritis, gastrointestinal disorders, and depression), who did not have other comorbidities (Wells et al., 1989). The impact of each condition on six health-related quality-of-life domains (physical function, role function, social function, mental health, self-perceived global health, and bodily pain) was assessed relative to a nationally representative sample of adults ascertained outside the clinic setting. The differences in scores on each of the six domains, relative to the nonclinic sample, show important differences in disease impact. These findings are shown in Figure 7.1.

The dotted line represents scores from the nonclinic sample, assigned a zero value for purposes of standardization. The figure shows that hypertension has little effect on reported function and well-being. People with the condition reported only poorer perceived health and a greater number of mental health symptoms, both in keeping with the disease label and need to take medication (which may itself have a quality-of-life impact). Arthritis and gastrointestinal (GI) disorders were roughly comparable in their effects on physical function, but GI orders were more burdensome on role, social function, and mental health domains, whereas arthritis was more burdensome in the bodily pain domain. Myocardial infarction had primarily physical effects, with very low scores in the physical and role performance domains.

Wells et al. (1989) point out the perhaps surprising result that outpatients meeting criteria for depression performed worse, not just on

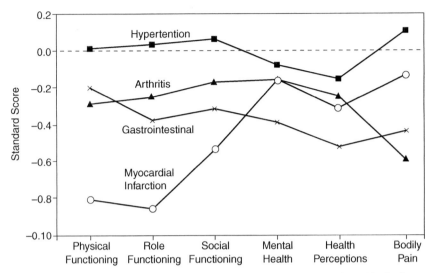

Figure 7.1 Health profiles for patients with four common conditions from Medical Outcomes Study.

Source: From "Functional Status and Well-Being of Patients With Chronic Conditions. Results From the Medical Outcomes Study," by A. L. Stewart, S. Greenfield, R. D. Hays, K. Wells, W. H. Rogers, S. D. Berry, et al., 1989. *Journal of the American Medical Association, 262*(7), 907–913. Reprinted with permission, *Journal of the American Medical Association.*

the mental health measures, as expected, but also on reports of physical function and role performance, in which they looked very much like the patients with myocardial infarctions. Wells concluded, "the functioning of depressed patients is comparable with or worse than that of patients with major chronic medical conditions."

Thus, the effect of mental disorders on daily life should not be underestimated. Below, we examine morbidity associated with depression and the role of depressive disorders in increasing the risk of future mortality and disability.

PRESENTATION OF MENTAL HEALTH SYMPTOMS IN LATE LIFE

Mental health symptoms seem to change with older age. For example, in later life depressive disorders fulfilling diagnostic criteria are relatively rare; "subthreshold disorders" are more common. Subthreshold depression, for example, includes symptoms of depression that are not severe, frequent, or disruptive enough to be labeled as clinical depression. In practice, people are said to have subthreshold depression when they report symptoms on a depression self-report measure that fall below standard thresholds for defining likely depression. In the case of the Center for Epidemiologic Studies-Depression Scale (CES-D), this would be a score above some minimum but below 16. In the case of the Geriatric Depression Scale (GDS) short form, this would be a score above 0 but below 10. In the case of the Patient Health Questionnaire (PHQ) (Spitzer, Kroenke, & Williams, 1999), it would be the endorsement of lack of interest and feeling down more than half the days of the week over the past 2 weeks, but endorsement of fewer than three other depression symptoms.

Rather than feeling depressed and reporting feelings of sadness or worthlessness, older people with depression may be more likely to report alternative clusters of symptoms, such as loss of interest in usual activities and somatic or cognitive symptoms, including fatigue, pain, sleep difficulties, and memory disorders. One study suggested that people at the oldest ages are more likely to report "delimited forms of distress," such as enervation, dysphoria, and sleep disturbances, rather than the anhedonia typical of younger cohorts (Newman, Engel, & Jensen, 1991). A similar process appears to be at work for anxiety, with greater likelihood of subthreshold anxiety disorders in later life.

Mossey and Moss (2002) reported a study of 600 community-dwelling elders aged 70 and older with a specific focus on subthreshold depression. They defined subthreshold depression by use of the CES-D (as well as additional questions assessing depressive symptoms) and found that 5.2% met criteria for depression and 22.2% for subthreshold depression. It was not surprising to find that people who met criteria for depression scored more poorly on measures of physical, functional, and social health, and were also likely to have more physician visits (22, compared with 13 in the group without depression) and spend a greater number of days in the hospital (12 versus 5.2 in the group without depression) during the previous year. An important result of this study was a set of similar findings for the subthreshold depression group. Older adults with subthreshold depression scored more poorly in measures of health and were also likely to have a greater number of physician visits and hospital days than the group without depression. Mossey and Moss (2002) conclude that "with a prevalence of 22%, the public health burden of an even modest impact of sub-threshold depression on life quality and functioning of older individuals is substantial."

It is also worth asking about the persistence and effect of mental health symptoms in older people after a diagnosis of depression. The natural history of depression in older adults was examined in the Longitudinal Aging Study, a cohort of older adults recruited in Amsterdam (Beekman et al., 2002). Within this large cohort, 277 were identified as depressed at baseline and were monitored for up to 6 years, with as many as 14 assessments in this period. Elders were assessed with the Diagnostic Interview Schedule (DIS), a clinical interview that allows diagnosis of depression and its subtypes. Use of the clinical diagnostic interview with such extensive follow-up is rare and allows insight on symptom duration, type of clinical course, and stability of diagnoses. In this group of older people who met criteria for depression at baseline, fewer than a fourth saw remission of their symptoms. On the whole, symptom levels remained high: 44% had an unfavorable but fluctuating course and 32% experienced a continuing severe chronic course. Older people with sub-threshold disorders were at risk for progression to more severe forms of depression. In this community cohort, the natural history of late-life depression turned out to be poor, with persistence and increasing morbidity as the most common outcome.

This brief review of research on the presentation of mental health symptoms in older adults suggests that symptom profiles in depression may be different, with less affective symptoms (i.e., feelings of worthlessness or sense that life is not worth living, crying, thoughts of suicide) and more somatic and cognitive symptoms. The result is a profile of symptoms short of the standard clinical syndrome. But subthreshold mental illness can also be consequential, with significant suffering, great health impact, and lost opportunities for productive aging. Clinical and service delivery staff who work with older adults will need to recognize these differences if they are to provide effective care and referral.

Given the reduction in the most severe forms of depression and anxiety with age, one wants to know why symptoms of this sort decline and come to be replaced by milder forms. Jorm, Christensen, Korten, Jacomb, and Henderson (2000) suggest that "ageing is associated with an intrinsic reduction in susceptibility to anxiety and depression." They ask for caution in this conclusion, because we have few longitudinal studies covering the adult life span and therefore cannot yet reliably distinguish aging from cohort effects. If this difference in symptom expression turns out to be reliably associated with age, they suggest that the reason may be decreased emotional responsiveness with age, increased emotional control, and a kind of "psychological immunization" to stressful experiences. Supporting the first of these hypotheses, Lawton, Parmelee, Katz, and Nesselroade (1996) reported lower self-reported frequency of many affects in cross-sectional comparisons of young, middle-aged, and older adults. Carstensen (1992) has also demonstrated less interest in novel stimuli and greater social selectivity with age as a way of conserving psychological resources and promoting well being. These changes are aspects of "gerotranscendence" (Torstan, 2005). These findings provide some support for reduced emotional expression and greater emotional control in later life and the "selective optimization with compensation" noted in Chapter 1.

These last points deserve special emphasis because they show again the pervasive link between life span processes and health. Emotional life changes across the life span. As a consequence, the experience of depression may also change. Depression is not trivial in late life, but it may take on a less florid form because of changes in emotional makeup. If one talks to older people and asks about the emotions, one is likely to hear statements about the decline of emotion: "the highs are not so high anymore, but the lows are not so low either." In our research, we find that older people speak wistfully of their more intense emotional life at younger ages but also report a good deal of relief at getting off that treadmill.

PREVALENCE OF MENTAL ILLNESS AT OLDER AGES

As mentioned above, syndromal depression, that is, severity and duration of symptoms that meet criteria for clinical diagnosis, is less common among older people than younger people. This is apparent in population surveys that query respondents on symptoms of depression, such as the National Health Interview Survey, 2000 (NHIS). "Severe psychological distress" in the NHIS was measured according to the frequency of six distress symptoms over the past 30 days. The six items formed a scale with a range of 0–24 (so that each item was scored 0–4), and a score of 13 or greater was used to define severe distress.

As Figure 7.2 shows, less than 2% of people aged 65 and older reported "serious psychological distress." In people aged 45–64, approximately 4% reported this level of distress, nearly twice as many. In the youngest age group, aged 18–44, the proportion was also higher, ap-

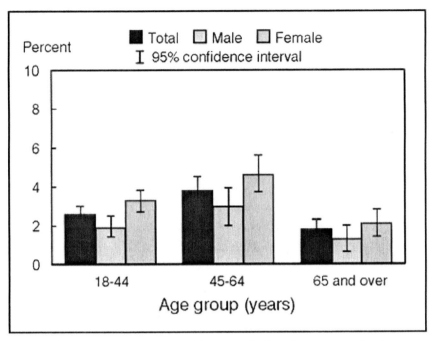

Figure 7.2 Percentage of adults aged 18 years and older who experienced serious psychological distress during the past 30 days, by age group and sex: United States, January–June 2002.

Notes: Six psychological distress questions are included in the Sample Adult Core component. These questions ask how often a respondent experienced symptoms of psychological distress during the past 30 days. The response codes (0–4) of the six items for each person are summed to yield a scale with a 0–24 range. A value of 13 or more for this scale is used here to define serious psychological distress.
Source: Based on data collected from January through June in the Sample Adult Core component of the 2002 National Health Interview Survey.

proximately 2.5%. Notably, in all age groups, women were more likely to report severe psychological distress than men.

A common measure of depression in late life, as mentioned earlier, is the Geriatric Depression Scale (Yesavage et al., 1983). The items cover dysphoria, sadness or lack of enjoyment (e.g., "Do you feel happy most of the time?" "Are you in good spirits most of the time?"); anhedonia, or lack of interest in activities that are usually sought out (e.g., "Have you dropped many of your activities and interests?" "Do you often get bored?"); somatic symptoms associated with depression (e.g., perceived memory problems, reduced level of energy); and demoralization or existential suffering (e.g., "Do you feel that your situation is hopeless?" "Do you feel that your life is empty?" "Do you often feel helpless?" "Do you feel pretty worthless the way you are now?") "Yes" responses to the 15 items are summed. In the short-form of the GDS, scores greater than 5 suggest possible depression and warrant follow-up. Scores greater than 10 are very sensitive for detecting syndromal depression.

Depression is usually assessed using self-report instruments of this sort, rather than clinical diagnostic interviews that allow for true diagnoses. This should be kept in mind when interpreting the diverse prevalence estimates of depression in older adults.

What then is the prevalence of depression in older people? A key consideration is what sort of older person: frail or hale, community resident or institutionalized, ascertained in a medical setting or not? Obviously, the prevalence of depression will be higher in people in medical settings or with extensive disability and chronic conditions than in a community sample of older people.

In one community study of people aged 65 and older, the Alameda County Study, 6.6% of men and 10.1% of women showed "symptoms of major depressive disorders." Once chronic conditions were controlled, the prevalence of depression of this severity did not increase with age. This is an important finding, consistent with what we have noted earlier. Depressive symptoms are much more closely associated with health status than with age. If the prevalence of depression appears to increase with age, it is entirely due to the increasing prevalence of chronic disease conditions with greater age (Roberts, Kaplan, Shema, & Strawbridge, 1997).

Compare this 5%–10% community prevalence with the much higher prevalence found in older outpatients. One study reported that 24% of an ambulatory care sample had "clinically significant depressive symptoms." However, even here, only 10% met criteria for major depressive disorder. Notably, only 1% of these people received treatment for a mental health problem (Borson et al., 1986).

The prevalence of depression in hospitalized and institutionalized older populations is even higher: 12%–45% in the hospital, and 15%–30% in skilled care facilities (Surgeon General, 1999). Likewise, the prevalence of depression in community-resident patients with the chronic diseases of late life is also quite high, 15%–20% in early Alzheimer's and perhaps 50% in Parkinson's disease.

MENTAL HEALTH IN A DISABLED OLDER POPULATION

The Women's Health and Aging Study, WHAS-I (Guralnik, Fried, Simonsick, Kasper, & Lafferty, 1995b) enrolled women with moderate to severe disability, representing the most disabled third of older women living in the community. Women were recruited from Medicare enrollee lists in the Baltimore, Maryland, area. Mental health in the sample was assessed with a variety of indicators, including the Geriatric Depression Scale (Yesavage et al., 1983), anxiety indicators from the Hopkins Symptom Checklist (Derogatis, Lipman, Riskels, Uhlenhuth, & Covi, 1974), the Perceived Quality of Life Scale (Patrick, Danis, Southerland, & Hong, 1988), and sense of control and efficacy from the Personal Mastery Scale (Pearlin & Schooler, 1978). The sample of over 1,000 women was divided into three age groups (65–74, 75–84, 85 and older) and three disability groups: women with "moderate disability" (limitations in upper extremity, lower extremity, or IADLs but no difficulty with ADLs), those with ADL difficulty without personal assistance, and those with ADL difficulty who received personal assistance.

Table 7.3 presents the mental health of women in WHAS-I. High levels of depressive symptoms, that is, symptomatology consistent with the clinical syndrome of major depression, were evident overall in 17.4% of the sample. Older people were less likely to report a high number of depressive symptoms: 14.3% of women aged 85 and older versus 18.6% of women aged 65–74. Disability, rather than age, was the stronger correlate. The proportion with symptomatology consistent with a diagnosis of depression was 13.1% in women with moderate limitations, 16.4% in women with ADL difficulty not receiving help, and 29.3% in women with ADL difficulty who received personal assistance.

Anxiety symptoms, unlike depression, increased with age: 2.8% in women aged 65–74, 4% in women aged 75–84, and 5.1% in women aged 85 and older. The relationship between disability and anxiety symptoms was less pronounced, increasing from 2.1% to 4.4% and 4.7% across disability severity categories.

Satisfaction with help received from family and friends was reported in approximately 80% of women, regardless of age or disability status (but note the gradient in satisfaction by severity of disability: 83.6%, 79.3%, and 74.8%). More pronounced are differences in the help these women feel they are able to provide to others. "Satisfaction with help

Table 7.3

MENTAL HEALTH INDICATORS: WOMEN'S HEALTH AND AGING STUDY, I

	AGE GROUP				DISABILITY STATUS		
	65-74	75-84	85+	MODERATE	ADL DIFFICULTY: NO HELP	ADL DIFFICULTY: HELP
High level of depressive symptomatology, %[a]	18.6	17.3	14.3	13.1	16.4	29.3
High level of anxiety, %[b]	2.8	4.0	5.1	2.1	4.4	4.7
Satisfied with help received from family & friends, %[c]	79.1	81.1	78.2	83.6	79.3	74.8
Satisfied with help you give to family & friends, %[c]	77.6	70.1	68.0	84.0	71.1	56.2
Satisfied with amount of variety in your life, %[c]	65.9	62.1	62.3	70.0	63.6	51.4
Satisfied with the meaning and purpose of your life, %[c]	76.4	75.8	75.7	79.7	74.8	72.1
I can do just about anything I really set my mind to do, % Strongly agree[d]	48.6	45.1	44.4	51.4	45.2	40.2
I feel helpless in dealing with the problems of life, % Strongly agree[d]	8.8	10.3	12.3	9.3	6.8	20.0

"Moderate disability": self-reported difficulty in two of three domains: upper extremity, lower extremity, or IADL.
Summarized from tables 8-1 through 8-5, "Lower-Extremity Function in Persons Over the Age of 70 Years as a Predictor of Subsequent Disability," by J. M. Guralnik, L. Ferrucci, E. M. Simonsick, M. E. Salive, & R. B. Wallace, 1995a. *New England Journal of Medicine, 332,* 556–561.
[a] High level of depressive symptomatology: Score ≥ 14, Geriatric Depression Scale, long form (Yesavage et al., 1983)
[b] High level of anxiety: maximum score ("extremely") on "felt nervous or shaky inside" during past week, Hopkins Symptom Checklist (Derogatis et al., 1974).
[c] Items from Perceived Quality-of-Life scale (Patrick et al., 1988).
[d] Items from Personal Mastery scale (Pearlin & Schooler, 1978).

provided to others" decreased from 84% in those with moderate limitations to 56.2% among women receiving assistance with ADL tasks.

"Satisfaction with variety in life" was also more strongly related to disability than age, approximately a 20% difference between women with moderate (70%) and severe disability (51.4%). But note also that half the women who received assistance with ADL tasks, and hence low scores on quality-of-life measures that emphasize function, still report satisfaction with variety in daily life. Note, too, that "satisfaction with the meaning and purpose of your life" was stable across age and disability categories; about three-quarters of these women, whatever their age or level of disability, reported satisfaction in this area.

Finally, this sample of women on the whole reported relatively low self-efficacy. Less than half reported confidence they could accomplish "anything I really set my mind to do." On the other hand, a minority of respondents reported "helplessness," less than 10% in the less severe disability groups and 20% in women receiving assistance with ADL tasks.

This inquiry suggests that disability has only a mild impact on mental health and general well being. This is an important result. Most of the women in this sample were able to maintain mental equipoise despite activity limitations. We should not underestimate the fundamental stability of mental health over the life span or the ability of older people to adapt to declines in the capacity to perform everyday activities.

OUTCOMES ASSOCIATED WITH MENTAL ILLNESS IN LATE LIFE

Depression in late life has been associated with an increased risk of mortality. The central question in this association is whether depression is a feature of disease and, for this reason, is artifactually associated with mortality, or whether depression is itself an independent risk factor for early death.

An accumulating set of evidence supports the latter hypothesis. For example, in the Cardiovascular Health Study (CHS), Schulz and colleagues showed that baseline depressive symptoms were associated with 6-year all-cause mortality in older persons (Schulz et al., 2000). The CHS consists of 5,201 people aged 65 and older from four communities across the United States. This study found a higher mortality rate (23.9%) in people with a greater number of depressive symptoms at baseline than in people with fewer depressive symptoms (17.7%). Depression in this study retained a significant association with mortality over 6 years of follow-up when controlling for sociodemographic factors, prevalent clinical disease, subclinical disease indicators at baseline, and biological or behavioral risk factors. In multivariate models that controlled for all of the factors, people with high depressive symptoms at baseline had a relative risk of 1.24 (95% CI, 1.06–1.46), about a 25% greater risk of mortality, compared with people with few or no depressive symptoms. Schulz (2000) suggests that "motivational depletion," lack of attention to self-care and treatment adherence and a more general loss of the will to live, may be responsible for this greater risk of death. Other research has confirmed this association, controlling as well for cognitive deficit (Rozzini, Sabatini, Frisoni, & Trabucchi, 2002).

Unutzer and colleagues (2002) reported a similar finding. They found that older adults with the most severe depressive symptoms had a significant increase in mortality risk, again after adjusting for demographics, health risk behaviors, and chronic medical disorders. The increased risk in mortality that was due to depression was comparable with mortality associated with such chronic medical disorders as emphysema and heart disease (Unutzer, Patrick, Marmon, Simon, & Katon, 2002b).

Mortality from suicide, in particular, is also a consequence of depression in late life. Suicide risk is highest in younger people and in people aged 85 and older. In fact, recent reports suggest that the highest suicide risk appears to be in White males aged 85 and older. The suicide rate for this group is 21 per 100,000, nearly twice the national rate of 10.6 per 100,000 (CDC, 2003).

One of the strongest tests of the clinical relevance of depression in older people is its role in predicting the onset of disability. In a review of 78 high-quality reports involving longitudinal studies (Stuck et al., 1999), depression was a consistently strong predictor of functional decline in older people. Depression predicted onset of activity limitations in studies that controlled for the presence of chronic conditions, behavioral risk factors, and cognitive status (Bruce, Seeman, Merrill, & Blazer, 1994). In one study, even the presence of depressive symptoms short of the severity or duration required for a diagnosis of depression ("subthreshold depression," described earlier) was a significant predictor of decline (Gallo, Rabins, Lyketos, Tien, & Anthony, 1997). Finally, there is also evidence that depressive symptoms are related to loss of underlying capacity in the pathway toward activity limitations (Penninx et al., 1998) (see Chapter 5).

These findings suggest that depression is a true cause of disability in older people, meeting many of the criteria for causality in epidemiology (Susser, 1997). Depressive symptoms can occur temporally prior to development of disability, appear to influence a link in the disablement pathway, and are consistently associated with disability across different age groups. Because treatment of depression is possible, this source of morbidity and disability should certainly be addressed in the care of the older person.

TREATMENT OF DEPRESSION IN LATE LIFE

We have already seen that depression is underappreciated and undertreated in older people, as it is younger people. The reasons for this neglect in late life are apparent from what we have already noted. The first reason has to do with the medical and psychosocial context of aging. Because most older people have a variety of medical conditions, it is tempting for physicians, families, and even elders themselves to assign symptoms of depression to these conditions. Similarly, it may be difficult, in some cases, to distinguish normal grief after the loss of a spouse, for example, from depression.

A second reason for underrecognition is the "softer" presentation of depressive symptoms, described above, and the greater prevalence of subthreshold disorders than of disease of accepted levels of clinical severity. The lack of affective symptoms in some cases, such as sadness, makes depression hard to diagnose for practitioners who do not have experience with geriatric mental health. The depressed elder may stress physical symptoms, reducing the likelihood of a mental health referral.

Finally, there is garden-variety ageism. Unfortunately, many providers and many older people themselves still think that misery is normal in late life. After all, the reasoning goes, late life is the time of decline in physical and mental health, so of course depression should be expected. This reasoning is absolutely fallacious, however, as we know from the studies of patients at the end of life. Depression is more common in terminal patients but far from universal. Even in these patients risk of depression appears to reflect life-long mental health more than illness and the dying process (Rabkin, Wagner, & Del Bene, 2000). Studies of people with severe neuromuscular disease approaching the end of life show only mild elevations in depressive diagnoses relative to primary care samples, and fewer than 20% express a wish to hasten dying (Albert et al., 2005; Rabkin et al., 2005). Most importantly, depression responds to treatment even in patients who are dying. Affective suffering should be considered a medical issue as significant as any other health indicator.

Treatment for depression in older people may rely on pharmacological agents, psychosocial interventions, or a combination of the two. Response rates in older people appear to be comparable with those in younger people, as both age groups respond in approximately 80% of cases (Surgeon General, 1999). However, older people may take longer to respond to therapy and may face a greater risk of relapse.

REDUCING THE RISK OF DEPRESSION AND ASSOCIATED MORBIDITY IN SENIORS

A pivotal randomized trial to improve outcomes among seniors with depression has provided important information on ways to reduce affective suffering in the primary care setting. PROSPECT (Prevention of Suicide in Primary Care Elderly-Collaborative Trial) examined whether a trained clinician can work in close collaboration with a primary care physician to implement comprehensive depression management and improve outcomes in older patients with depression (Mulsant et al., 2001). In PROSPECT, primary care practices in three regions were randomly assigned to either an intervention arm involving depression health specialists or an active control arm consisting of depression screening and assessment services without the health specialist. The choice of this control arm is important, because such screening and assessment is considered state-of-the-art but has been associated with high rates of suicide in older people related to untreated or undertreated depression.

One key outcome in the trial was "suicidal ideation," thoughts of suicide. Rates of suicidal ideation declined faster in intervention patients compared with usual-care patients. Resolution of suicidal ideation was faster among intervention patients. Intervention patients also had a more favorable course of depression relative to severity of symptoms and time to remission (Bruce et al., 2004). Further results revealed that the intervention offered more diffuse mental health benefits as well (Alexopoulos et al., 2005). Results from PROSPECT suggest that the integration of more active depression care in primary geriatric care is an important opportunity for addressing risk of depression and reducing morbidity from mental health disorders.

Another productive area for intercepting depression among seniors is to harness community-based agencies that provide aging services. These agencies have regular contact with vulnerable elders and are sometimes the only source of such contact. For example, virtually all aging services providers (see Chapter 3) provide social visiting or other "check-in" services, in which agency staff or volunteers call seniors who receive services to stay in contact and unobtrusively determine new needs. These kinds of contact may uncover mental health needs and could be harnessed explicitly for assessment of depressive symptoms and, when needed, referral. But the challenges of developing such programs are not trivial. How should staff or volunteers, who often lack mental health training, be trained? What kind of supporting staff needs to be attached to agencies in case of need for mental health services? What kind of referral pipeline would best link aging services providers to mental health services?

A number of such programs have recently been developed and assessed in randomized trials. Three have achieved status as evidence-based approaches, according to the National Council on Aging Services. It is instructive to look at each program to distinguish alternative approaches to assessment and service delivery.

■ PEARLS, the *P*rogram to *E*ncourage *A*ctive, *R*ewarding *L*ives for *S*eniors (Ciechanowski et al., 2004) is designed for seniors with subthreshold depression. It involves problem-solving treatment, social and physical activation, and potential recommendations to patients' physicians regarding antidepressant medications. Patients receiving the PEARLS intervention were more likely to have reduction in depressive symptoms and to achieve complete remission from depression than patients in a control education condition. They were also more likely to report improvements in health-related quality of life. The program is delivered by trained counselors in a participant's home, and the cost to implement PEARLS is approximately $630 per patient.

■ Healthy IDEAS (*I*dentifying *D*epression, *E*mpowering *A*ctivities for *S*eniors) (Quijano et al., 2007) delivers depression care through agency case managers who receive mental health training through the program. Depression care involves behavioral activation, promoting involvement in meaningful, positive activities. The start-up cost for an agency is approximately $2,500.

■ IMPACT (*I*mproving *M*ood-*P*romoting *A*ccess to *C*ollaborative *T*reatment for *L*ate *L*ife *D*epression) (Lin et al., 2003) uses a team approach designed to integrate treatment of depression within primary care. In the IMPACT model, a nurse, social worker, or psychologist works with the patient's regular primary care provider to develop a course of treatment. The cost of implementing IMPACT is approximately $500 per patient per year.

The three programs differ in their integration with medical providers, level of mental health training for agency staff, site of care, and combination of counseling and use of psychiatric medication. We are unaware of attempts to roll out these programs outside the confines of demonstrations or clinical trials. Thus, an important area for research would include investigation of the following issues:

- Whether treatment on site versus referral off site has greater benefit;
- How to tailor programs like IMPACT, designed for primary care, for social service agencies;
- How the organizational structures of agencies may lend themselves to different kinds of interventions;
- How sensitive and specific depression screening is in this setting;
- What sorts of follow-up are required to pre-empt depression among people who screen positive;
- How to ensure that mental health services offered by agencies are reimbursable; and
- How to build linkages between social service agencies and medical providers, such as federally qualified health clinics.

We anticipate increasing research and demonstration activity in this area, or perhaps a major community-based prevention trial that will harness aging services providers for this effort. This approach follows recommendations of the Institute of Medicine report, *Retooling for an Aging America* (2008), that emphasize the importance of new, flexible models to meet the public health burden of depression and other chronic illnesses in older Americans.

NEGLECT AND ABUSE

Victimization of older people takes many forms and extends across a continuum of behavior (Nerenberg, 2007). On one extreme of this continuum we might place neglect of the older adults, whether self-neglect or inattention to an elder's needs by others. On the other extreme, we might place active physical abuse and exploitation. Somewhere in the middle lies purposeful neglect designed to injure or coerce. These are often lumped within a single category of "mistreatment," which is defined differently across surveys. Adult Protective Services, municipal agencies defined to assess and intervene in the case of victimization of older people, define three forms of mistreatment (Lachs, Williams, O'Brien, & Pillemer, 2002):

> *Abuse:* Willful infliction of pain or mental anguish, or purposeful withholding of resources necessary to meet basic needs;
> *Neglect:* Failure of an elder to satisfy basic needs (food, shelter, medication management, medical care) either because of incompetence in the elder or because another person charged with care for the elder fails to meet these needs (abandonment, poor supportive care);
> *Exploitation:* Taking advantage of an elder to steal or dispossess the elder of money, wealth, or valued goods.

Over an 11-year period, the cumulative incidence of abuse in the New Haven component of the Established Populations for Epidemiologic Studies of the Elderly (EPESE) was 7.2% (202 of 2,802). These 202 people came to the attention of the Connecticut Ombudsman and Elderly Protective Services. Of the 202, 44 were verified as cases of abuse and 120 as cases of self-neglect; 38 were nonverified allegations. Thus, the incidence of abuse was 1.6% (44 of 2,802) and self-neglect was 4.3% (120 of 2,802) over this 11-year period. If we take the total incidence of 7.2% and convert it to a yearly estimate, the annual incidence is about 6.5 cases per 1,000 per year (.072/11 per 1,000). We can compare this estimate with the 32 per 1,000 reported in a random sample prevalence survey (Pillemer & Finkelhor, 1998). This suggests that about one in five cases of abuse, neglect, or exploitation comes to the attention of protective services.

A variety of research is now available on the correlates of elder mistreatment. Using the merged EPESE-protective services dataset described earlier, Lachs and colleagues have shown that elders referred to protective services were at an increased risk of mortality, a threefold increase in the case of abuse and nearly a twofold increase in the case of self-neglect (Lachs, Williams, O'Brien, Pillemer, & Charlson, 1998).

This excess risk was calculated in models that adjusted for many predictors of mortality, including sociodemographic characteristics, chronic disease status, functional and cognitive status, social networks, and depressive symptoms.

Elders referred to adult protective services also face an increased risk of nursing home placement. In the same EPESE cohort monitored for 11 years, 31.8% of elders not referred to protective services were admitted to skilled care facilities. In elders referred to protective services for abuse, the rate was 52.3%; and for elders referred for self-neglect, the rate was 69.2% (Lachs et al., 2002).

What factors predispose elders to mistreatment? In the case of self-neglect, key risk factors are cognitive impairment and depression, although one study identified additional risk associated with living alone, poverty, male gender, and a particular profile of chronic conditions, such as stroke and hip fracture (Abrams, Lachs, McAvay, Keohane, & Bruce 2002). Elder self-neglect is associated with poorer physical function (Dong, Mendes de Leon, & Evans, 2009), whereas abuse may be more highly associated with cognitive impairment (Cooper et al., 2009).

Thus, abuse and self-neglect involve both elder and family features. Elders with cognitive impairment and greater needs in care because of disability are more likely to be abused or experience neglect (and less likely to report it). Family caregivers with substance abuse problems, mental and physical health symptoms, lower socioeconomic status, and poor coping and caregiving skills are more likely to abuse vulnerable elders.

SOCIAL ISOLATION

One result of poor mental health is social isolation, which, in turn, is associated with poor outcomes in a variety of areas, including greater risk of suicide, poor medication management, inferior nutrition, overuse of laxatives and other over-the-counter medicines, and poor living environments (i.e., greater risk of exposure to extremes of heat and cold). The connection between comorbid disease, poor mental health, social isolation, and these additional negative outcomes has been called a "spiral of deterioration" (Alexopoulos et al., 2002).

Yet, it also seems that social isolation in itself is a risk factor for poor outcomes. In one study, for example, poor health, physical disability, and social isolation were all independently associated with depression. Once controlling for these factors, the association between depressive symptoms and lower socioeconomic status was no longer significant, leading the authors to suggest that "money cannot buy happiness" in older adults (West, Reed, & Gildengorin, 1998).

Social isolation and loneliness also increase the risk of nursing home admission, even when the effects of other predisposing factors (such as age, education, income, mental status, physical health, morale, and social contact) are controlled (Russell, Cutrona, de la Mora, & Wallace, 1997). Why should loneliness or social isolation predict nursing home admission? Russell and colleagues suggest that this association may indicate that some lonely and isolated older adults in this rural Iowa sample may have sought out nursing home admission as a strategy to gain social contact.

BROADER CONSIDERATIONS OF ENVIRONMENTAL INFLUENCES ON HEALTH

Exposure to extreme heat and cold causes more deaths among older people than the natural disasters that usually make the headlines, such as earthquakes and floods. An important study by Klinenberg (2004) shows the critical role of social isolation for risk of hyperthermia, that is, heat death. Isolation, which we usually think of as problems for individuals, turns out to depend heavily on features of communities. Findings from the Chicago heat wave described by Klinenberg have unfortunately been replicated in France, Italy, and other countries over the past two decades.

How many people died of hyperthermia as a result of the July 1995 Chicago heat wave? The answer is not an obvious one. The official heat-related death toll was 465 for July 14–20, the week where the heat reached its maximum, and 521 for the month as a whole. But this count depends on the integrity of case ascertainment and a particular definition of heat death. A more careful look at mortality for the week of July 14–20 relative to deaths in prior years showed an excess of 739 deaths among older people. This is the more likely toll of this terrible heat wave. Beyond mortality, we are unaware of studies that have quantified excess hospitalizations, emergency room visits, or other morbidities in the weeks of the heat wave.

Mortality among older adults was not uniform across socioeconomic status or community residence. Victims were primarily older, poorer, African American, and isolated. In age-adjusted analyses, three

African American elders died for every two Whites, just as men were more likely to die than women. Figure 7.3 shows mortality by race, stratifying by age. Among people aged 85 and older, nearly twice as many African Americans were likely to die compared with Whites.

Klinenberg (2004) reviews the many arguments city and health officials made to explain this disparity. Differences in individual health status, such as the presence of cardiovascular disease, is one possibility. And, indeed, CDC case-control studies did note that cardiovascular disease was more prevalent among decedents relative to age-matched elders living in the same buildings. But this does not account for the racial difference. Socioeconomic factors are also likely to be relevant, but Klinenberg shows that similarly impoverished communities did not bear the same brunt of heat mortality. For example, North and South Lawndale, contiguous communities with equal proportions of both older people and older people living below the poverty level, differed by a factor of 10 in heat deaths. The difference, Klinenberg argues, is in community social capital, of health resources related to social ties. South Lawndale's predominantly Latino community was economically vibrant, less crime-ridden, more densely populated, and had active civic organizations. North Lawndale, predominantly African American, stood out among Chicago communities for loss of population over the prior 30 years, crime, decaying housing stock and, most critically,

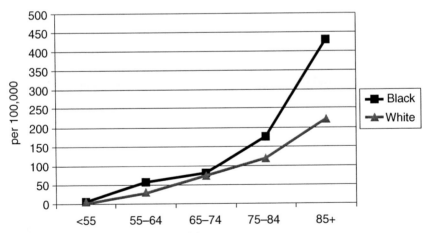

Figure 7.3 Heat mortality: Chicago, 1995.

Source: From *Heat Wave: A Social Autopsy of Disaster in Chicago,* by E. Klinenberg, 2004, Chicago: University of Chicago Press.

absence of economic activity and civic organization. Isolated elders in North Lawndale were most at risk of heat death. They lived in fear of crime and nailed windows shut. They feared opening doors to city social workers sent to check up on them. Even if they ventured outside, they had no place to go because there were few stores, parks, or community gathering places to seek cooler air or information about services. Most critically, they had no one to check up on them as part of the normal course of daily life.

As with this contrast in communities, so went the city. Figures 7.4 and 7.5 show the relationship between risk of heat death among older people and broad macrosociological factors, such as proportion of population lost over the prior 30 years and crime rank. We plot the position of the 12 communities with the highest heat mortality and the 12 with the lowest. The patterns are striking. Weak neighborhoods lead to greater risk of isolation, which in turn increases the risk of a wide variety of negative health outcomes, including risk of heat death. The Chicago heat

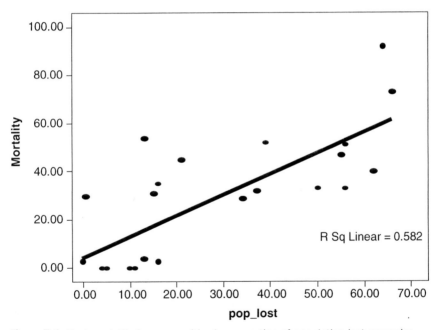

Figure 7.4 Heat mortality in communities by proportion of population lost over prior 30 years.

Note: Twenty-four communities with lowest and highest heat mortality deaths.
Source: From *Heat Wave: A Social Autopsy of Disaster in Chicago*, by E. Klinenberg, 2004, Chicago: University of Chicago Press.

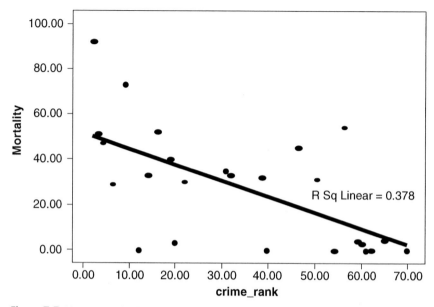

Figure 7.5 Heat mortality in Chicago communities by Community Crime Rank

Note: Twenty-four communities with lowest and highest heat mortality deaths.
Source: From *Heat Wave: A Social Autopsy of Disaster in Chicago*, by E. Klinenberg, 2004, Chicago: University of Chicago Press.

deaths make clear the health protective properties of social networks and more diffuse community solidarity.

These aspects of social capital are an active area of research in aging and public health. Social capital may be involved in quite distal health processes, such as likelihood of recovery from coronary disease (Scheffler et al., 2008). Similarly, measures of community integration that appear quite remote from health processes, such as the proportion of people in a community performing volunteer service, may turn out to be critical resources for healthy aging. Even more striking, what we see in risk of heat death or other extreme health events may apply to a far more general range of health behavior and outcome. Wight and colleagues (2006) used data from the Health and Retirement Survey, merged with community ecological indicators (i.e., census tract indicators of median levels of education or income) to show that community status and individual cognitive health are related. Levels of community educational attainment, apart from individual education, may explain variance in MMSE scores. This relationship is shown in Figure 7.6.

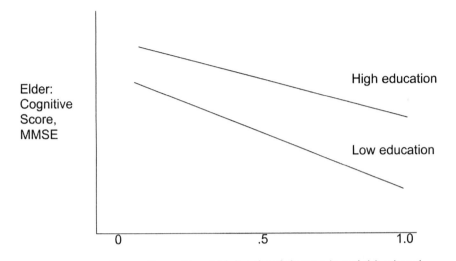

Proportion without high school degree in neighborhood

Figure 7.6 Neighborhood effects on relationship between individual education and cognitive performance.

Source: Adapted from "Urban Neighborhood Context, Educational Attainment, and Cognitive Function Among Older Adults," by R. G. Wight, C. S. Aneshensel, D. Miller-Martinez, A. L. Botticello, J. R. Cummings, A. S. Karlamangla, et al., 2006, *American Journal of Epidemiology, 163*, 1071–1978.

The proportion of people in a community with a high school education helped predict individual MMSE performance independently of individual education. Thus, although people with greater education performed better on the test, people with the same educational achievement did better if they lived in communities where most people had completed high school. Wight et al. (2006) advance a number of potential explanations. Low-education communities have (a) greater exposure to chronic stressors and low social resources that hinder engagement in physical and cognitive activities (walking places, social support); (b) fewer cognitively stimulating or supportive resources (physicians, libraries), and (c) higher tolerance for illness and untreated chronic disease that may affect cognition. These are productive areas for further research and suggest that community-level interventions to improve social resources may offer strong benefit to elder cognitive and physical health.

SUMMARY

Burden of Mental Illness. The effect of mental disorders on daily life should not be underestimated, in the young as in the old. By any measure, whether a national estimate of lost productivity or reports of daily symptoms, mental illness is as debilitating as physical illness.

Presentation and Prevalence of Mental Health Symptoms in Late Life. Mental health symptoms appear to change with older age. In later life, depressive disorders fulfilling diagnostic criteria are relatively rare; "subthreshold disorders" are more common. Subthreshold depression, for example, includes symptoms of depression that are not severe, frequent, or disruptive enough to be labeled as clinical depression. In the National Health Interview Survey, 2000, less than 2% of people aged 65 and older reported "serious psychological distress," less than half that reported by people aged 45–64. However, evidence is now available to suggest that subthreshold depression is a risk factor for poor outcomes, including declining function, increased disability, cognitive impairment, and death.

Mental Health in an Older Population With Disability. In the most limited subsample of women in WHAS-I, mental health is related to severity of disability, but mental health is, on the whole, well preserved. This speaks to adaptation in late life and psychological resiliency, and reminds us again that mental and physical health are separate but related spheres.

Outcomes Associated with Mental Illness in Late Life. The Cardiovascular Health Study showed that people with pronounced depressive symptoms were at risk for higher mortality (23.9% versus 17.7% in people with few depressive symptoms). This finding persisted when analyses controlled for other factors that increase mortality risk. Similar findings have been reported for depression, and risk of disability, cognitive decline, nursing home placement, suicide, and a host of other negative public health outcomes.

Treatment of Depression in Late Life. Evidence suggests that older people respond to treatment at rates comparable with younger people, although differences in metabolism, polypharmacy, and the presence of other chronic conditions complicate treatment. A major obstacle is an ageist expectation that affective suffering is a part of late age and frailty.

Neglect and Abuse. Despite difficulty in defining these domains, it is now clear that self-neglect is more common than outright abuse, that the most vulnerable older adults are most often victims, and that both forms of mistreatment have major public health consequences.

Social Isolation. Older people desire less novelty in social life than younger people do and may be more comfortable with a smaller set of friends. Yet isolation is a public health issue to the extent it is associated with medication misuse, poor nutrition, and greater risk of depression and suicide.

Broader Considerations of Environmental Influences on Health. Social capital, the health benefit associated with social networks and strong communities, may have powerful effects on health risk at old ages, ranging from risk of heat death to cognitive performance.

Aging, Public Health, and Application of the Quality-of-Life Paradigm

8

Research on "quality of life" actually involves two distinct domains, which unfortunately are not always clearly distinguished (Albert, 1997; Albert & Teresi, 2002; Spilker & Revicki, 1999). One domain is *health-related quality of life*, or more simply, "health status assessment," which emerged from efforts to develop measures of disease impact that would be useful across a variety of clinical trial and program evaluation settings. The other is not a health measure but rather an indication of the effect of personal resources or environmental factors on daily experience. This might be called *nonhealth* or *environment-based quality of life*. This second set of measures emerged from efforts to identify community-level indicators of well-being and belongs to the "social indicators" or "social ecology" research tradition.

Maintaining this distinction is important. Health-related quality-of-life domains—older adults' reports of functioning, discomfort, pain, energy levels, social engagement—will track more closely with clinical measures of disease status than non-health-related QOL indicators, such as the capacity to form friendships, appreciate nature, or find satisfaction in spiritual or religious life. The latter are also quality-of-life domains, and severe health limitation will ultimately affect these as well, but they are less related to clinical indicators of health. Health-related QOL will therefore be correlated with clinical indicators, whereas non-health-related personal or environmental indicators of QOL may or may not be.

Recognizing this distinction eliminates much of the confusion about the "idiosyncracy" or instability of QOL ratings (Leplege & Hunt, 1997). In this chapter, we briefly define the two quality-of-life fields and assess their relevance for research on public health and aging.

This inquiry is important because gains in quality of life remain a key objective of *Healthy People 2010.* "Healthy People 2010 focuses on how changes in health status and activity limitations affect Americans at the population level."(*Healthy People 2010*, Executive Summary). Indicators of quality of life used in Healthy People 2010 include:

- Self-assessments of overall health status by individuals or their proxies.
- Composite measures that include multiple dimensions of health.
- Measures that combine death rates and health, such as years of healthy life.

Other QOL measures that appear in *Healthy People 2010* include "expected years in good or better health," "expected years free of activity limitation," and "expected years free of selected chronic diseases."

In a first look at these indicators using data from 2001–2002, individuals in the United States could expect to live 68.6 years in good or better health, 65.5 years without activity limitation, and 47.5 years without selected chronic diseases. Expected years in good or better health and expected years free of activity limitations appear to be increasing, but expected years free of selected chronic diseases may be declining (see Chapters 4 and 5).

These measures, although imperfect in many ways, will likely continue to be important as indicators of population health, useful for tracking trends over time and for comparing national health systems. For this reason it is useful to examine the foundations of these measures.

IDENTIFICATION OF QOL DOMAINS

Health-related QOL encompasses domains of life directly affected by changes in health. Jaeschke, Singer, and Guyatt (1989) provide a good thumbnail test of whether a domain falls within the category of health-related QOL. They ask, if a patient is successfully treated by a physician, what aspects of his or her life are likely to improve? These are health-related QOL domains. In other words, if a patient reports changes in status that lead a care provider to seek a different medication or a change in a care environment, these changes are likely to fall within the realm of health-related QOL (Berzon, Leplege, Lohr, Lenderking, & Wu, 1997).

What features of daily life or changes in status are likely to be medically relevant in this sense, and hence count as health-related QOL? Obvious candidates include *functional status* (i.e., disability, whether a patient is able to manage a household, use the telephone, or dress independently); *mental health, affective status, or emotional well-being* (i.e., depressive symptoms, positive affect); *social engagement* (i.e., involvement with others, engagement in activities); and *symptom states* (i.e., pain, shortness of breath, visual acuity, fatigue).

Non-health-related QOL domains, by contrast, include features of the natural and built environment (such as economic resources, housing, air and water quality, community stability, access to the arts and entertainment), as well as personal resources (such as the capacity to form friendships, appreciate nature, or find satisfaction in spiritual or religious life). These factors clearly affect quality of life but, unlike health-related QOL domains, are less likely to be the target of medical care.

The two components of QOL differ in other ways as well. Non-health-related QOL is more heterogeneous, with less consensus about the range of domains that should be included in the measure. For example, consider a health-related QOL state. No one would suggest that severe abdominal pain is preferred to a runny nose. The question is how much better. In fact, research on ratings of the severity of health conditions are remarkably consistent across age groups and in cross-national research (Patrick, Sittampalam, Somerville, Carter, & Bergner, 1986), although people with disease conditions appear to rate their health-related QOL somewhat higher than nonpatients asked to rate the same health state (Torrance, 1987). Consensus of this sort is harder to establish for spirituality, friendship, or access to the arts.

As an illustration, consider the question, "on a scale of 1–100, how would you rate your health today?" One of us (SA) has fielded this question with over 10 classes of students studying quality-of-life assessment. Each class has 12–15 students with a mean age of about 25. Students are not given a definition of health. Remarkably, each replication produces approximately the same mean and standard deviation, 85 ± 8. The range is typically from 65–70 to 99 (very rarely does someone give himself or herself a perfect score). How can this be? At least among a healthy sample attending universities, we share the same bodies (more or less), same experience of symptoms and wellness (more or less), and same appreciation of the disabling quality of symptoms.

It is valuable to obtain information on both health- and environment-related QOL, but health-related QOL has received more attention in public health efforts involving older adults for several reasons. First, older people are at risk for chronic conditions, and effective disease management in large part consists of finding treatments that minimize the QOL impact of disease. Second, measurement efforts for health-related QOL are further advanced than efforts related to non-health-related QOL. Finally, although housing, air quality, and other components of the environment are clearly important features of QOL, such factors cannot be addressed easily by a clinician, but instead require attention at the community level. However, it is important to recognize the link between the two. Lawton (1991) reminds us that the two are sometimes hard to separate: successful treatment by a physician may improve one's capacity to make friends, for example.

As mentioned earlier, health-related QOL as a field of inquiry emerged from research on "health status." Early measures, such as the Sickness Impact Profile (SIP) (Bergner, Bobbit, Pollard, Martin, & Gleason, 1976), sought to identify common domains affected by disease that would allow clinicians to gauge the impact of diverse clinical conditions. This goal was a major motivation of development of more recent measures as well, such as the Medical Outcomes Study (MOS) short-form QOL questionnaires (Stewart et al., 1989) and FACT battery (Cella & Bonomi, 1996).

A key element of the SIP, and also of almost all QOL measures that have followed, is that patients themselves rate how impaired they are. This subjective element is the essential feature of health-related QOL, for who can better report on the QOL impact of a medical condition than the patient (Gill & Feinstein, 1994)? Indeed, health-related QOL is sometimes called "patient-reported outcomes" (PRO) to stress this subjective focus. The SIP identified 12 health-related QOL domains: ambulation, mobility, body care and movement, communication, alertness behavior, emotional behavior, social interaction, sleep and rest, eating, work, home management, and recreation. The MOS identified a different set of domains: health perception, pain, physical function, social function, mental health, role limitation from physical causes, and role limitation from mental health causes. Others, such as the Health Utilities Index (HUI), stress still different domains; in this case, a "within the skin" approach to health status, that is, domains that are more closely connected to clinical conditions. Thus, the HUI Mark II measure includes sensation, mobility, emotion, cognition, self-care, pain, and fertility (Feeny, Furlong, Boyle, & Torrance, 1995).

Apart from differences in the specification of QOL domains, the measures also differ in the ways they are used to derive a global health state or health-related QOL score. In the MOS, for example, domains are grouped according to their primarily "physical" or "mental" health basis, as established in factor analysis. Pain, physical function, and role limitation-physical form a "physical health component," and mental health and role limitation-emotional form a "mental health component." Scores within each set of domains are aggregated. Keeping the two separate as distinct indicators or dimensions of health-related QOL is appropriate because studies show that the correlation between mental and physical health is about 0.50, only a moderate correlation.

Other measures cross-walk health states and respondent-rated global reports to derive a single score. For example, the EuroQOL (Dolan, Gudex, Kind, & Williams, 1996) contains five domains (mobility, self-care, usual activity, pain/discomfort, and anxiety/depression), each with three levels. If each combination of the five domains were a distinct state, even this simple five-domain categorization would generate, 3^5 or 243 unique groupings. Not all of these combinations are possible (for example, it is impossible to be "confined to bed" on the mobility dimension and have "no problems with self-care" on the self-care dimension). After eliminating these empirically null states, a more manageable (but still large) number remain. Global scores can be assigned to the states by having respondents with the state rate their global health on a visual analog scale (ranging from 0 to 100). More complicated generation of global scores from QOL domains is also possible. In the HUI, each domain is weighted, and global scores reflect the combination of domain weightings and levels reported for each domain. Still other approaches obviate the need for deriving global scores by having respondents rate themselves directly, for example, on a visual analog scale ranging from 0 to 100.

Interest in assigning scores to subjective reports of health-related QOL draws on early research in psychophysics. Early on, psychologists noted that ratings of a subjective state (e.g., pain) corresponded to the intensity of a stimulus (e.g., increasingly cold temperature). These investigations suggested that subjective ratings were reliably associated with objective states. Thus, to return to our earlier example, people consistently give a worse score abdominal pain on a measure of discomfort or interference with work to "severe abdominal pain" than to "runny nose." The challenge is to determine how much worse.

In fact, large-sample investigations have allowed researchers to estimate how much worse one state is relative to another. For example, suppose we establish two numeric anchors: 1.0 for the state of no symptoms/no daily limitations and 0.0 for death (recognizing, however, that some people consider certain health states, such as coma or intractable pain, as states worse than death). Kaplan's Quality of Well-Being/General Health Policy Model (Kaplan & Anderson, 1996) subtracts 0.17 for the state of "runny nose"; thus, someone with a runny nose alone is at approximately 83% of optimal health. "Sick or upset stomach, vomiting" is associated with a subtraction score of −0.29; someone with this condition alone would therefore be at approximately 71% of optimal health. The difference between the two ratings is a measure of how much worse "abdominal pain" is compared with "runny nose." These numerical ratings are derived from respondents who rated descriptions of a wide variety of health states, but who often did not necessarily experience those states first hand. Nevertheless, such ratings are used to establish the impact of one health state compared with another in terms of health-related QOL.

The underlying metric for these evaluations is abstract. It is essentially a measure of how preferred or "dispreferred" one health state is relative to another, in other words, a "utility." An alternative tradition in QOL measurement avoids specification of numeric values on such an underlying dimension. This tradition relies on experiential indicators of morbidity or disability. Thus, Sullivan (1966) early on developed an index of morbidity, or health state, based on disability. Living arrangement (nursing home or community), severity of mobility impairment, ability to perform major age-appropriate roles (school, work, home maintenance, personal self-maintenance), and limitation in usual, daily activities formed a natural hierarchy of disability. This mutually exclusive classification generates five health-impact or QOL states, ranging from institutional residence at one end to community residence without disability or limitation in daily activities at the other.

Another approach intermediate between these two is to seek a single, common measure of health impact in terms of some other dimension of daily life. These dimensions include time use (Albert & Logsdon, 2001; Moss & Lawton, 1982), mood states (Larson, Zuzanek, & Mannell, 1993), or mental health stress (Testa & Simonson, 1996). The Behavioral Risk Factors Surveillance System (BRFSS) used by the Centers for Disease Control adopts this approach. It relies on reports of "not good health days," days when a component of health is adversely affected (Hennessey, Moriarty, Scherr, & Brackbill, 1994; CDC, 2000). Respondents are asked, "Thinking of the past 30 days, how many days were there when your physical health was not good?" Other questions ask about mental health, sleep, energy, anxiety, and related domains in the same format. This approach allows a conjoint measure of "healthy days" (30 minus the sum of "not good physical health days" and "not good mental health days") (Hennessey et al., 1994), which can serve as a global health-related QOL indicator. Thus, someone reporting 3 not good physical health and 4 not good mental health days would have a total of 7 not good days, or 23 healthy days. (Following BRFSS conventions, we adopt the conservative approach of a sum, allowing that the same day may have been a "not good" day in both physical and mental health.) Someone reporting this profile over the last month would have a global QOL score of 23/30 (0.77), or 77% of optimal health-related QOL.

The Centers for Disease Control and Prevention has assessed healthy days in the period 1993–2007 in its Behavioral Risk Factors Surveillance System. These repeated cross-sectional surveys show slight increases in unhealthy mental health days over the past 15 years but stability in physical health and activity limitation. To get a feel for the quality-of-life impact of aging (that is, the effect of the accumulation of chronic disease and increasing senescence), we can compare people aged 18–24 with those aged 75 and older. The proportion reporting 14 or more "not good" physical health days in the past 30 days (or 2 weeks over the past month) was 20% among people age 75 and older and 4% among people aged 18–24. The proportion reporting 14 or more days of activity limitation was 10% among people aged 75 and older and 4% among people aged 18–24. By contrast, the proportions are reversed for mental health days; 6% of older people and 11% of younger people report 14 or more days of not good mental health (see Chapter 7).

The different approaches converge on a common normative question. Can we determine *how much* better life is at a higher level of health than at a lower level? Or, more starkly, how much better than death is a state of compromised health? Patrick and Erickson (1993) stress these questions when they define health-related QOL as "the *value* assigned to the duration of life, as modified by impairment" (page 22, emphasis added). The goal of measurement of health-related QOL is first to define health states, that is, to develop measures that capture the impact of changes in health. The second goal is to assign plausible numeric indicators for such changes. Although this second task may seem difficult, and even inappropriate, people already express preferences for different health states and in doing so implicitly assign values to health changes. People evaluate symptom states every day and make treatment decisions based on their judgment of the likely impact of treatment or nontreatment. The QOL paradigm attempts to formalize this process.

It is also worth noting what the QOL paradigm does not assess. Health-related QOL measures do not tell us what puts quality into life. They have the much more limited goal of establishing the effect of changes in health on everyday life. Nor do QOL measures tell us anything about the value of life, or what makes someone attached to living. We know that many people with very low scores on QOL measures find life satisfying and meaningful. For example, they may score very high on measures of mental health despite very severe limitations in physical status. Or they may even score poorly on physical and mental health measures and yet still express strong attachment to life. The QOL score only specifies the degree of *health impact*. It is not a measure of attachment to life or the perceived value of life.

As a final illustration of the position of QOL domains relative to other indicators of health, it is worth comparing clinical outcomes with health-related QOL outcomes. Take, for example, a randomized clinical trial in cancer therapy. Clinical outcomes for this trial would include survival time, disease-free survival time, tumor response, and perhaps treatment-associated toxicities (which together might be used to generate a "Q-Twist measure," time without symptoms or toxicity). By contrast, QOL outcomes for this trial would capture the effects of treatment and disease on someone's ability to function in everyday life, which might include productivity at work, independence in self-care tasks, emotional stability, and engagement in valued activities. Ware and Stewart (1992) summarize the differences this way: "Clinical measures of functioning do not characterize human functioning well. They reveal little about how well the individual functions in everyday life or how that person feels, both of which are affected by disease and treatment."

CLINICAL SIGNIFICANCE OF QOL MEASURES

How much must a QOL indicator change for us to be confident that an intervention has produced a meaningful improvement in patient status? Lydick and Epstein (1993) remind us that this question is a problem for all clinical research, not just research in health-related QOL. They describe a therapy for benign prostatic hypertrophy that increased urine flow 3 ml/sec compared with urine flow in a placebo group. By itself, this effect is hard to interpret. Could this degree of change fall within normal variability? This question became clear only when an epidemiologic study showed that urine flow rates decline 0.2–0.3 ml/sec per year of life. A 3-ml/sec improvement is thus equivalent to about 15 years of "urinary aging." Thus, an improvement of 3 ml/sec is indeed a clinically meaningful change.

An alternative way to establish clinical significance in this case would have been to ask men with slower urine flow rates if urination is a problem for them. Do men with slower urine flow rates find urination more uncomfortable, more time-consuming, or more embarrassing? Are men who differ by 3 ml/sec or more in urine flow more likely to report such problems? This would be an alternative indicator of clinical significance and may be required for definitive proof of clinical significance, even in the presence of age differences in urinary flow.

These thoughts suggest a view of clinical significance in terms of a "minimal clinically significant difference" (Jaeschke et al., 1989). This, as we stated above, is a change in patient-reported status that would lead a care provider to seek a different medication or a change in a care environment. Otherwise stated, these are changes that would lead a clinician to make a change in patient management ("in the absence of troublesome side effects and excessive cost"). Again, patient behavior is a good guide here. If patients report such changes to a clinician, and the clinician is not impressed enough to alter management, patients are apt to go elsewhere.

To identify this minimal clinically significant difference, we can rely on distribution-based statistical tests or external criteria to anchor these differences. The basic distribution-based test to assess clinical significance is effect size. This approach examines the importance of a change by comparing the magnitude of the change in some measure with variability in the measure in a group at baseline, before implementation of the intervention. This ratio gives an indication of change over and above normal variation.

Anchor-based indicators are probably more useful for establishing the clinical significance of changes in QOL measures. The most obvious anchor is the patient's global rating of change in quality of life (Jaeschke et al., 1989). That is, do patients who report improvements of a certain magnitude in a particular QOL domain (for example, pain or fatigue) also report improvements in global quality of life or well being? The minimal clinically significant difference in the pain or fatigue measure would be the score change associated with a difference in the global rating. The global rating of cognitive change mentioned in Chapter 7 follows this line of reasoning and is used to anchor changes in cognitive test performance.

Other anchors include life events or mental health stress. These are perhaps most useful for measures of mental health. A mental health score difference of 3 points, for example, was shown to be equivalent to the effect of a major life event, such as losing a job. Testa and Simonson (1996) have generalized this approach.

But the most straightforward and perhaps most meaningful anchor for assessing changes in quality of life may be age. Given age-related declines in function and increases in chronic conditions, age provides a natural metric for assessing the QOL effects of clinical interventions. If we know that an intervention improves quality of life by 5% on some scale, and also that a 5% difference is typical of two age strata (say, ages 75 and 80) for this measure, then the intervention is associated with a 5-year "reduction" in age. To establish clinical significance requires that we have QOL or clinical norms for different age groups, which are not always available. Still, age offers a natural scale for this sort of investigation, as we show below.

THE QUALITY-OF-LIFE PARADIGM IN AGING

Introduction of a quality-of-life focus in research on aging was pioneered by Katz et al. (1963) and Lawton (Lawton & Brody, 1969; Lawton, 1991), with their focus on functional status and behavior, which is now universal in gerontology and geriatrics. Lawton summarized the QOL emphasis for care of older people very well when he wrote, "function and behavior, rather than diagnosis, should determine the service to be prescribed" (Lawton & Brody, 1969). The common, final pathway of different diseases is their impact on functional ability and other domains of QOL; thus, the focus in later life should be development of strategies, both clinical and environmental, to minimize these effects and work with the strengths that older people continue to retain.

However it is measured, health-related QOL declines with age. This is a central, inescapable consequence of the increased prevalence of chronic disease with greater age and the effects of senescent changes in many physiological domains. Senescence, as we have seen, is evident in a variety of changes across biological systems: for example, declines in working memory, psychomotor speed, touch sensibility, vision, and hearing; loss of skeletal muscle and strength; and reduction in joint range of motion. These changes affect health-related QOL: for example, pain in arthritic joints leads to circumscription of choice in daily activities; lower-extremity weakness means difficulty climbing stairs or standing up long enough to prepare a meal; and slowing of psychomotor skills may mean inability to drive safely. Older people adjust their daily lives to accommodate these decrements, and adjustment strategies may reduce the effects of such decrements on health-related QOL.

Still, cross-sectional studies show strong declines in health-related QOL with increasing age. The effect of age on the "healthy days" measure of the BRFSS, described above, is shown in Table 8.1. The mean number of days over the past month in which respondents reported problems with physical health increases monotonically with age, from 1.8 in the 18- to 24-year-old group to 6.2 in people aged 75 and older. Differences are small between the younger adjacent age strata (1.8 vs. 2.1 in people aged 18–24 and 25–44, respectively). These differences increase in later ages, from 3.5 in people aged 45–64, to 4.7 in people aged 65–74, and finally to 6.2 in the oldest age group.

Mental health shows the opposite trend, consistent with results from Chapter 7. The youngest group reports the greatest number of "not good" mental health days, 3.4 of the last 30 days, and this number declines with age until it reaches its low, 1.9, among people aged 75 and older.

The composite "healthy days" measure declines from 25.1 in the youngest age group to 23.0 in the oldest. Using the convention described above, these values represent global health-related QOL values of 83.7 and 76.7 on a scale of 0–100, a fairly small difference. As an indicator of clinical significance, people (of all ages) unable to work because of a health condition reported a mean of 10.7 healthy days, or 35.7 on the same transformed 0–100 scale.

An alternative indicator of the effect of age on health-related QOL is the "well year" equivalent developed by the National Center for Health Statistics to track progress toward the *Healthy People 2000* goal of increasing active life expectancy (Erickson, Wilson, & Shannon, 1995). This measure uses two items from the National Health Interview Survey (NHIS) to define QOL states. Self-ratings of health (excellent, very good, good, fair, poor) are cross-classified with self-reports of activity

Table 8.1

HEALTHY DAYS BY AGE, BEHAVIORAL RISK FACTORS SURVEILLANCE
SYSTEM (BRFSS), 1993

AGE GROUP	N	GOOD HEALTH DAYS	NOT GOOD PHYSICAL HEALTH DAYS	NOT GOOD MENTAL HEALTH DAYS
18–24	4,279	25.1	1.8	3.4
25–44	19,756	25.2	2.1	3.1
45–64	11,445	24.6	3.5	2.8
65–74	4,975	24.2	4.7	1.9
75+	3,064	23.0	6.2	1.9

Data based on 21 states and District of Columbia. "Not good days" represent mean number of days in the last 30 where component of health was "not good." "Good health days" is the subtraction of sum of "not good physical and mental health days" from 30, with the restriction that this sum cannot be negative. From "Current Trends Quality of Life as a New Public Health Measure," *Morbidity and Mortality Weekly Report,* May 27, 1994, p. 378.

limitation (not limited, limited in some activity but not major activity, limited in major activity, unable to perform major activity, limited in IADL, and limited in ADL). Self-reported health serves as a subjective global summary of health, whereas self-rated activity limitation reflects a more clearly behavioral indicator of health and performance. The 5 × 6 cross-classification yields 30 QOL states, ranging from the state of excellent health with no activity limitation to the state of poor health with ADL limitation.

The weaknesses of this approach are many: for instance, the measure does not contain a mental or cognitive component (except insofar as they figure in to global ratings of health) and it does not contain information on the many domains that go into people's ratings of their health and participation in activity. Still, as a blunt summary measure, it offers the advantage of brevity, broad application, and availability from a large, national survey. Every American can be assigned to one of the 30 states based on answers to the two questions. The distribution of the American population in 1990 across the 30 QOL states is shown in Table 8.2.

The largest proportion of Americans assigned themselves to the state of excellent health and no activity limitation, 38.1%. Another 26.3% and

Table 8.2

PERCENTAGE OF PERSONS IN THE CIVILIAN NONINSTITUTIONALIZED U.S. POPULATION, BY HEALTH STATE DEFINED IN TERMS OF ACTIVITY LIMITATION AND PERCEIVED HEALTH STATUS, NHIS, 1990

ACTIVITY LIMITATION	PERCEIVED HEALTH STATUS				
	EXCELLENT	VERY GOOD	GOOD	FAIR	POOR
Not Limited	38.1	26.3	18.2	3.3	0.3
Limited: Other	0.6	1.1	1.8	1.3	0.4
Limited: Major	0.5	0.7	1.3	0.7	0.2
Unable: Major	0.1	0.2	0.5	0.6	0.5
Limited in IADL	0.1	0.2	0.5	0.6	0.6
Limited in ADL	<0.1	0.1	0.2	0.3	0.5

18.2% assigned themselves to the no activity limitation category but with "very good" and "fair" health, respectively. The next largest group, 3.3% assigned themselves to the no activity limitation category but with "fair" health. Thus, these four health states accounted for 85.9% of the American population. This distribution is welcome to the extent that it indicates high health-related QOL among a large majority of Americans. It is unwelcome, however, from a measurement point of view. It suggests that the "no activity limitation" anchor for this dimension does not differentiate QOL states well. That is, large proportions of people with vastly different ratings of health all endorse "no limitation" in activity. This suggests a ceiling effect in the activity limitation dimension, that is, the need for additional differentiation of the state of "no activity limitation."

Note in Table 8.2 that each of the other states contains less than 2%, and in most cases less than 1%, of the U.S. population. The category of poor health and ADL limitation, is endorsed by just 0.5%. Because the NHIS excludes institutional populations, this, as we have seen, is an underestimate of the proportion of people with low health-related QOL. Note, too, the off-diagonal cells (left- and rightmost corner cells of the table). A very small number, less than 0.1%, rate their health as excellent yet report maximum limitation in activity, that is, limitation in ADL; 0.3% report poor health yet no limitation in activity. Are these QOL states possible, or should we assume error in people's answers? Can we imagine scenarios in which these answers would be plausible?

The small number who rate their health as excellent yet report maximum limitation in activity may include people with severe disability but nonprogressive disease, such as the quadriplegic who relies on personal assistance but is able to work in an adapted environment. On the other hand, this person may also be among those reporting no activity limitation. The group reporting poor health yet no limitation in activity may represent people forced to be active despite their poor health, the "obligatorily active" (Draper & Harpending, 1990). Or this group may truly face no current limitation in activity but face a poor prognosis in the near future, such as persons whose cancer was diagnosed recently.

We can assess the effect of age on the likelihood of falling into one or another of these categories by re-examining Table 8.2, limiting the cross-classification this time to people in the oldest age groups. Table 8.3 presents a similar table for people aged 85 and older. Remember that these older people are also community-resident, which is true for the NHIS sample generally, and therefore not representative of the oldest old (see below).

We see a great migration to cells downward and to the right, reflecting an increased prevalence of poorer health-related QOL. In 1990, only 7% of the community-resident 85 and older population fell within the category of excellent health status and no activity limitation. Almost as many, 6.5%, fell into the category at the other extreme (poor health-ADL limited). Note that the same ceiling effect demonstrated for all ages is apparent in self-reports from the oldest old: people with very different self-rated health states were still all able to endorse the "no activity limitation" category. Overall, among people aged 85 and older all the health states were well populated. The modal health state was "good health-no activity limitation," rather than "excellent health-no activity limitation," which was the modal state in the population as a whole.

Researchers have extended the 30-state model by assigning QOL values or utilities to each state, shown here as Table 8.4. The most healthful state was assigned 1.0, the least healthy state 0.10, reserving 0.0 for death. (Sensitivity analyses varying the 0.10 utility did not change differences between other states in large ways [Torrance, Erickson, Patrick, & Feldman, 1995].) The values were established in the following way. First, a statistical technique was applied to determine differences between levels of the self-rated health and activity limitation dimensions. For this

Table 8.3

NATIONAL CENTER FOR HEALTH STATISTICS: NATIONAL HEALTH INTERVIEW SURVEY; POPULATION AGED 85 AND OLDER, 1990

	EXCELLENT	VERY GOOD	GOOD	FAIR	POOR
Not limited in major activity	7.0	11.7	16.4	6.3	2.0
Limited: other activity	1.9	2.6	4.7	4.1	1.0
Limited in IADL	2.3	3.1	7.0	6.8	3.1
Limited in ADL	1.2	1.6	4.9	5.8	6.5

Entries are proportion of noninstitutionalized U.S. population, aged 85 and older, weighted to represent U.S. population.
Courtesy of Ronald Wilson, Office of Analysis, Epidemiology, and Health Promotion, National Center for Health Statistics.

effort, correspondence analysis showed that levels of self-rated health and activity limitation were not equally spaced (for example, "very good," "good," and "fair" had values of 0.85, 0.70, and 0.30, respectively). Consistent with the utility estimation approach, these values specify numeric differences between states on a common scale of utility, how much more or less one state is preferred to another. Second, survey data were used to assign a value to one of the off-diagonal cells (using the Health Utilities Index). Finally, the two sets of values were combined in a multiplicative model to assign values to each joint state.

The final results, shown in Table 8.4, show that the state of excellent health-no activity limitation (1.0) is 0.08 units greater than the state of very good health-no activity limitation (0.92) and 0.19 units greater than the state of excellent health-limited in major activity. The latter difference suggests that being limited in a major life activity reduces health-related QOL by approximately 20%. In contrast, someone reporting good health and a limitation is assigned a score of 0.67, or 33% less than someone reporting excellent health and a limitation.

Researchers have attempted to make these abstract values more concrete by interpreting them as percentages of a full year of healthy life. For someone in the excellent health-no activity limitation state, which is assigned a utility of 1.0, a year of life would be equivalent to a year of healthy life. For someone in the state of very good health-no activity

Table 8.4

VALUES FOR HEALTH STATES DEFINED IN TERMS OF ACTIVITY LIMITATION
AND PERCEIVED HEALTH STATUS

ACTIVITY LIMITATION	PERCEIVED HEALTH STATUS				
	EXCELLENT	VERY GOOD	GOOD	FAIR	POOR
Not limited	1.00	0.92	0.84	0.63	0.47
Limited: other	0.87	0.79	0.72	0.52	0.38
Limited: major	0.81	0.74	0.67	0.48	0.34
Unable: major	0.68	0.62	0.55	0.38	0.25
Limited in IADL	0.57	0.51	0.45	0.29	0.17
Limited in ADL	0.47	0.41	0.36	0.21	0.10

limitation, with its utility score of 0.92, a year of life would be equivalent
to 0.92 years of healthy life (Erickson et al., 1995). Each year lived by
someone in good health but with limitation in major activity would be
equivalent to 0.67 years of healthy life.

Each age group will have a distribution across the 30 QOL states
and therefore a mean health-related QOL value. These values give a
health-related QOL prevalence at each age and can accordingly be used
in life table calculations to estimate a healthy life expectancy, analogous
to the disability-free life expectancy method of Sullivan (1971). For the
noninstitutionalized population covered in the NHIS, mean QOL state
values in 1990 were 0.77 for people age 65–70, 0.75 for age 70–75, 0.72
for age 75–80, 0.67 for age 80–85, and 0.60 for age 85 and older. People
aged 40–45, by contrast, had a mean of 0.86 (Erickson et al., 1995).

To generate health-related QOL scores for age groups in the entire
U.S. population, institutional populations must be included and values
assigned to these groups, which include prisoners (mean value of 0.74:
very good health, limited in major role), nursing home residents (mean
value of 0.21: fair health, ADL limitation), long-term hospital residents
(mean value of 0.45: good health, IADL limitation), residential care facilities (0.72), and the military (1.0). The inclusion of these populations
(with these imputations of mean QOL state) lowers scores slightly in
each of the older age groups. For the total U.S. population covered in

1990, mean QOL state values in 1990 were 0.76 for people age 65–70, 0.74 for age 70–75, 0.70 for age 75–80, 0.63 for age 80–85, and 0.51 for age 85 and older.

These values are entered in the life table model to convert person-years lived by people in given age intervals to "healthy person-year" equivalents. Thus, people born in 1990 who reach age 85 contribute an additional 193,523 person-years to this birth cohort's total years of life before they die. However, because the mean QOL value for this age group is 0.51, these 193,523 person-years are equivalent to 98,697 (193,523 × 0.51) healthy years. Summing up these quality-adjusted years across all age groups yields the cumulative sum (T_x) we have seen in Chapter 2. If we divide the cumulative sum at each age interval by the number of people entering this age interval, the result is healthy life expectancy, the quality-adjusted analog to life expectancy.

In 1990, healthy life expectancy in the United States for men and women combined was 64.0 years and life expectancy was 75.4 years. People born in 1990, then, had a "healthy proportion of life expectancy" of 84.9% (64/75.4), that is, approximately 85% of life in the state of excellent health with no activity limitation. This proportion of life remaining that can be expected to be lived in that state shrinks with advancing age: 68.5% at age 40–45, 57.2% at age 65–70, and 37.3% at age 85 and older.

Thus, the increasing prevalence of chronic conditions and senescent changes lower mean QOL scores (by increasing the proportion of people in other states), which means fewer years of healthy life in later age intervals, and a smaller proportion of remaining years of healthy life. These trends differ by socioeconomic status. Healthy life expectancy at birth in 1990 was 65.0 among Whites, 56.0 among African Americans, and 64.8 among Hispanics. The three groups had very different life expectancies: 76.1 for Whites, 69.1 for African Americans, and 79.1 for Hispanics. The proportion of total years in which individuals in each race-ethnicity group could expect to be in optimal health reflects both life expectancy and healthy life expectancy. This proportion was 85.4% for Whites, 81.0% for African Americans, and 81.9% for Hispanics in 1990. These are important findings, as they suggest the important public health goal of eliminating a health disparity and also the need to improve the experience of all groups.

These results are based on life table methods and do not follow a sample of people as they actually age. In fact, there are few studies that track changes in quality of life as people age. Longitudinal studies of quality of life in old age are challenging because of deaths, which remove people whose QOL has declined most. One study that addressed this problem assessed Health Utilities Index (HUI-Mark 3) scores in a population-based sample of Canadian seniors over 10 years, 1994–1995 to 2004–2005 (Orpana et al., 2009). In the HUI-3, scores range from –0.36 to 1.00, with 1.00 indicating perfect health. Changes of 0.03 or more are considered clinically significant. The measure computes QOL as a weighted score based on ratings in eight domains: vision, hearing, speech, ambulation, dexterity, emotion, cognition, and pain-discomfort. In this sample of nearly 8,000 people, aged 40 and older in 1994–1995, approximately 1,600 died over the 10-year follow-up period. At the 1994–1995 baseline, scores ranged from 0.88 in people aged 40–49 to 0.44 in people aged 90 and older. Over the 10 years, HUI scores remained high and stable until about age 70 in both men and women. QOL in men begins to decline precipitously after age 75. For women, declines in QOL accelerate later, after age 80. These growth model results include the effects of mortality and nursing home placement.

GENERALIZATION OF THE QUALITY-ADJUSTMENT PARADIGM

We have seen that health-related quality-of-life research depends on two key assumptions: specification of plausible, discrete health states, and assignment of numeric values to these states. The first assumption implies clear boundaries between health states and the ability to calculate survival in particular health states. The second implies reasonable consensus on how much worse one health state is relative to another. These distinctions can be difficult to draw for health states that are similar and are fraught with imprecise judgments. Thus, if we return to Table 8.4, we note that adjacent health states sometimes differ by only a few units on the utility scale. Such similarities may be interpreted as "indifference" between health states that are more or less equivalent.

If we can accept these assumptions, then utility- or quality-adjusted life-year (QALY) can be a useful tool for public health and aging research. Let us examine a simple example. Table 8.5a presents data for a hypothetical individual who died at age 80. He occupied four health states during his life. From birth to age 60, his QOL state was valued at 1.0. Thus, the healthy-year equivalent for this state of health was 60 years. At age 60, he suffered a heart attack, which prevented him from working, his major activity. The utility for this state was 0.80. He lived in this state for 5 years, resulting in a healthy-year equivalent of 4 years (0.80 × 5). At age 66 he suffered a second major health event. He was given a diagnosis of Parkinson's disease, was forced to take a set of extensive medications, alter his daily activity (for example, limiting driving), and begin to think himself as an old person in relatively poor health. The utility for this state was 0.60 and the duration of the state was 10 years, resulting in a health-year equivalent of 6 years. Finally, at age 76 he was given a diagnosis of dementia secondary to Parkinson's disease. The QOL valuation for this state was 0.40, and he lived 5 years in this state before death, resulting in a healthy-year equivalent of only 2 years. If we sum down the columns in Table 8.5a, we see that he lived 80 years, but an equivalent of only 72 healthy years.

Looking across the 80 years he lived, we see that the proportion of life in the highest health state was 90% (72/80) (alternatively, his mean QOL value across the life span was 0.90). But note the very different picture in later life beginning at age 66. The proportion of life lived in from age 6 the highest health state 6 until death was only 53% (8/15), and his mean QOL state during this period was 0.53, quite low, equivalent, as we have seen, to the mean state for people age 85 and older.

If we look now at Table 8.5b, we can demonstrate the effect of a health intervention by use of the same quality-adjusted model. In this simple model, some kind of health intervention, say, an effective disease management program for his Parkinson's disease begins at age 66, state 3a. This program involves better pharmacotherapy (less adverse effects from his medication, easier dosing schedule and better adherence, better management of tremor and slowness). The QOL value for this state is 0.65, rather than 0.60 and he gains an additional year of life in this state because the drug therapy also delays onset of Parkinson's dementia. He lives in this state 11 years, the equivalent of 7.15 years (11 × 0.65). He reaches the dementia milestone at age 77, but with excellent supportive care and perhaps moderation of dementia progression because of his prior drug therapy, the QOL state is valued at 0.45, rather than 0.40. He lives 6 years in this state for a healthy-year equivalent of 2.7 years (6 × 0.45).

With these interventions, the man lived 82 years, the equivalent of 73.85 healthy years. This is again 90% (73.85/82) of the life span, no different than the prior model. Interventions often add years to life, which must be considered in calculated benefit. The true benefit is seen in the last years of life. From age 66, when the intervention was introduced,

Table 8.5

CALCULATION OF YEARS OF HEALTHY LIFE (YHL)

A. WITHOUT INTERVENTION

AGE SPAN	HEALTH STATE	DURATION	HQOL VALUE	YHL
0-60	1	60	1.00	60
61-65	2	5	.80	4
66-75	3	10	.60	6
76-80	4	5	.40	2

DEATH

		____		____
		80		72

B. WITH INTERVENTION

AGE SPAN	HEALTH STATE	DURATION	HQOL VALUE	YHL
0-60	1	60	1.00	60
61-65	2	5	.80	4
66-76	3a	11	.65	7.15
77-82	4a	6	.45	2.70

DEATH

		____		____
		82		73.85

HQOL = health quality of life.

to death, he lived 17 years, the equivalent of 9.85 years of healthy life. Thus, the proportion of life lived in a healthy state from age 66 on was 58% (9.85/17), an improvement of 5% over the nonintervention model. Through this intervention, our hypothetical individual lived an additional 2 years at a higher mean QOL (0.58 vs. 0.53).

Is this a large difference? Should we be impressed by a 5% improvement in mean QOL? This speaks to the issue of the clinical relevance of change in QOL scores, discussed above. A difference of 0.05 in mean

QOL scores is equivalent to about a 5-year age difference in late life. For example, the mean QOL score for people aged 70–75 is 0.74 and for people aged 75–80 it is 0.70. The intervention, then, brought about a change roughly equivalent in magnitude to the difference in QOL between people aged 70–75 and 75–80.

Even with benefit measured on the scale of age, one can still ask if such an intervention is worth mounting. How does this benefit compare with the costs of implementing such a program? The quality-adjusted model can be used to develop a ratio of cost to utility helpful for answering such questions. This ratio answers the question: "What does an extra year of healthy life cost?"

To answer this question, we need the cost of care with the intervention and the usual cost of care. Let's say that the cost of current, nonintervention care for this man was $5,000 a year, and the cost with the intervention $7,000 a year. These costs, incurred over the duration of the intervention, serve as the numerator for the cost-utility ratio. To return to the examples shown in Table 8.5 (a and b), the numerator is (7,000 × 17) minus (5,000 × 15), i.e., 17 years of life with the intervention ($119,000) versus 15 years of life without ($75,000), or $44,000. The denominator is the additional years of healthy life provided by the intervention. With the intervention, the man lived the equivalent of 9.85 years of healthy life; without it, he lived only 8 years in this state. The difference, then, is 1.85 years. Given these values, the cost-utility ratio would be calculated as 44,000/1.85, or $23,784. Thus, this program of effective disease management provides an additional year of healthy life at a cost of $23,784. (More complex calculations would include a discounting factor to control for the effect of inflation over long periods.)

Whether this intervention is "worth" the cost is in part an ethical issue (see Chapter 11). But one way to assess its incremental cost is to compare it to other interventions. This illustration might be considered a reasonable investment since it is comparable to the cost of an additional healthy life-year in hypertension management programs (Patrick & Erickson, 1993).

HEALTH-RELATED AND ENVIRONMENT-RELATED QOL IN OLD AGE

In contrast to health-related QOL, environmental or nonhealth QOL may remain high throughout life and may even improve with greater age. With retirement, for example, older people have greater leisure time; and with children gone, houses paid for, and potentially success-ful investments, they may have greater disposable income as well. As a result, older people have increased opportunities to develop interests and create satisfying environments. These freedoms and opportunities counterbalance declines in health-related QOL and may be responsible for the great resiliency older people show in the face of declining health and impending death. Because person- and environment-based QOL do not decline with age, older people may have advantages in building environments that promote QOL.

Lawton (1991) has expressed the relevance of nonhealth, environment-based QOL for old people very well. He asks, "do frail people do better if they have a loved spouse, a fulfilling relationship with a child, an area of expertise that can be applied despite the illness, a sphere of life where autonomy can still be exercised, or an ideology that organizes the meaning of pain, suffering, life, and death?" The answer, of course, is yes. In the presence of declining health and declines in health-related quality of life, these factors may become even more im-portant. They become the basis for continuing attachment to life and play a role in effective adjustment to limitations in health and maximiza-tion of health-related QOL.

SUMMARY

Differences Between Health-Related and Environment-Based Quality of Life. Health-related and environment-based quality of life must be distinguished. Health-related quality of life is inexorably linked to age and shows clear declines across the life span, in keeping with senescent processes and increased susceptibility to chronic disease. Nonhealth or environment-based quality of life is not a health impact measure but rather registers the effect of personal resources or environmental fac-tors on daily experience. The two come together in the ability of older people to modify environments in ways that limit the QOL impact of poor health.

Identification of QOL Domains. A good test of whether a domain falls within the category of health-related QOL is to ask what aspects of a person's life are likely to improve if a patient is successfully treated by a physician. These are health-related QOL domains, which typically include measures of physical, affective, and social function, along with symptom states.

Measuring QOL. Can we determine *how much* better life is at a higher level of health than at a lower level? Patrick & Erickson (1993) define health-related QOL as "the *value* assigned to the duration of life, as modified by impairment" (emphasis added). The goal of measurement of health-related QOL is to develop measures that capture the impact of changes in health and to assign plausible numeric indicators for such changes. Although this second task may seem difficult or even inappropriate, we should remember that people already implicitly assign values to these health changes. Every day people evaluate symptom states and make treatment decisions based on their judgment of the likely impact of treatment or nontreatment.

"Minimal Clinically Significant Difference" in QOL. Clinical significance in self-reported QOL is identified by a change in patient-reported status that would lead a care provider to seek a different medication or a change in a care environment. Otherwise stated, these are changes that would lead a clinician to make a change in patient management. Patient behavior is a good guide here. If patients report such changes to a clinician, and the clinician is not impressed enough to alter management, patients are apt to go elsewhere.

Age as an Anchor for Assessing Change in Health-Related QOL. Given the pervasive effect of age on quality-of-life states because of senescence and the increasing prevalence of chronic conditions, age provides a natural metric for assessing the QOL effects of clinical interventions. Quality-of-life changes can be referenced to norms at different ages, allowing one to associate changes in a health-related QOL domain to age equivalents. Thus, increasing urine flow 3 ml/sec in men with benign prostatic hypertrophy is equivalent to lowering their "urinary age" 10–15 years.

Health-Related QOL and Healthy-Year Equivalents. In the *Healthy People 2000* "years of healthy life" measure, health states are defined by the cross-classification of self-rated health and reported activity limitation. These states are assigned QOL values on a 0–1.0 scale. Given one's QOL state and its assigned value, the number of years lived in this state can be converted to a "healthy years equivalent," or the number of years lived in excellent health with no limitations. This is a quality-adjusted measure. Thus, 5 years of life in a health state with a value of 0.80 would be equivalent to 4 years of healthy life (5 × 0.80).

For the total U.S. population covered in 1990, mean QOL state values in 1990 were 0.76 for people age 65–70, 0.74 for age 70–75, 0.70 for age 75–80, 0.63 for age 80–85, and 0.51 for age 85 and older. The increasing prevalence of chronic conditions and senescent changes at later ages lowers mean QOL scores (by increasing the proportion of people in less healthful states), which means fewer years of healthy life in later age intervals, and a smaller proportion of remaining years in healthy life.

These trends differ by socioeconomic status. Healthy life expectancy at birth in 1990 was 65.0 among Whites, 56.0 among African Americans, and 64.8 among Hispanics. The three groups had very different life expectancies: 76.1 for Whites, 69.1 for African Americans, and 79.1 for Hispanics. The proportion of total years in which individuals in each race-ethnicity group could expect to be healthy years was 85.4% for Whites, 81.0% for African Americans, and 81.9% for Hispanics in 1990. This difference suggests the important public health goal of eliminating a health disparity and also the need to improve the experience of all groups.

Health-Related and Environment-Related QOL in Old Age. In contrast to health-related QOL, person- and environment-based QOL do not decline with age. Older people can use this to their advantage in building environments that promote QOL even in the presence of chronic conditions.

9 Aging, Public Health, and Long-Term Care

Is long-term care an appropriate topic for public health and aging? We think so, although some investigators limit public health and aging efforts to healthier elders who do not make use of supportive care services. This limitation is artificial for a number of reasons. First, older people increasingly move between states of ability and disability, in which they may require long-term care services for some period of time and later recover function. Early work from the National Long Term Care Survey showed substantial movement over 5 years toward both decline and improvement in elders with limitations in household competencies (the IADLs: cleaning, cooking, shopping, laundry, medication management, handling money, using the telephone) and isolated ADL limitations (such as limitations only in bathing) (Manton, 1992). More recent work has shown great dynamism in states of disability in old age (Gill et al., 2002; Hardy & Gill, 2004). Second, it is artificial to truncate public health efforts according to elder function or disability. A theme running throughout our account of the field is the need to acknowledge the full spectrum of health and function in old age, as well as the unity of risk factors and the potential for intervention across the life span. Finally, an increasing body of research shows that prevention of excess morbidity is critical among even the most frail and that the potential for gain through population-based prevention efforts is as strong here as in other populations.

Given the focus on allowing people with disabilities to live in maximally integrated settings (a step beyond the former goal of "the least restrictive setting"), we use "long-term" or "supportive" or "residential" care rather than "custodial care," a term that has appropriately and increasingly dropped out of the professional lexicon. This chapter reviews what long-term care is, provides an overview of recent trends in use and spending, and delves into the major types of long-term care: home- and community-based services, personal assistance services, family caregiving, and residential care settings. We then take up the question of how public health efforts might enhance long-term care and review several research topics that have recently gained interest: recognizing older people's care preferences, upgrading home attendant and nursing assistant care, and expanding options for supportive care and housing for older adults.

WHAT IS LONG-TERM CARE?

"Long-term care" includes the complete spectrum of services and supports required to meet health and personal care needs over an extended period of time. It is distinguished from medical care in that it is supportive rather than curative and is designed to maximize independence in daily living among people with health limitations. It is distinguished from acute or subacute care in that it is not rehabilitative. Rather, long-term care provides services that allow older people to meet personal self-maintenance needs (such as bathing, dressing, using the toilet, and the other ADLs; (see Chapter 6). Older people receiving long-term care are not expected to improve in function (although this may occur), and, in fact, elders receiving long-term care are likely to require increasing levels of supportive care, moving from help initially with transportation and household tasks (such as cleaning or cooking), to help with medication management and ADLs, and finally to help with the most basic ADL tasks, such as toileting, transfer, and feeding. The latter are supportive care needs consistent with skilled nursing facility care.

Thus, long-term care covers a wide spectrum of services and settings. It may involve activity programming for elders with dementia in an adult day program, ADL support from a home care agency, medical supplies or assistive technology from a vendor that contracts with a local Area on Aging, residence in a nursing home, home-delivered meals from a church, congregate meals in an assistive living facility, or case management to secure such services.

Consistent with the preference to maintain vulnerable seniors in their homes and a health-financing system that favors medical rather than supportive care (see Chapter 6), family members necessarily provide the vast bulk of long-term care services. However, with the increasing availability of home- and community-based services, family caregivers are now more likely to share long-term care with formal paid providers. Families thus have increasing contact with a wide variety of providers and payers. These include Medicare in the case of ADL support linked to rehabilitation following a hospitalization, Medicaid for nursing home care, paraprofessional or informal nonfamily caregivers who are paid out-of-pocket, Medicaid waiver programs that allow payment to family caregivers for ADL support, and Medicare-Medicaid programs that link medical and long-term care, such as the Program for All-Inclusive Care for the Elderly (PACE). Medicaid waiver programs allow states increasing latitude in bundling long-term care services for lower-income elders and younger people with disabilities.

Finally, in some cases, it is genuinely difficult to tell where long-term care services begin and end. For example, visiting nurses and other home health care rehabilitative services are normally linked to posthospital care and are limited by Medicare to 90-day cycles. But in many cases these services serve as long-term care placeholders until families are able to put other services in place, as families recognize that the discharged elder can no longer function independently in the home. Likewise, programs that combine medical and supportive care blur these boundaries. In some municipalities, as in New York City, Medicaid-eligible seniors can receive home health care nursing services along with separate paraprofessional ADL-based home care on a long-term basis. Even families may be unclear whether they are providing long-term care. Although family members can identify when they began to provide ADL support (Albert & Brody, 1996), they are not always able to distinguish when they stopped providing occasional help and became "caregivers."

OVERVIEW: TRENDS IN LONG-TERM CARE USE AND SPENDING

Spending on long-term care in the United States for all ages reached nearly $200 billion in 2004; approximately half of this amount was paid by Medicaid. Approximately 20% was paid by Medicare, another 20% through out-of-pocket payments, and the remainder through health insurance (including long-term care insurance) and other public sources (Komisar & Thompson, 2007). From 1990 to 2004 national long-term care expenditures grew at an annual rate of 7.4%, somewhat higher than the 7.0% average annual growth rate for all personal health care spending. Two important trends in long-term care payments include a growing share of public funding and a shift away from spending on institutional care toward home- and community-based services. These trends show increasing public sector commitment to long-term care and recognize the public's preference for care in the home or community, whenever possible. Spending on noninstitutional care was 19% of Medicaid's long-term care spending in 1995, but it reached 37% in 2005 and continues to increase (Komisar & Thompson, 2007).

Approximately 9 million people over age 65 need assistance with one or more personal self-maintenance activities, such as bathing or dressing (ADLs) (U.S. DHHS National Long Term Care Clearinghouse, www.longtermcare.gov/LTC/Main_Site/index.aspx). As we analyze in more detail (Chapter 6), these 9 million represent approximately 25% of older adults. In 2005, approximately 1.5 million of these people received care in nursing homes (approximately 4.6% of people aged 65 and older), again pointing to the many other components of the long-term spectrum and the many different ways older adults manage to meet these most basic needs.

Skilled nursing home use is clearly only the tip of the iceberg of long-term care. Even among older adults with ADL limitations, for every one receiving nursing home care, seven others receive long-term care in the community. Of course, nursing home care is reserved mostly for the oldest and most severely dependent elder, but it is notable that residence in skilled nursing homes among older adults continues to decline. The rate per 1,000 was 54.0 in 1985, 46.4 in 1995, and 34.8 in 2004 (Federal Interagency Forum on Aging-Related Statistics, 2008). Still, the need for long-term care is a feature of aging. Approximately 70% of individuals over age 65 will require some type of long-term care services during their lifetimes, and over 40% will spend at least some time in a skilled nursing facility (Kemper, Komisar, & Alecxih, 2005). Someone aged 65 in 2005 is likely to need long-term care services for 3 years of his or her remaining life span.

As mentioned earlier, families provide the bulk of long-term care services. Approximately three of four caregivers of older adults with long-term care needs are family members. Half of these family members provide help daily, and two-thirds live with care recipients. Although the hourly investment in caregiving is linked to elder needs, most of these informal, unpaid caregivers provide 1–5 hours of care daily (Johnson, Toohey, & Wiener, 2007). Important emerging trends in family caregiving include increases in the proportion of husbands and sons providing care, and reductions in the proportion of households in which a middle-generation caregiver is "sandwiched" between the demands of elder and child care.

HOME- AND COMMUNITY-BASED SERVICES

For an appraisal of access to paid or "formal" home- and community-based services, it is helpful first to examine the residential arrangements of older people, because people living in supportive housing may receive some services by virtue of residence. Table 9.1 shows the proportion of older adults living in different kinds of residential settings in 2005. Data on older people living in "naturally occurring retirement communities" (NORC), which may also be a site for long-term care services, are harder to come by because their definition is less clear and they vary greatly in access to long-term care services (Ormond, Black, Tilly, & Thomas, 2004). In Table 9.1, "community housing with services" includes assisted living, board and care homes, and senior citizen housing that provides support for household maintenance activities. Long-term care facilities are Medicare- or Medicaid-certified entities that provide full-time personal assistance care.

Table 9.1

RESIDENTIAL ARRANGEMENTS OF OLDER ADULTS, 2005

	65+	65–74	75–84	85+
ALL SETTINGS (1,000'S)	**33,394**	**16,116**	**12,703**	**4,575**
Residential type, %				
Traditional community	93.0	98.0	92.6	76.3
Community housing with services	2.4	0.7	3.1	6.8
Long-term care facilities	4.6	1.3	4.3	16.9

From *Older Americans 2008: Key Indicators of Well-Being,* by Federal Interagency Forum on Aging-Related Statistics, 2008, Table 37a. Retrieved September 15, 2009, from http://www.agingstats.gov/chartbook2008/default.htm.

As expected, we see a clear association between age and residence in supportive housing. Whereas nearly all elders aged 65–74 reside in traditional community housing, only three fourths of people aged 85 and older live in the community. Use of nursing home care increases from 1.3% in people aged 65–74 to 16.9% in people aged 85 and older. The proportion without disability is 63.6% among community-dwelling elders, 39.6% in people living in community housing with services, and 5.8% in people living in long-term care facilities (the latter include spouses of more impaired elders and people who reside in these facilities for lack of alternative housing). In the group residing in community housing with services, over 80% receive prepared meals and housekeeping services and nearly half receive help with medications.

For elders living outside supportive housing settings, in-home services are provided by both Medicare and Medicaid, as noted earlier. The rate of Medicare home health care visits in 2005 was 2,770 per 1,000, or about 2.8 home health care episodes for each older adult. This is in keeping with the high rate of hospitalization among older people (350 per 1,000) (Federal Interagency Forum on Aging-Related Statistics, 2008, Table 29a). Use of Medicare home health care is again strongly related to age. The rate per 1,000 in 2005 was 1,333 for people aged 65–74, 3,407 for people aged 75–84, and 6,549 for people aged 85 and older (Federal Interagency Forum on Aging-Related Statistics, 2008, Table 29b).

Medicaid home- and community-based services are far more extensive and vary considerably by state and, in some cases, by county. Medicaid provides personal care services through an optional state plan benefit (Title XIX) and the more common 1915(c) waiver. For further information on the relevant Medicaid services, see the Web site of the Centers for Medicare and Medicaid Services (http://www.cms.hhs.gov/ MedicaidStWaivProgDemoPGI/). State commitment to personal care services for the elderly and adults with disabilities varies dramatically. In 2001, Medicaid personal care participants per 1,000 people ranged from 7.33 to 0.04 per state, and per capita expenditures ranged from $91.21 to $0.02 (LeBlanc, Tonner, & Harrington, 2001).

The diversity of Medicaid home- and community-based services is impressive. In New York City, 10 different programs are available. These include Traditional Personal Care, Consumer-Directed Personal Assistance, Long-Term Home Health Care, Medicaid Managed Long-Term Care, the Program for All-Inclusive Care for the Elderly (PACE), Certified Home Health Agency Services, Medical Adult Day Health

Care, the Traumatic Brain Injury Waiver, the Nursing Home Transition and Diversion Waiver, and Medicaid Advantage Plus. Two-thirds of these programs require nursing home levels of need for eligibility. In New York City in 2007, approximately 166,000 people received in-home services through Medicaid programs (compared with 81,000 receiving nursing home or assisted living services). Of the $12.3 billion spent on Medicaid long-term care services in New York City 47% went to these home- and community-based services (Hokenstad & Shineman, 2009).

A survey of older adults receiving Medicaid waiver personal care services in Virginia suggests that the program meets the needs of recipients, and that recipients are on the whole very satisfied with aides and care delivery (Glass, Roberto, Brossoie, Teaster, & Butler, 2008–2009).

PERSONAL ASSISTANCE SERVICES AND PUBLIC HEALTH

Across the different programs that deliver formal, paid home- and community-based services, 1.2–1.5 million Americans receive personal assistance services (PAS) (LeBlanc et al., 2001). Recipients receiving PAS require long-term help with bathing, dressing, and other activities of daily living, receive this support from nonmedically trained providers, and would otherwise require nursing home residence to meet their needs (Kitchener, Carrillo, & Harrington, 2003; LeBlanc et al., 2001). PAS is not designed to manage a client's clinical needs, but rather to manage disability and support independence at home. Thus, PAS is *not* a skilled care intervention, as in the case of the Medicare home health benefit, which stresses rehabilitation, but it may have beneficial health consequences by effectively managing disabilities that would otherwise put people at risk for poor outcomes. We have shown that PAS is associated with a potential health benefit, even though its primary purpose is to provide support for independent living at home (Albert, Simone, Brassard, Stern, & Mayeux, 2005b). Thus, PAS may have important public health significance. However, little research is available on the measurement of effective PAS delivery and its health and quality-of-life consequences.

Increases in the prevalence of PAS are expected, given the substantial growth in Medicaid programs that provide PAS, an aging population, declines in the nursing home population, and legislative efforts (e.g., the *Olmstead* decision, in which the Supreme Court in 1999 upheld elements of the Americans With Disability Act that mandate the most integrated setting for people with long-term care needs; see *Olmstead v. L. C.* (98-536) 527 U.S. 581, 1999). In addition, consumer-directed PAS is now a popular option, with elders and their families taking control of the hiring and training of PAS providers or, in some cases, serving as paid PAS providers themselves. Thus, examination of outcomes associated with PAS is critical for an accurate appraisal of the conditions under which elders and their families can best benefit from the program.

Studies of PAS outcomes are complicated by two key factors. First, the number of PAS hours per week that elders receive (service intensity) is based on the severity of disability (need). More severe disability will be associated with unfavorable outcomes, even when PAS is delivered effectively. Second, informal care arrangements complicate assessment of PAS outcomes. Family caregivers may supplement paid PAS to different degrees (or develop variable kinds of division of labor), making it difficult to assess the effect of PAS on outcomes. Careful designs will be required to disentangle these confounding factors.

Some initial evidence in this area is available from "cash and counseling" demonstrations. Medicaid has allowed waiver programs for PAS that encourage consumer-directed care, in which families may hire (and fire) home care providers. In these programs, certified home care agencies may vet home attendants or handle payroll and other administrative duties, but families supervise PAS and work out hourly arrangements with home care attendants. The Arkansas Cash & Counseling Demonstration (Independent Choices) suggests that suboptimal delivery of PAS is a concern (Foster, Brown, Phillips, Schore, & Carlson, 2003).

In this demonstration, Medicaid-eligible elders were randomly assigned either to a consumer direction arm, in which they were able to use a monthly allowance to purchase PAS services (as well as assistive equipment), or to standard agency care. Elders able to direct PAS care were more likely to report that providers completed tasks and that household and transportation needs were met. But these simple indicators reveal considerable variation in how effectively PAS was delivered, even when families were able to hire relatives or friends as PAS providers. For example, 65.8% of elders in the consumer direction arm reported that PAS providers "always" completed mandated care plan tasks, compared with 47.2% in the standard agency care arm. Thus, PAS delivery by this simple measure was effective in only about half to two-thirds of cases across the two groups.

Despite only partially effective delivery of PAS, elders in the consumer direction arm were more likely to report they were "very satisfied with the way they spend their life these days" (55.5% vs. 37.0%).

Also, "treatment group members were somewhat less likely than control group members to report some kinds of health problems that might indicate they received inferior or insufficiently frequent personal assistance" (Foster et al., 2003). These findings suggest that effective delivery of PAS may be associated with health benefit.

Thus, an important area for public health inquiry in home- and community-based services is direct investigation of features of PAS delivery that promote desired outcomes. Does PAS allow elders to meet basic provisioning, hygiene, mobility, and nutrition needs? And does effectively meeting these needs in turn promote desired short-term health and functioning outcomes, such as fewer falls, better skin integrity, weight maintenance, and lower extremity strength, which may in turn influence well being?

It is clear as well that personal assistance care does not occur in a vacuum. Whereas family care without paid assistance is still the most common caregiving arrangement, the proportion of families that combine formal and informal care has grown to encompass about a third of caregiving arrangements (Federal Interagency Forum on Aging-Related Statistics, 2008). Thus, a second line of inquiry should be to examine the relationship between family caregivers and paid providers because this might affect PAS delivery and outcomes.

Table 9.2 illustrates a public health approach to assessment of PAS and suggests linkages between delivery of PAS and relevant indicators of health and functioning.

Table 9.2

DOMAIN-SPECIFIC INDICATORS OF EFFECTIVE PAS DELIVERY AND OUTCOMES

PERSONAL ASSISTANCE TASK	INDICATOR OF EFFECTIVE DELIVERY	CLINICAL STATUS INDICATOR
PAS provider report: ADL		
Bathing: frequency, comfort performing task, difficulty	Personal cleanliness	Skin integrity
Dressing: frequency of clothing changes, elicitation of elder preferences	Clothing comfort, variety	

(Continued)

Table 9.2

DOMAIN-SPECIFIC INDICATORS OF EFFECTIVE PAS DELIVERY AND OUTCOMES (*Continued*)

PERSONAL ASSISTANCE TASK	INDICATOR OF EFFECTIVE DELIVERY	CLINICAL STATUS INDICATOR
Toileting: presence of toileting schedule; comfort with task	Availability of commode; report of availability of prompt toileting & cleanliness	
Grooming: frequency	Satisfaction with appearance	
Eating: recognition of dietary restrictions & limitations posed by dentition	Foods appropriate to dentition & swallowing status; verbal/physical prompting; report of variety & satisfaction	Weight maintenance, dehydration; appetite
PAS Provider Report: Mobility		
Transfer & mobility support: frequency, difficulty	Presence of assistive devices, provider ability to lift elder; report of fear of falling during transfer, opportunity to move, access to rooms	Lower extremity strength & balance performance; opportunity to change environment
PAS Provider Report: IADL		
Meal preparation: concern for elder meal preference and schedule	Regularity of meals and snacks, sufficient food in home; enjoyment of social and physical setting of eating	
Laundry: frequency	Cleanliness of clothing & linens	Relocation of elder over follow-up
Housework: frequency	Cleanliness of household, clutter; appliances in good repair; trash removal; comfort, satisfaction with living quarters	
Shopping, errands: frequency	Adequate food & household supplies, timely replacement	

FAMILY CAREGIVING

In its most expansive definition as unpaid help with household tasks and care management for a chronically ill, disabled, or aged family member or friend, more than 50 million Americans can be considered caregivers in any given year (National Family Caregivers Association, www. thefamilycaregiver.org). Limiting the definition to people who provide unpaid ADL or IADL care lowers the yearly prevalence (in 2004) to 44.4 million (National Caregiver Alliance and AARP, 2004). With these definitions, family caregivers are active in approximately 20% of U.S. households. Note that these estimates do not separate caregiving to older and younger adults with disabilities.

These surveys suggest the following profile of the typical family caregiver: she is 46, married, and employed; and she is caring for a widowed mother who does not live with her (National Caregiver Alliance and AARP, 2004). This profile is in keeping with the greater likelihood of women as caregivers (60%) and the lower likelihood of spousal caregiving (30% of family caregivers are themselves aged 65 or older). The economic value of family caregiving is substantial and has been estimated at over $300 billion yearly, nearly twice as much as the total costs incurred by the formal long-term care sector of paid home care and long-term care facilities (AARP, 2006). Given the growing rate of people over age 65 (projected to increase at 2.3% annually) and much slower rate of growth in younger people likely to provide care (0.8% annually), shortfalls in family caregiving can be expected, along with a greater cost burden for the formal long-term care sector (Mack & Thompson, 2001).

The high prevalence of such caregiving has led the CDC to develop a caregiver module for its ongoing Behavioral Risk Factors Surveillance System (BRFSS). In the BRFSS, caregiving is established with the following question: "People may provide regular care or assistance to a friend or family member who has a health problem, long-term illness, or disability. During the past month, did you provide any such care or assistance to a friend or family member?" The module will be fielded nationally in 2009 and will provide the first state-level estimates of caregiver prevalence.

In an initial statewide survey in North Carolina using the BRFSS module, the prevalence of caregiving was 15.4% (DeFries, McGuire, Andresen, Brumback, & Anderson, 2009). Approximately 75% of caregivers were providing help to people aged 60 and older. By respondent self-report, 41.5% of care recipients were cognitively impaired. Caregivers in this survey provided a mean of 20.2 hr/wk in the case of cognitively impaired care recipients and 16.6 hr/wk for other care receivers. Mean duration of caregiving was just under 4 years for people with cognitive impairment, and just under 3 years otherwise. Not surprisingly, care recipients with cognitive impairment were older, as were their caregivers.

The associations between family caregiving and various outcomes, both negative and positive, have been extensively documented. On the negative side, family caregiving is associated with lost wages and work absenteeism, lower work productivity, and greater risk of poverty (Schulz & Martire, in press). Strained caregivers face an increased mortality risk (Schulz & Beach, 1999) and an increased risk of depression, anxiety, substance abuse, and other chronic conditions (Cannuscio et al., 2002). On the positive side, caregiving is associated with gains in personal mastery, family continuity, and, in some cases, new careers in aging and health services.

While only 17% of family caregivers provide 40 hr/wk of care or more (National Caregiver Alliance, 2004), less intensive caregiving can be associated with a variety of negative outcomes, in particular, with the caregiver's health. These associations were explored in a sample of 17,000 U.S. employees from a large corporation who completed health risk appraisal questionnaires on the job (National Caregiver Alliance and MetLife Mature Market Institute, in press). In this sample, 11.6% of employees reported they provided care to an older person. Employees reporting elder care responsibilities reported poorer health than noncaregivers in a variety of domains:

- Caregivers were more likely to report fair or poor health. For example, among female employees aged 50 and older, 17% of caregivers reported fair or poor health compared with 9% among noncaregivers.
- Employees providing elder care were significantly more likely to report depression symptoms and diagnoses of diabetes, hypertension, and pulmonary disease. For example, in models adjusting for age, gender, and work type, caregivers were 26% more likely to report diagnoses of diabetes.
- Female employees with elder care responsibilities reported more stress at home than noncaregivers in every age group. Stress at home appears to affect younger female employees most. Caregivers were more likely to report negative influences of personal life on work.

- Elder care demands were associated with greater health risk behaviors. For example, smoking is higher among male caregivers, especially among young men. Smoking is also higher among caregivers relative to noncaregivers among white collar employees. Among blue collar workers, alcohol use is higher among caregivers.

- Employee caregivers find it more difficult than noncaregivers to take care of their health. For example, among women, caregivers were less likely to report annual mammograms.

- Employees with elder care responsibilities were more likely to report missed days of work. Overall, 8.5% of noncaregivers missed at least 1 day of work over the past 2 weeks because of health issues compared with 10.2% of caregivers. Differences were mostly driven by the much higher absenteeism among younger caregiver employees.

In addition, this study found that the greater prevalence of chronic disease among caregivers and related challenges to health maintenance is costly. Imputing the average cost of a series of sentinel health conditions, employees with elder care responsibilities cost employer health plans 8% more per year more than noncaregiver employees. Excess employee medical care costs associated with elder care were highest among younger, male, and blue collar employees.

A recent study (Amirkhanyan & Wolf, 2006) raises questions about whether these associations are the result of the stress of caregiving per se, or from having a parent who needs care, irrespective of one's role in providing care to that parent. Using panel data from the Health and Retirement Study, the authors estimated models of mental symptoms of 3,350 men and 3,659 women. They found that female, but not male, caregivers whose parents needed care exhibited adverse mental health symptoms. However, both male and female noncaregivers whose parents needed care were also more likely to report such symptoms than noncaregivers. In other words, adverse psychological outcomes related to having a parent with care needs may be dispersed throughout the family and not just to those providing hands-on care. The authors conclude that the focus on caregivers, and not other family members, may be underestimating the social burdens of disability at older ages.

This brief treatment of family caregiving shows the central public health significance of this component of long-term care. First, families provide perhaps two-thirds of the supportive care elders with disabilities require. Even when formal paid care is involved, as in nursing home care or home health care, family caregiving does not end. Families are nearly always partners in these efforts. The contribution of family caregiving to elder health, hard to quantify, is clearly substantial, as are the effects of caregiving on other family members of having an older relative with care needs, including both caregivers and noncaregivers. Second, family caregivers face the substantial health consequences of caregiving, visible in virtually every domain of health and well-being. Finally, family caregiving affects the ramifying networks of these caregivers: employers, children, spouses.

A productive area for public health and aging is better coordination of formal services and family caregiving. In a study of the end of paid home health care for people discharged from hospitals with stroke, we found substantial family caregiving involvement during this period, which lasted, on average, approximately 7 weeks. Between a third and a half of these family caregivers were not adequately prepared for the case closing. Although clinicians reported that they informed patients and family caregivers that the service would be limited and short-term, agencies did not have a systematic or consistent way of preparing caregivers for case closing and referrals to community resources (Levine et al., 2006).

LONG-TERM RESIDENTIAL CARE ARRANGEMENTS

In 2005, the United States had approximately 16,000 certified nursing homes and 35,000 assisted living residences (Alecxih, 2006; U.S. DHHS National Long-Term Care Clearinghouse). These serve approximately 1.5 million and 900,000 people, respectively. The difference between the two is slowly disappearing. Despite the requirement that new admissions to assisted living sites be mobile or not meet criteria for dementia, these people age in assisted living sites and develop such disabilities, and they are now often maintained on site without transfer to skilled nursing facilities. Assisted living facilities are now likely to offer dementia-specific services, such as Alzheimer's special care units. Research suggests that the prevalence of disability and cognitive impairment in the two settings is not as different as might be expected (Zimmerman et al., 2005). Nursing homes are far more regulated than assisted living facilities are, and this convergence in services and populations suggests that assisted living will ultimately need to be similarly monitored and regulated.

Variation within the two residential settings is important. Skilled nursing facilities may be freestanding or linked to hospital systems; also, the national and state Veterans Administration and now even prison systems administer nursing homes. Physicians may or may not be based on site. Nursing facilities may or may not offer hospice beds and differ in the proportion offering "Medicaid beds." Almost all now contain wings for subacute rehabilitative care, short-stay posthospital care for people unable to return to their homes even with home health care.

Assisted living facilities may contain skilled nursing units on site, as in the case of continuing care retirement communities. They also differ in their opportunities for community integration, privacy, likelihood of aging on site given increasing disability, and spectrum of services offered.

Concern for the quality of residential long-term care services is long-standing. After exposure of the industry's inadequacies in the 1980s, the Institute of Medicine proposed quality standards that were later incorporated into the 1987 Nursing Home Reform Act. This legislation aimed to ensure that residents of nursing homes receive high-quality care designed to promote the "highest practicable" physical, mental, and psychosocial well-being. To achieve this aim, nursing homes were required to provide a consistent and wide spectrum of services, including nursing, social services, rehabilitation, pharmacy, and nutrition. Larger nursing homes were required to have a full-time social worker, and many now include additional staff, such as activity therapists. The 1987 Nursing Home Reform Act also required periodic assessment and a linked comprehensive care plan for each resident. These were formalized in the Resident Assessment Instrument (RAI), which includes a Minimum Data Set (MDS) that is now collected by all nursing homes, and which is transmitted electronically to the Centers for Medicare and Medicaid Services. MDS information is used to generate Resident Assessment Protocols (RAPs) that are used to personalize care. Initial versions of the MDS involved only nurse and therapist ratings, which were ideally integrated and qualified in quarterly (and sometimes monthly) meetings with families and, when possible, residents. The newest version of the MDS (3.0) now includes an opportunity to collect information from residents themselves on key quality-of-life domains.

A 2001 Institute of Medicine report reexamined quality of care in long-term care settings and noted some improvements in nursing homes (such as declines in chemical and physical restraints for agitated residents), but continued concerns for undertreatment of pain, high rates of pressure ulcers, under- and malnutrition, and other shortfalls in quality supportive care (Wunderlich & Kohler, 2001). Assisted living facilities came under fire for inadequate concern for resident privacy and inadequate staffing. The IOM report also stressed the need for greater consumer access to information about particular long-term care sites to make informed choices.

This review led to the launch of Nursing Home Compare in 2002, a Web site in which consumers can examine quality and staffing indicators for any certified nursing home according to region or other search criteria. The Web site integrates data from the Online Survey, Certification and Reporting system (OSCAR), which captures complaints, facility-level staffing, and MDS resident-level information. Quality indicators currently tabulated in Nursing Home Compare include the proportion of residents who fail to meet particular benchmarks, such as receiving a flu vaccination, having moderate to severe pain, being physically restrained, feeling depressed or anxious, using an in-dwelling catheter, losing mobility, having a urinary tract infection, or losing a significant amount of weight.

This model was later expanded to cover Medicare home health care agencies in the Home Health Compare Web site. Again, consumers choosing home health care providers can examine performance of particular agencies on a variety of quality indicators, such as the proportion of clients who gain in mobility, who see progress in restoration of ADL function, and who are readmitted to hospitals. Home Health Compare is based on data collected in OASIS, the Outcome and Assessment Information Set, used in all Medicare-certified home health care agencies.

Access to real-time information about the performance of nursing homes and home health care agencies represents an important step in promoting empowerment of consumers and accountability of providers. One may quibble with the appropriateness of particular indicators or the reliability of data, insist on the need to visit sites or make personal inquiries in any case, or question whether consumers appreciate the limitations of such information. This level of engagement in long-term care choice and planning is a central development likely to lead to important change in how families obtain long-term care services. We can expect to see expansion of this approach to Medicaid services and perhaps aging services, in general, as the aging services system adopts a common dataset (SAMS, see Chapter 3) and a new focus on outcomes and quality indicators.

Finally, it is important to note that disparities extend to long-term care services. Evidence suggests that nursing home care is currently a two-tiered system (Mor, Zinn, Angelelli, Teno, & Miller, 2004). The bottom tier consists of facilities that provide care to Medicaid residents almost exclusively. This 15% of nursing homes has fewer nurses, lower occupancy rates, and more health-related deficiencies. As a result, these nursing homes face a greater risk of decertification from the Medicaid-Medicare program. They are mostly found in poor counties and are more likely to serve African American residents. This disparity is of a piece with disparities in access to high-quality medical care and requires appropriate changes in financing and policy.

ENHANCING LONG-TERM CARE

Kane and Kane (2000) have specified goals for supportive care populations, such as people with Alzheimer's disease or severe psychiatric illness, or people dependent on extensive medical technologies. For these populations, rehabilitation or cure is not a reasonable goal, nor, in some cases, is extended survival. That is, for an individual with severe dementia receiving formal home care services, or the older patient receiving ventilator care in a nursing home, excellent supportive care should be the goal but will most likely not extend survival or lead to regained function. What, then, are the goals for enhanced supportive care? What outcomes would be reasonable targets for interventions in these populations? Table 9.3 shows supportive care goals for these populations.

These goals, for example, dignity, privacy, a sense of security, or the opportunity to participate in meaningful activity or reciprocal social relationships, are the essence of sensitive treatment of any person. The goals are no different than ones we set for ourselves and expect in daily activity. Thus, an important conclusion from research with supportive care populations is that the same goals apply. Privacy is as important in the nursing home as anywhere else. Allowing someone to maintain individuality, perhaps through the use of personal objects or "memory cases," is appropriate in institutions just as it is in homes. "Meaningful activity" is a goal even for someone with severe memory impairment and even if attempts at such activity strike the observer as terribly primitive or unsatisfying.

In fact, one additional conclusion from Kane's approach is that we cannot presume to know, without detailed investigation, the valence of behaviors for people with severe dementia. Agitation is almost always a negative behavior (patients appear distressed, risk injuring themselves, and elicit negative responses both from caregivers and other patients). Likewise, a patient's demonstration of a preference, or assertion of continuity with the past, or clear pleasure in activity is easily recognized as positive behavior (as indicated by facial expressions of happiness, contentment, or interest) (Lawton et al., 2001). But the valence of other behaviors is less clear (see Chapter 7). Wandering, perseveration, delusions, and vocalizations are disturbing to observers but may represent sources of pleasure or engagement to the person with severe dementia (Albert, 1997).

For supportive care populations, the following areas have recently become topics of research: recognition of older people's care preferences and designing care regimens that respect such preferences; upgrading home attendant and nursing assistant care; developing special care units for people with Alzheimer's disease; expanding options for supportive housing; and supporting family caregivers. We examine each below.

Table 9.3

GOALS FOR ENHANCED SUPPORTIVE CARE

- Sense of security and order
- Enjoyment
- Meaningful activity (opportunity to accomplish goals)
- Social relationships (opportunity for reciprocity)
- Dignity
- Privacy
- Individuality (identity with past)
- Autonomy (opportunity to express preferences)
- Spiritual well-being
- Functional competence
- Physical comfort

From "Expanding the Home Care Concept: Blurring Distinctions Among Home Care, Institutional Care, and Other Long-Term Care Services," by R. A. Kane, 1995, *The Milbank Quarterly, 73*(2), 161–186.

Recognizing and Taking Older People's Care Preferences Seriously

Are family caregivers, even when they are in daily contact with patients with dementia, good judges of patient preferences? Reason for doubt on the accuracy of caregiver perceptions is evident in Logsdon's finding of high correlations between caregiver mental health, particularly depression, and caregiver ratings of a patient's quality of life (Logsdon, Gibbons, McCurry, & Teri, 2001). Depressive symptoms in caregivers were associated with lower ratings of patient quality of life, suggesting that caregivers are not accurate reporters, but rather transfer their own negative perceptions on to patients.

A related result is shown in Figure 9.1, which displays patient reports of enjoyment in activity, caregiver perceptions of patient enjoyment in activity, and the relationship between each of these reports and *patient* reports of depressive symptoms. The figure is based on reports from 161 patient-caregiver pairs in a clinical cohort of Alzheimer's patients with mildly dementia. Patient reports of enjoyment in activity were correlated with patient depressive symptoms. Caregiver reports of patient enjoyment were less clearly related to patient depressive symptoms. Thus, at least in the case of enjoyment of activity, patient reports may be more accurate than caregiver reports.

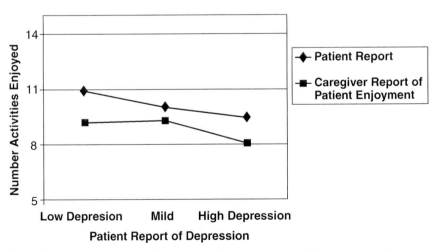

Figure 9.1 Mild dementia: Patient reports of enjoyment in activity correlated with patient-reported depressive symptoms. $n = 161$, ratings from patients with mild dementia and caregivers.

This situation contrasts with other domains of patient experience, in which caregiver reports may, in fact, be more accurate than patient reports. In the same Columbia clinical cohort, for example, caregiver reports of the *frequency* of patient activity were significantly correlated with the patient's Mini-Mental State Examination score. Patient reports of activity frequency were not related to patient cognitive status. Thus, for these elders with mild dementia, reports of affective experience (enjoyment in activity) are likely to be more accurate than reports of the frequency of behaviors or symptoms.

Examining the care and more general psychosocial preferences of community-dwelling elders has become an important focus of research. As Carpenter and colleagues point out, "just as people have unique wishes about the medical care they receive, they may have unique wishes about the personal care they receive as they become more dependent" (Carpenter, van Haitsma, Ruckdeschel, & Lawton, 2000). Documenting these preferences is useful for the concurrent delivery of care, but may also be useful for establishing an "advanced psychosocial directive," a statement about preferred care delivery and living situation that can be consulted when a person is no longer able to state these preferences. This approach would likely encourage individualized care planning rather than current standard service plans.

In a pilot concept-mapping approach to psychosocial preferences, Carpenter and colleagues (2000) found that preferences for care and caregiving formed a well-defined cluster, distinct from other domains (such as "growth activities," "leisure," or "self-dominion"). On a scale of 1–5 to indicate importance, preferences in this domain ranged from 4.35 ("caregivers should know about my medical conditions and treatment") to 1.90 ("caregivers should address me by my first name"). Midrange preferences included "having friends involved in my care," "using alternative medicine providers," "having caregivers call me by a particular name," and "accepting restrictions for my safety." The investigators have developed an extensive inventory to assess daily preferences, the Preferences for Everyday Living Inventory, and fielded it in a large sample of elders in different care settings.

One of us (SA) used a modified version of this preference inventory to examine concordance between family and formal caregivers on the perceived preferences of people with dementia for particular activities. For this study, patients with mild to moderate dementia who were attending an adult day care program at a senior center were enrolled. The primary family caregiver (the person making sure the needs of the patient were met, either directly or by arranging services) was identified. The formal caregiver in every case was a home attendant who provided care in the patient's home and also accompanied the elder to the adult day care program. The families and home attendants in this study spoke Spanish. Concordance between the two different types of caregivers was assumed to be an indicator that patients with mild to moderate dementia were able to communicate preferences (even if they could not state them in an interview or research questionnaire). Each type of caregiver was asked to rate how important particular behaviors or activities were to the patient on a 4-point Likert scale (very, some, little, or no importance).

Concordance between family and formal care providers was quite good. The proportion of patients for whom family caregiver and home attendant maximally disagreed (i.e., where one said the activity was "very important" and the other said "no importance") was low. For activities with low frequency, pairs were discordant in less than 15% of instances. These preferences included the wish to be left alone, to have a challenging task, to talk about worries, and to keep to a particular routine. For more commonly preferred activities, such as choosing what clothes to wear, hearing the news, spending time outside, and having visitors, discordance was also relatively uncommon and was again about 15%. This level of agreement between different types of caregiver suggests that patients with mild to moderate dementia can express preferences, as evident in the joint recognition of such preferences by people who spend time with these elders.

Upgrading Home Attendant and Nursing Assistant Care

As we have seen, home care paraprofessionals are an important element in the long-term care spectrum. They provide in-home support for elders with ADL needs severe enough to require nursing home levels of care. These paraprofessionals do not have medical training and are barred from providing help with prescriptions or medical equipment. In New York City's Home Care Services Program, a Medicaid waiver program, 65,000 low-income elders received ADL support from home attendants in 2005, and the number is increasing each year. New York City continues to have the highest percentage of Medicaid recipients using home care services and the highest expenditures for such services, as well as the highest state spending for Medicaid services (Centers for Medicare and Medicaid Services /Office of Research, Development, and Information [ORDI], 2008).

Nearly a third of the elders receiving home care through the New York City program have moderate to severe dementia and have some degree of cognitive impairment (Hokenstad, Ramirez, Haslanger, & Finneran, 1997). In fact, in a study of elders with Alzheimer's disease living in the community, more than half of the sample received ADL support from home care paraprofessionals. Moreover, a quarter of the sample received *all* ADL care from such paraprofessionals (Albert et al., 1998).

Home care paraprofessionals are typically referred to as "home attendants" (HAs). Older adults with disabilities who meet income requirements are eligible, and an algorithm used by the New York City Health Resources Administration assigns blocks of hours according to severity of ADL limitation, medical conditions, and availability of informal care. Home attendant time is allocated in 4-, 8-, 12-, or 24-hour blocks, with weekly visits from a visiting nurse service and quarterly reevaluation of the elder by the subcontracted home care agency. Home care agency care coordinators supervise groups of attendants, and HAs are required to meet in-service requirements on a regular basis.

The difficulty of the HA-client relationship is apparent in a number of ways: HAs are family and not family; they perform roles typically assumed by family but are also performing a job. They may care for more than one client at a time, sometimes in "cluster care" arrangements. They are often asked to perform tasks outside the scope of their duties. They have to get along with other family members. They are isolated for a large part of the day with a person who has some authority over them but is also dependent on them.

Albert's interviews with 70 home attendants from two home health care agencies provide insights into their situation. These were seasoned paraprofessionals; inclusion criteria required that they had at least 1 year of experience. The interviews revealed that HAs in New York City were almost exclusively female, members of minority groups, and largely immigrants. Their median age was 49 years, and the median length of time they had been in the United States was 17 years, suggesting that these women were well-established breadwinners for their families. They had worked as HAs for a median of 9.5 years, and most were working full-time (with overtime) in this capacity. The median number of clients they had been assigned over time was 12, and one of every four clients was reported to have dementia.

In their current situation, the median number of hours spent with the index client was 55.0 per week over a median of 4 days per week.

The high number reflects the large number of HAs spending 24 hr/day with clients for 3–4 days per week. (More recently, the NYC Human Resources Agency that administers the program has begun to reduce 24-hour shifts.) The large number of hours per HA also reflects the low-wage nature of the work and the need for these women to work extremely long hours. In fact, 44% of the HAs had another client, and the median number of hours for such second clients was 12.0 per week.

The median age of their clients was 82, of whom 86% were women. HAs reported that more than half the elders showed signs of depression and that approximately 40% had Alzheimer's disease or stroke. Symptoms of poor health were highly prevalent among clients. About a third were reported to have dyspnea, difficulty swallowing, or severe pain. Cognitive symptoms were also highly prevalent: 62% were reported to have a memory problem, 32% were said to be disoriented, and 5% were said to be vegetative. HAs provided help with bathing, dressing, and outdoor mobility in almost every case, and the majority of clients were also receiving aid in toileting, indoor mobility, and bed/chair transfer. Half of the client sample was incontinent, a third were limited to bed or chair, and 16% could not be taken outside. Thus, these elders were receiving support equivalent to nursing home care.

Home attendants were also asked to rate how difficult it was to provide care for their clients so that correlates of these ratings could be examined. The strongest correlate of perceived "easiness" was client emotional status. "Easy" clients were reported to demonstrate positive affects more frequently than other clients ($r = 0.40$, $p < .01$). They were also seen as more satisfied with the care provided by the HA ($r = 0.30$, $p < .05$). The presence of daily medical symptoms was associated with greater difficulty in providing care ($r = -0.27$), but none of the other indicators of poor function or general medical status achieved statistical significance. Severity of functional deficit was not strongly associated with HA judgments of client difficulty, suggesting that HAs view this aspect of their work as a "job," without the emotional valence family caregivers attribute to such care.

Almost all training sessions ("in-services") for home attendants stress the physical demands of care, and not help with practical issues that might mitigate the more emotionally charged challenges of home care. Albert and colleagues have developed a manual, based heavily on their interviews with home attendants, to remedy this gap (Albert, 2002). To give the flavor of this approach, Table 9.4 provides an excerpt from the manual.

Developing training in this practical approach to the dilemmas of home care would go a long way to improve the experience of home care

Table 9.4

EXCERPT: HOME ATTENDANTS SPEAK ABOUT HOME CARE

WHAT YOU DO . . . WHEN YOU FEEL YOU CAN'T HANDLE THE JOB BUT FEEL YOU CAN'T GIVE THE JOB UP

Sometimes conditions in a home or with a particular client are just not acceptable. You can notify the agency and complain, or give up the job. But because of the wait to get a new long-term client assignment, you may be reluctant to complain or leave.

One home attendant reported that she did put up with a terrible home situation, where they would not even let her use the toilet, because she did not feel she could afford to give up the job. Another mentioned that she did not report neglect of the client to the agency for the same reason. She was afraid the agency would call the family, and that the family would dismiss her. As she put it, "You cannot tell them. You have to walk into that house everyday. You don't know what they will do to you."

But other home attendants disagreed. "If you feel the family might threaten you or something, you don't want to be there. You don't go back there." Or, as another said, "I am not going to put myself in that kind of predicament. I will tell the agency that they better take me out of there." Even home attendants who had put up with terrible conditions in the past because they felt they needed a job now agreed that it was not a good strategy. Better to quit the job than face abuse.

One complication, though, is concern for neglected or abused clients. "If I see something like that, I don't stay on the job but you feel sorry for the client." Still, no one benefits, neither you or the client, if you keep quiet about a situation of neglect or abuse. The welfare of clients requires that you report the problem to the agency. This allows the agency to arrange for the proper intervention.

How do you let the agency know about a problem with a client or home? Using the telephone in the home may be a problem because of privacy. Clients and families may listen in. One solution is to call while you are out doing errands: "When I call the agency to speak to the coordinator, I always try to call when the client sends me to the store. So I call when I am out in the street."

From Speaking from Experience: Home Attendants Speak about Home Care (Albert, 2002)

for both caregivers and care receivers. A second approach would be to "credentialize" paraprofessional care, that is, make it more of a profession, with standardized training, licensure, and opportunity for continued training leading to nursing degrees. This would likely result in wage increases and improvement of work conditions.

Similar challenges appear to be at work among certified nursing assistants (CNAs), who provide the bulk of care, as we have seen, in nursing homes. They provide almost all "bed and body work" for residents and, as a result, have the most daily contact with residents. New efforts are underway to take advantage of the CNA's greater contact with residents to improve resident care, especially in the setting of special care units for people with Alzheimer's disease (see below).

Do CNAs view residents in the same way as nurses or nurse managers? Or does their greater contact with residents lead them to rate residents differently? Albert and colleagues examined this issue in a pilot study. Forty CNAs were asked to nominate a "difficult" and an "easy" resident under their care. They then completed eight questions regarding these residents' behaviors, which were drawn from the nursing home Minimum Data Set form (see above). CNA ratings were compared with the nurse-rated MDS record within the same month.

On the whole, agreement between CNA ratings and MDS scores was low. For example, in the case of verbal abuse, 24 of 40 CNAs reported verbal abuse from the resident, which was recorded in only one MDS chart for this set of residents. On almost every indicator, CNAs reported more symptoms (depressive mood, memory problems, dependence in daily tasks, and physical abuse) than the MDS record. These findings need to be investigated further. It may be that CNAs use different criteria when completing MDS questions, or, more likely, daily contact with residents allows them to identify greater deficits. If CNA ratings were incorporated into MDS records, different resident assessment protocols would be triggered and perhaps more intensive care plans initiated.

Schnelle and colleagues (2009) have developed standardized training and observation protocols to demonstrate that opportunities for more effective care delivery are often missed in the nursing home, and also that specific training for nursing home staff in ADL care, mobility, and psychosocial support result in improved outcomes. Standardized observation protocols also show that many MDS measures recorded by staff do not fully capture resident experience. For example, in one study of standardized observation of ADL care, staff failed to offer residents choices for at least one of three care activities in all 20 nursing homes in the study. In morning ADL care, staff did not offer choices to residents in when to get out of bed (11%), what to wear (25%), and location of breakfast dining (39%). Only two of the 20 nursing homes were cited for this deficiency in formal surveys (Schnelle et al., 2009). In randomized trials of carefully designed training protocols for care delivery by

CNAs, a feeding assistance intervention led to increases in caloric intake and weight gain (Simmons et al., 2008). Similar benefit was evident for continence, mobility, and pain recognition interventions, in some cases with family members noting benefit (Cadogan et al., 2004; Levy-Storms, Schnelle, & Simmons 2007). Related efforts have shown that training CNAs in behavioral management techniques may reduce agitation episodes during ADL care (Burgio al., 2002). These interventions require careful attention to behavior streams to establish relationships between resident and aide behavior (Roth, Stevens, Burgio, & Burgio, 2002). Relationship building is especially relevant for "culture change" efforts in nursing homes, that is, a movement in which nursing homes are attempting to increase the quality of care provided and quality of life for their residents by shifting the focus from being solely responsive to regulatory requirements to placing the resident and staff's needs at the center of care concerns.

Special Care Units for People With Alzheimer's Disease

Freiman and Brown (1996) point out that "today's nursing home population is more functionally and cognitively disabled and requires more skilled and/or specialized care than ever before." Special care units (SCUs) for Alzheimer's disease have been developed to meet this need. The 1996 Medical Expenditures Panel Study (MEPS) found that over 10% of nursing homes in the United States had an Alzheimer's unit, at that time a total of 73,400 SCU beds in just over 2000 homes. SCUs tend to be relatively small, in keeping with the greater staff time and more specialized staff assignments typical of the units. The MEPS survey found that Alzheimer's units contained a mean of 34 beds (Freiman & Brown, 2001).

Despite the growth in specialized care for Alzheimer's disease, at this point there is still no standard definition of an SCU. Units called "SCUs" differ considerably in environmental design, physical separation from other units in nursing homes, specialized dementia care training for staff, staffing ratios, and activity programming (Morris & Emerson-Lombardo, 1994; Teresi, Holmes, Ramirez, & Kong, 1998). This variation has posed difficulties for the assessment of the SCU as a superior approach in Alzheimer's care.

Outcome studies have not found an SCU benefit in slowing the trajectory of functional or cognitive decline (McCann, Bienas, & Evans, 2000; Phillips et al., 1997). The SCU setting, however, may offer benefit in promoting participation in activity (as measured by behavior stream real-time observation) and resident well-being (as observed in ratings of resident affective expression) (Holmes, Teresi, & Ory, 2000). SCU care differs in important but unexpected ways from non-SCU care in residents with similar physical and cognitive status. SCU residents in one study were less likely to be tube fed and more likely to have more extensive care plans, but did not differ in physical restraints and actually were more likely to be prescribed psychotropic medications (Gruneir, Lapane, Miller, & Mor, 2008).

Although results to date have been mixed for SCU evaluations, the evaluation effort has been useful in drawing attention to features of environment and staffing that affect resident well-being. One finding of interest is that environmental simplification for residents with Alzheimer's disease, in the absence of increased staffing, may have negative effects (van Haitsma, Lawton, & Kleban, 2000). On the other hand, changes in lighting may affect sleep patterns, which in turn may affect agitation behaviors (Kutner & Bliwise, 2000). Low levels of light, excess glare, and noise may be environmental sources of excess morbidity for patients with Alzheimer's disease that can be altered easily (Sloan, Mitchell, Calkins, & Zimmerman, 2000). Changing staff assignments so that particular CNAs are assigned to particular residents may also promote resident participation in organized activity (Lindeman, Arnsberger, & Owens, 2000).

The role of nursing home staff, in particular, the CNA, as an agent of resident well-being is only now being fully appreciated. Innovations in the delivery of nursing home care are now underway, and undergoing evaluation, to see whether giving staff greater latitude to change the way they deliver care offers benefit to residents. For example, in one labor-management partnership in New York City, staff on certain demonstration units is free to assign more time to certain activities (such as bathing or feeding), based on their understanding of resident needs and unit dynamics. In another nursing home, CNAs are being encouraged to upgrade clinical skills, communicate information they have obtained about resident health, and participate in comprehensive care-planning meetings for residents. The role of labor-management partnerships in this effort is critical.

Expansion of Options for Supportive Care and Housing

Kane (1995) has identified a series of policy challenges for home care that would give adequate scope to the preference of frail older people to live in homes, rather than institutions, and that would also give greater flexibility to service providers to cross current, fixed service categories. She urges policymakers to think beyond the rigid service categories that have been linked to particular living environments, such as home care, board and care or assisted living care, and nursing home care.

This change has already begun. "Home care" paraprofessionals now assist clients outside the home, as they travel, shop, go to physician appointments, attend adult day care, or simply go outside for exercise or entertainment. "Home care" paraprofessionals also provide ADL care and housekeeping support to frail older people who do not live in "homes" in the traditional sense, but who instead reside in group settings, such as board and care homes, low-income housing, or single-room occupancy hotels (that have become de facto sites for long-term care). This is a welcome development, for it suggests that people can hold on to "home" despite severe ADL needs, and that providing ADL support can be made flexible enough to accommodate different kinds of home settings and preferred personal lifestyles.

Implicit in this expansion of the home care concept is recognition that the nursing home is mostly a residence rather than a site for medical or nursing care. The 24-hour care designation of nursing home care is a fiction. As Kane (1995) points out, "These prescribed settings provide remarkably little nursing care." One study of nursing home care, reported by Kane, showed that 39% of residents received no care from a registered nurse in a 24-hour period. The mean duration of nursing care over this 24-hour period was quite small: for RN care, 7.9 minutes; for LPN care, 15.5 minutes; and for CNA care, 76.9 minutes. Thus, the nursing home is mainly a residence, and care of this sort or degree could be brought into homes, although not necessarily in as cost-effective a manner. "This modest amount of care cannot be replicated at home for the same price because the nursing home efficiently provides stand-by assistance and can meet unscheduled, quickly arising needs" (Kane, 1995). PACE has developed models, however, that allow cost-effective home care service in lieu of nursing home care, provided that housing services are altered to create more easily serviced groups of elders.

While extending what we mean by "home care," it is also worth thinking about ways to extend the flexibility of "service provision." A number of such efforts are underway. One is to allow greater delegation of nursing skills in home care settings. Traditionally, only nurses could administer medications, care for wounds, monitor vital signs, perform catheter or ostomy care, or suction patients who are on ventilators. Kane (1995) reminds us that families have always performed these tasks, and that family members learn these skills from nurses. There really is no reason why less skilled formal caregivers, such as home care paraprofessionals, cannot take on these tasks. It would mean an upgrading of their skills, a boon to family members, and a significant cost savings.

A second development in the expansion of services is a shift in the balance of authority between home care providers and families. The "consumer-directed care" movement, as mentioned earlier, allows elders and their families to use funds assigned for a home care benefit (such as the Medicaid personal assistance home care benefit) to hire, train, and employ home care aides as they think best. In practice, families are helped by home care agencies in this process. The agencies suggest lists of potential workers, provide training and counseling on how to be an employer, and usually manage disbursement of funds.

Finally, families are now being trained to take a more active role in planning for hospital discharge or the end of home health care services. New Web sites, "caregiver navigation programs," and greater emphasis on family involvement in discharge planning will probably place greater emphasis on improving care transitions, which have proven to be one of the greater challenges in long-term care.

SUMMARY

What Is Long-Term Care? "Long-term care" includes the complete spectrum of services and supports required to meet health and personal care needs over an extended period of time. Long-term care primarily provides services that allow older people to meet personal self-maintenance needs, such as bathing, dressing, using the toilet, and the other activities of daily living.

Trends in Long-Term Care Use and Spending. Need for long-term care is best indexed by the proportion of older people with ADL limitations who require personal assistance services. These services are provided in a variety of settings, ranging from the certified nursing assistant in a skilled nursing facility to unpaid family in their homes. In the United States, Medicaid is the primary payer, accounting for about half of these costs for the 9 million older people with ADL limitations and the 1.5 million receiving paid personal assistance services.

Home- and Community-Based Services. In between skilled nursing homes and family care is the wide spectrum of services and providers elders need for supportive care. These include home health care, personal assistance care, adult day care, provision of assistive and medical equipment, and even home modification. States continue to innovate in bundling long-term care services by use of Medicaid waiver options.

Personal Assistance Services and Public Health. Personal assistance services may have beneficial health consequences by effectively managing disabilities that would otherwise put people at risk for poor outcomes. An important area for public health inquiry in home- and community-based services is direct investigation of features of PAS delivery that promote desired health and functioning outcomes. Does PAS allow elders to meet basic provisioning, hygiene, mobility, and nutrition needs? And does effectively meeting these needs, in turn, promote fewer falls, better skin integrity, weight maintenance, and increases in lower extremity strength? Do these outcomes in turn influence well being?

Family Caregiving. Fifteen to 20% of U.S. households provide family caregiving support. Family caregivers face severe challenges in maintaining their own health and well-being under this strain, with consequences on employment and other spheres of life. Yet the contribution of families to elder supportive care is central to elder health and forms the backbone of long-term care delivery in the United States.

Long-Term Residential Care Arrangements. In 2004–2005, the United States had approximately 16,000 certified nursing homes and 35,000 assisted living residences, which served approximately 1.5 million and 900,000 people, respectively. Nursing homes have a national standard for data recording and quality assurance, and this information is available to consumers who need to choose nursing home care. Similar standardization and public access is available now for home health care and may extend to other aging services as well.

Enhancing Long-Term Care. For the individual with severe dementia receiving formal home care services, or the older patient receiving care in a nursing home, dignity, privacy, a sense of security, and the opportunity to participate in meaningful activity or reciprocal social relationships are the essence of sensitive treatment. To reach this goal, we need to take the care preferences of older people seriously, upgrade home attendant and certified nursing assistant care, continue to redesign care environments (such as special care units for people with Alzheimer's disease), and introduce greater flexibility in home care and service delivery, making families partners whenever possible.

10 Mortality and End-of-Life Care

Mortality has already appeared in prior chapters, first as one of the five "faces" of aging, second as a key factor driving population aging and, more generally, the age structure of populations. We also examined historical change in the age distribution of deaths, in life expectancy, and in the distribution of causes of death. Still, mortality requires more detailed treatment. It is clearly a central outcome in aging and public health, but it is also more complex than usually recognized. Dying in late life almost always includes frailty, multiple diseases, and additional intervening medical events. Once we move beyond simple counts of total or cause-specific mortality to measurement of mortality as a sequence of events over a potentially long period, we are forced to recognize that it is often difficult to state when dying begins and what someone actually died of.

Lynn and Adamson (2003) discuss changes in the end-of-life experience in the United States that have occurred over the past century. They highlight five major changes. First, in 1900 life expectancy was only 47 years. That is, a very small percentage of people lived into the 70s, 80s, or beyond. By 2000, this figure had reached 75 (and it is over 77 years today). Second, in 1900 most people died at home. Today, the most common site of death is a medical facility or institution, although in recent years a slight trend away from dying in institutions has been observed. Third, most medical expenses in the last year of life were paid by the family in 1900; today, Medicare pays for the majority of care in the last year of life. Fourth, the types of conditions from which individuals die have shifted from primarily acute conditions in 1900 toward three major chronic conditions: heart disease, cancer, and stroke. Finally, the period of disability prior to death in 1900 in general was very brief, amounting to weeks or at most months, whereas today individuals live on average for 2 years with activity limitations in the years prior to death. These macrolevel changes set the stage for thinking about how Americans die today and the changing role of public health in creating the condition under which individuals, in particular, older adults, experience a good death.

CAUSES OF DEATH

People die of something, and this "something" is listed on death certificates. Terminology around these causes has shifted in the past decade as many states have begun to adopt the latest (2003) version of the death certificate. Death certificates now distinguish among "immediate causes," "underlying causes," and "other significant conditions" that contribute to death. Immediate causes include proximal conditions that lead immediately to death whereas underlying causes are part of the chain of events that lead to the immediate cause. In contrast, other significant conditions are more tangential than the immediate and underlying causes, for example, longstanding chronic conditions that complicate recovery and therefore play a role in the death that is caused by another condition. Prior to 2003, the certificate distinguished only between "primary" causes of death (those proximal to death, similar to immediate) and "contributory" causes (those more distal, likely encompassing both underlying and other significant conditions). Accordingly, public health surveillance of mortality makes use of the terms immediate and underlying causes, as well as primary and contributory causes, for attributing deaths to disease and tracking changes in cause-specific mortality.

The revised death certificate also includes information on age, race, whether the decedent is of Hispanic origin, sex, and residence. Age is rarely missing; well under 1% of death certificates lack information on age at death (Pickle, Mungiole, Jones, & White, 1996). Every death in the United States is recorded on these certificates, which are sent to local departments of health and then to the National Center for Health Statistics. For example, the number of deaths recorded in the United

States in 2006 was 2.4 million (NCHS, 2009). Heart disease (25% of deaths), cancer (24%), and stroke (6%) were the leading causes of death, together accounting for 55% of all deaths (NCHS, 2007). These causes, all chronic diseases that predominantly affect older people, should be contrasted with external causes of death, such as injuries (including motor vehicle accidents), suicide, and homicide. Together, these account for just 7.2% of deaths in a year (5%, 1.4%, and 0.8%, respectively).

The quality of cause-of-death information on death certificates appears to be good, although some problems have been identified. Currently, a computerized algorithm is used to apply World Health Organization coding for all medical conditions reported. Indicators of quality of cause-of-death information suggest that the system works reasonably well. Exercises in which experts code medical information show high agreement with algorithm assignments. Also, the proportion of certificates with unclassifiable causes of death (residual or nonspecific category of the International Classification of Disease [ICD-9 categories 780–799]) has declined considerably, whereas the number of medical conditions reported on death certificates has increased, suggesting increased specificity.

Still, while underlying cause information in death certificates agrees well with hospital records, the validity of cause-of-death information is less certain for deaths outside of medical settings (Pickle et al., 1996), some 54% of all deaths in 2004 (NCHS, 2006). More generally, when the person completing cause-of-death information does not have a detailed understanding of a person's medical condition, "underlying" and "contributing" causes of death may be confused. Pickle et al. (1996) illustrate this problem in the case of long-term diabetics. People with diabetes are at high risk of death from stroke and heart disease, which are likely to appear on their death certificates. Diabetes, however, is underreported on the death certificate for people who died of stroke or heart disease. The result is an underestimate of the mortality burden of diabetes.

Hadley (1992) has pointed out the difficulty of maintaining the distinction between "underlying" and "contributing" causes of death for the older population. It may not be possible to identify what is "underlying" and what is "contributory" in older people, where multiple pathologies are common and chronic conditions interact in complex ways. What should be listed as the underlying or contributory cause of death in a person who died of a fall or pneumonia but also had longstanding diabetes and osteoporosis and a recent stroke? The more important question is to determine how this set of chronic conditions may have led to the fall or pneumonia, or how these conditions may have made this fall or pneumonia lethal.

More generally, we can ask why longstanding chronic conditions ultimately kill older people. Is the death simply the result of continued progression of the disease? Or is the death the result of greater vulnerability to pathology of a given severity because of frailty or some other chronic condition? Or, finally, is the death actually the result of some new pathology that has emerged because of the person's chronic disease status? It may be difficult to separate these factors in death certificates, which have traditionally not listed chronic conditions as contributory causes of death, or in autopsy series, which are not representative of the universe of deaths.

Alzheimer's disease is a case in point. It has a long latency period, perhaps even 20–40 years, over which brain lesions develop. These are the characteristic neuritic plaques and neurofibrillary tangles that obstruct amyloid clearance, which are evident in neuropathological studies (autopsy confirmation of the disease). At some point in disease progression, these neuropathological changes begin to affect cognition and motor function. The characteristic cognitive changes include deficits in short-term memory and language, and typical motor findings include extrapyramidal signs (slowness, rigidity, tremor). When these symptoms become severe enough to interfere with the performance of ordinary daily tasks, such as work, household maintenance, or shopping, the patient has reached a new milestone in disease progression. We say that the patient has made the transition from subclinical to clinical disease; indeed, it is only at this point that a patient typically presents to the internist or neurologist and is given a diagnosis, perhaps after neuropsychological testing and brain imaging to rule out other causes of dementia. The patient then goes home to live another 7–8 years, on average, before dying, along the way crossing additional milestones of progressively more severe disability (Stern et al., 1994). The patient finally dies during a hospitalization, let's say, after being transferred from a nursing home. He or she may have been transferred to the hospital because of a pneumonia that did not respond to oral antibiotics, but by this point the patient probably had already developed a wasting syndrome, severe weakness in the lower extremities, poor skin integrity, and exacerbation of intercurrent heart disease.

Did this patient die of pneumonia or wasting, Alzheimer's or heart disease, or some broader complex of aging-related disease? The answer is not obvious.

MORTALITY RATES: KEY TRENDS AND PATTERNS

The National Center for Health Statistics' annual mortality data *Deaths: Final Data* and *Deaths: Leading Causes* (both National Vital Statistics Reports) are key documents for understanding mortality in the United States (see Chapter 2). NCHS combines vital statistics from death certificates with estimates of the size of the population, either from the Census or from postcensal estimates prepared in cooperation with the Census Bureau. Postcensal estimates are derived by updating the resident population in the Census by drawing upon several measures of population change, including births and deaths, immigration, and migration within the United States.

Mortality Trends by Age and Sex

Figure 10.1 presents death rates by age and sex, from 1955 to 2005. The graph shows declines in death rates per 100,000 population for nearly all age groups. Striking are the declines in infant mortality (under 1 year), but also the fact that declines in deaths at ages 65–74, 75–84, and even 85 and older have continued.

If one were to redraw the graph for 2005 with the x axis age and y axis rate per 100,000 population, the age-specific mortality curve would show a clear "check-mark" or "j" shape. That is, the death rate is high in the perinatal period and first year of life, reaches its nadir at about age 10, and then increases steadily. The death rate per 100,000 is currently less than 20 for ages 5–14 and increases to nearly 20,000 for ages 85 and older. There is, of course, considerable variation across sex and race, with White women having the lowest rates and Black men the highest; but the relationship between age and mortality risk is consistent across the groups.

This j-shaped pattern is sharply defined for many of the cause-specific mortality plots. Heart disease, many of the cancers (for example, lung, prostate, and breast), stroke, pneumonia/influenza, and perhaps liver and chronic obstructive pulmonary disease (COPD) all follow this pattern. Death from these diseases (and also incidence) is strongly related to age and increases across the entire life span. A variant of this pattern is evident for mortality from some of the cancers and liver disease. Mortality from these causes appears to plateau in the sixth decade and perhaps even decline at older ages. Finally, the very different pattern for external, accidental causes of death, and the special case of suicide is notable. Mortality from unintentional injuries, motor vehicle accidents, homicide, and

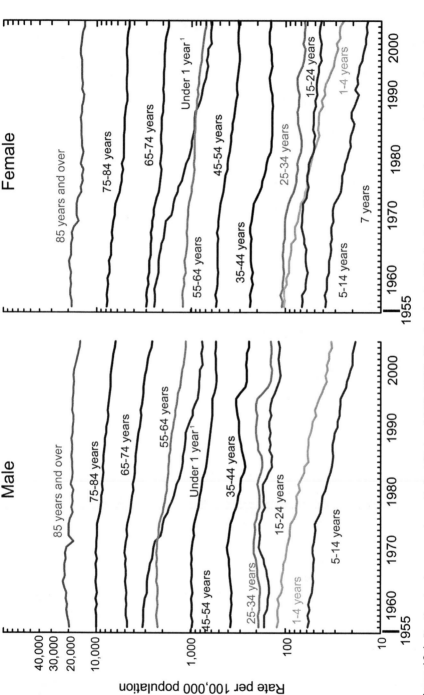

Figure 10.1 Death rates by age and sex: United States, 1955–2005. [1]Death rates for "Under 1 year" (based on population estimates) differ from infant mortality rates (based on live births). From CDC/NCHS, National Vital Statistics System, Mortality: http://www.cdc.gov/nchs/deaths.htm.

Source: From "Deaths: Final Data for 2004," by A. M. Miniño, M. Heron, B. L. Smith, and K. D. Kochanek, 2004. Retrieved September 15, 2009, from http://www.cdc.gov/nchs/data/nvsr/nvsr56/deaths04.htm.

suicide is highest for young people and reaches its peak at approximately age 20. Mortality from these causes may continue to increase over the life span (unintentional injuries), remain more or less flat (motor vehicle accidents, suicide, firearm suicide), or decline (homicide, firearm homicide). These broad patterns once again confirm the centrality of age for chronic disease mortality.

Crude Versus Age-Adjusted Trends

Figure 10.2 shows trends in the crude and age-adjusted death rate over the past half-century or so. The trend in the crude death rate, while declining, vastly underestimates the reduction in mortality in the United States since the 1960s. Because the U.S. population grew increasingly older over the century (and because age is a risk factor for mortality), it is necessary to standardize the population in each year to ensure that populations of similar age structure are being compared. The age-adjusted death rate includes this correction factor and shows that annual mortality has declined by half over the century, from approximately 1,300 in 1960 to approximately 800 per 100,000 people in 2005.

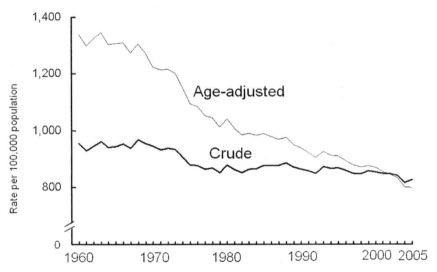

Figure 10.2 Crude and age-adjusted death rates, United States, 1960–2005.

Source: From "Deaths: Final Data for 2005," H.-C. Kung, D. L. Hoyert, J. Xu, & S. L. Murray, April 24, 2008, *National Vital Statistics Report, 56*(10). Retrieved September 15, 2009, from http://www.cdc.gov/nchs/data/nvsr/nvsr56/nvsr56_10.pdf.
Note: Crude death rates on an annual basis per 100,000 population; age-adjusted rates per 100,000 U.S. standard population; see "Technical Notes."

An alternative way of measuring this mortality reduction is to look at declines in the years of life lost to disease, given declines in cause-specific mortality. Years of potential life lost before age 75 is a measure of premature mortality. Information from eight separate age groups (<1, 1–14, 15–24, and five 10-year age groups from 25–34 through 65–74) is used in calculating the measure. The number of deaths in each age group is multiplied by the difference between age 75 years and the mid-point of the age group. For example, the death of someone in the 65- to 74-year-old age group counts as 75–69.5 or 5.5 years of life lost. The total years of potential life lost is calculated by summing years of life lost over all age groups.

With declines in cause-specific mortality, the number of years of life lost to disease should also decline. The age-adjusted years of life lost to disease was 10,448 in 1980, 9,086 in 1990, and 7,300 in 2005 (Health, United States, 2008).

This decline in years of potential life lost before age 75 is consistent across diseases and extends to unintentional injuries, suicide, and homicide. Evidently, improvements in health and environment across the life span have pushed the risk of death from disease out to later and later ages, resulting in lower death rates and fewer years of life lost to disease. Also, changes in safety standards (seatbelts, traffic patterns, law enforcement, occupational health efforts) may have helped reduce years of life lost to unintentional injuries. Finally, it may be that the decline in the mortality burden of suicide (392 to 347 years of life lost per 100,000 between 1980 and 2005) may be due, at least in part, to improved mental health services and broader changes in help-seeking patterns.

Trends in Causes of Death at Older Ages

In 1980, 1,341,848 people aged 65 and older died. The 10 most prevalent causes of death were heart disease, cancer, stroke, pneumonia and influenza, chronic obstructive pulmonary disease, atherosclerosis, diabetes, unintentional injuries, kidney disease, and liver disease. Heart disease, cancer, and stroke together accounted for 74.5% of these deaths.

In 2005, 1,788,189 people aged 65 and older died (remember that there were many more people aged 65 and older in 2005 than in 1980, so that this absolute increase actually represents a smaller proportion of people aged 65 and older). As shown in Figure 10.3, the 10 leading causes of death were much the same, with heart disease, cancer, and stroke now accounting for far fewer, but still most of the deaths (now,

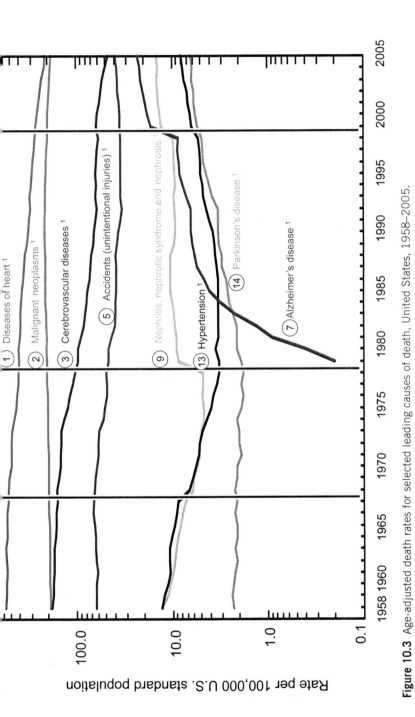

Figure 10.3 Age-adjusted death rates for selected leading causes of death, United States, 1958–2005.

Source: From "Deaths: Final Data for 2004," by A. M. Miniño, M. Heron, B. L. Smith, and K. D. Kochanek, 2004. Retrieved September 15, 2009, from http://www.cdc.gov/nchs/data/hestat/finaldeaths04/finaldeaths04.htm.

Note: Circled numbers indicate ranking of conditions as leading causes of death in 2005.
[1] Age adjusted rates per 100,000 U.S. standard population. ICD is International Classification of Disease. From CDC/NCHS, National Vital Statistics System, Mortality.

57.6% of deaths). However, atherosclerosis and liver disease no longer appear as leading causes of death in 1999. They were replaced by Alzheimer's disease (seventh place) and septicemia (tenth place).

It is hard to know what to make of these changes. Surely, people had, and died of Alzheimer's disease in 1980. Part of the change can be attributed to the revision in coding conventions (the shift from ICD-9 to ICD-10 coding between 1980 and 1999), and part to public recognition of Alzheimer's disease as a cause of death in its own right. These nonmedical factors must be considered when interpreting vital statistics. Nevertheless, as Lynn and Adamson (2003) point out, over the longer term, the shift from acute to chronic conditions as causes of death is one that has literally changed the face of death in America.

A similar conclusion was reached by Manton (1992) who analyzed birth certificate information from successive birth cohorts to show that mortality from specific diseases, whether indexed by underlying cause or total-mention data, has been declining in some cases even at very late ages. Mortality rates for six White male cohorts, all born between 1884–1888 and 1909–1913, were plotted against age group. In this way, he examined differences in mortality in people of the same age who were born at different times. Declines in mortality at late age in these birth cohorts may indicate changes in exposure to risk factors earlier in life. Manton (1992) suggests that these changes may also indicate changes in the basic disease process, for example, slower progression.

Figure 10.4a reproduces Manton's cohort plot for total-mention occurrences of cerebrovascular disease, and Figure 10.4b for underlying cause occurrences. The plots show lower mortality from cerebrovascular disease at each age across the successive birth cohorts. For example, people born in 1899–1903 and 1904–1908 reached ages 75–79 in 1974–1978 and 1979–1983, respectively. Mortality from cerebrovascular disease was much lower in the more recent cohort, as the figures show. This trend is true for other adjacent birth cohorts who reached comparable ages.

These results suggest that cause-specific mortality is truly declining for some (but, of course, not all) of the major diseases of late life. The results imply that deaths from these conditions are being postponed to later ages, either because people contract the disease at later ages or because they are living longer with it. Or it may be that people are dying of other causes, but again these deaths also appear to be postponed to later ages, because most of the major diseases show similar reductions in mortality across adjacent birth cohorts. Of course, postponement of

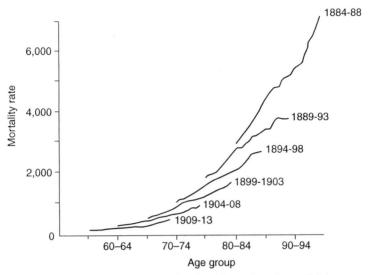

Figure 10.4a Cohort plot, mortality for six white male cohorts. Total-mention occurrences, cardiovascular diseases.

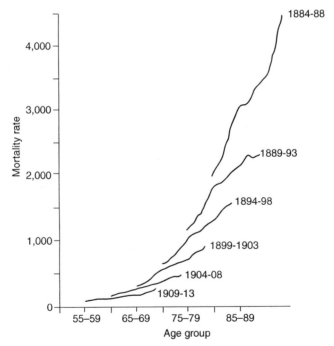

Figure 10.4b Cohort plot, mortality for six white male cohorts. Underlying-cause occurrences of cerebrovascular disease.

Source: From The Oldest Old, edited by Suzman, Willis, & Manton. Fig. 8-3a, 8-3b (c) 1992 by Oxford University Press, Inc. By permission of Oxford University Press, Inc.

disease to later ages is preferable to living longer with disease. Both outcomes are consistent with reduction in mortality in late life and longer life expectancy. Investigation of this issue requires a careful look at disability and active life expectancy, as we covered in Chapter 5.

Flow and Location of Older People Before Death

Location of death is important to the extent that it may influence the quality of end of life, including services received. Figure 10.5 maps the flow of older persons through the health care system as they move from community residence to hospital or nursing home care, and finally to death, and gives an indication of the magnitude of each pathway to death for 1990.

Of the 1,966,000 deaths of noninstitutionalized older people tracked in 1990 (6.7% of the total noninstitutionalized population), approximately 60% died in hospitals (about half of those in the intensive care unit), another 22% died after nursing home placements, and the remainder died in home settings, with or without hospice care. The figure simplifies the flow of older people as they approach death in a number of ways. First, nursing home deaths follow two routes. One route involves admission to nursing homes from the community followed by death, with or without hospitalization. In 1990, 697,000 older people (2.4%) entered the nursing home directly from the community, while another 1,334,000 (4.6%) entered nursing homes from hospitals. The two streams together yield

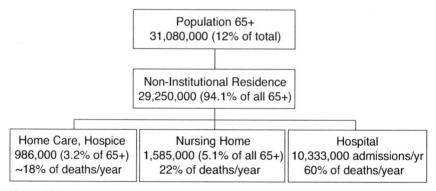

Figure 10.5 Flow and location of older people with death as end point, United States, 1990.

Source: From NCHS, Vital and Health Statistics, Series 13, No. 112, 1990.

2,031,000 people entering nursing homes in the year. However, about a quarter of these admissions was temporary, with elders returning to community-based care or independence after short-stay respite or rehabilitation.

A second simplification involves hospital admissions. The noninstitutionalized population had approximately 10,333,000 admissions in the year, which followed a total of some 159,490,000 visits to physicians. Thus, approximately 6.5% of physician visits, or 1 in 20, were followed by hospitalization. Of these admissions, 1,180,000 died in the hospital, so that approximately 1 in every 10 admissions was followed by death in the hospital. The number is obviously higher if we add deaths among patients transferred to hospitals from nursing homes.

On the other hand, it is reassuring to examine the complement of the figures described above. Over 93% of noninstitutionalized elders did not die in the year. A similar proportion avoided spending any days in nursing homes. The vast majority of physician visits were not followed by hospitalization, and the vast majority of hospitalizations were followed by discharges back into the community.

Pulling the 1990 data together was no easy task; some 10 different data sources were consulted in composing the preceding paragraphs! However, there is no other way to get a sense of the complex flow of people and settings as death approaches. In an attempt to update these figures at least in the aggregate, we examined mortality data from the National Center for Health Statistics, 2004. Of the 1.7 million deaths in people aged 65+ (of 2.4 million deaths in total), about 760,000 deaths occurred in the hospital, 500,000 in the nursing home, 400,000 in homes, 10,000 in hospice, and less than 100,000 in other settings.

If we compare the 1990 and 2004 mortality data, we see declines in the proportion of deaths in the hospital (from 60% to 45%) and an increase in deaths in nursing home (22% to 29%), and increases in the proportion dying at home. The low proportion of older adults recorded as dying in a hospice facility in 2004 bears comment because it is so low. For example, of people who died at age 85 and older in 2004, less than 3 per 1,000 died in a hospice facility. This number is undoubtedly lower than the number of older people who died while receiving hospice care, since many hospice services are provided at hospitals, nursing homes, and at home through home-care agencies, rather than in free-standing hospice facilities. Exactly how many older adults are receiving hospice services at the time of their death is not known from death certificate data; however, Medicare program statistics suggest that approximately

800,000 beneficiaries used the hospice benefit in 2004, and this figure has been steadily increasing (Centers for Medicare and Medicaid Services, 2007).

DISPARITIES IN MORTALITY RISK

Educational attainment, typically measured by how many years of school someone has completed early in life, as well as other indicators of socioeconomic status (SES) (income, wealth, occupation), are strong predictors of disparities in late-life disability, health status, and mortality risk. What is true for education applies to other socioeconomic indicators.

The association between early educational attainment and mortality can be gleaned from statistics reported by the National Center for Health Statistics for people aged 25–64; the yearly report of U.S. mortality does not provide this breakdown for people aged 65 and older because of errors in the reporting of education on death certificates for this group. Mortality per 100,000 people is provided for all-cause mortality by educational groups: people who did not complete high school (<12 years), for people who completed high school (12 years), and for people who had schooling beyond high school (13+ years). The most recent year presents such data stratified by the type of death certificate used in a given state; we therefore rely on data from 2002 to make the point that mortality in the under-65 age group is strongly related to educational attainment. People who had completed one or more years of post-high school education had a mortality rate of approximately 209 per 100,000, whereas those with 12 years of education died at a rate of 516 per 100,000, and those with less than 12 years of education had an even higher rate (616 per 100,000). In short, the risks of dying for someone with more than a high school education are now one-third the risks of someone with less than a high school education. We previously reported this ratio to be one-half in 1998, suggesting that the disparity between more highly and less highly educated individuals has increased.

This difference in risk appears for all three of the cause-specific mortality measures (see Figure 10.6). This risk difference, evident across such very different sources of mortality, suggests that education lowers mortality in some general way. It is associated with reductions in risk behaviors (i.e., smoking, multiple sex partners, driving while intoxicated) linked to all three sources of mortality, with more effective health-seeking

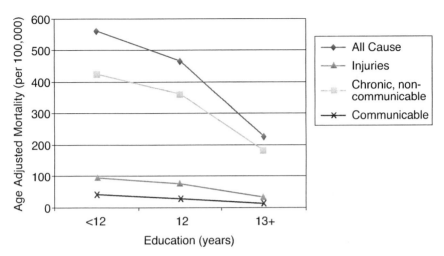

Figure 10.6 Education and cause-specific mortality, 1998, ages 25–64.

Source: From "Deaths, United States, 2000," by Centers for Disease Control and Prevention, 2000a. *National Vital Statistics Reports, 48*(11). Hyattsville, MD: National Center for Health Statistics.

behaviors once disease becomes apparent, and with greater wealth and hence access to medical care. This difference in mortality risk by educational attainment persists despite a more general decline in U.S. mortality. Indeed, mortality has declined for all three of the education groups, but the gap between the groups has not narrowed.

Elo and Preston (1996) have shown that this relationship holds in late life as well, although it is slightly attenuated. They examined death rates per 1,000 in the period 1979–1985, breaking out mortality risk by age (25–64, 65–89) and gender. They treated education more carefully than most studies. The plots for the older age group are shown as Figure 10.7, which show age-standardized adjusted risk.

These results clearly show the protective effect of early education on late-life mortality. Women have an advantage at every education level, but men and women each face lower mortality risk with increasing education. An education gradient applies across the entire range of education but becomes most pronounced with completion of high school and more advanced schooling.

Not shown is the comparable figure for people aged 25–64. At younger ages, however, the education effect is even stronger, as might

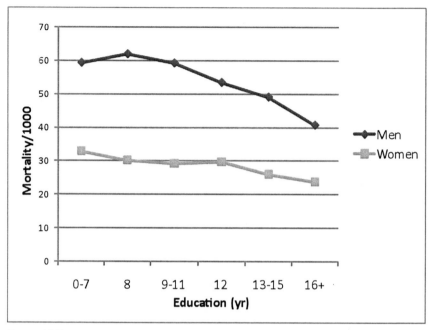

Figure 10.7 Mortality risk, United States, ages 65–89, 1979–1985.

Source: From "Educational Differentials in Mortality: United States, 1979–85," by I. T. Elo and S. H. Preston, 1996, *Social Science and Medicine, 42*, 47–57.

be expected because education has greater scope to affect death rates (which, on the whole, are much lower). Relative to men with high school education, men in the younger age group with 16+ years of school face a mortality risk of 0.67 and men in the older age group a mortality risk of 0.76. For women, the comparable risk ratios are 0.84 and 0.80, respectively. These data show that the protective effect of education is indeed attenuated in late life.

Still, given the great significance of education for mortality risk and the increasingly educated older population, it is interesting to imagine postponement of mortality from this factor alone, apart from improvements in medical care. Figure 10.8 shows the increasing proportion of women who have completed high school, by birth cohort. As the figure shows, over 30 years (comparing women born between 1916–1925 and 1946–1955), the proportion completing high school increased from 55% to 85%. We can expect an increasingly educated older population to have a very different experience of health and dying in coming decades.

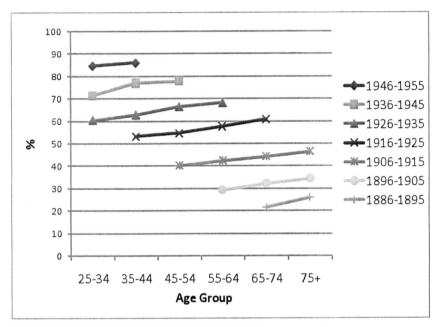

Figure 10.8 Proportion completing high school, by birth cohort, U.S. women.

Source: Data from Spain & Bianchi (1996), Table 3.1.

Not only has the older population been experiencing increased levels of educational attainment, but it has also become—and will continue to shift in the future toward being—more racially and ethnically diverse. Consideration of racial and ethnic disparities in mortality is thus in order.

Figure 10.9 shows mortality rates from 1960 to 2006 for Blacks and Whites and from 1997 to 2006 for individuals of Hispanic origin. These rates have been age adjusted so that the populations' age structures are assumed to be identical. It is noteworthy that the mortality rates of all three groups have declined over time, but mortality rates for Blacks remain the highest and the gap has not changed appreciably over time.

The exceptionally low mortality risk of Hispanics, despite their higher risk socioeconomic profiles, has come to be known as the "Hispanic Paradox" (Markides, Rudkin, Angel, & Espino, 1997; Palloni & Morenoff, 2001). A review published in 2001 (Franzini, Ribble, & Keddie, 2001), concluded that the paradox was apparent in mortality especially for older adults and among infants, but that the causes of the paradox remained largely unknown. Three possible explanations were posed, two related to immigration: a healthy immigrant effect (that immigrants tend to be

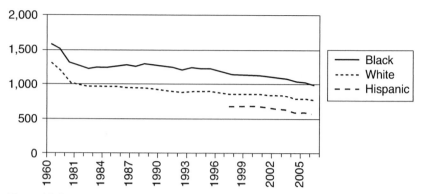

Figure 10.9 Age-adjusted mortality rates 1960–2006, by race and ethnicity.

Source: From Heron, Hoyert, Murphy, et. al., (2009). Deaths: Final Data for 2006. National Vital Statistics Reports 57(14), Tables 1-2.

a selected group that is healthier than average than the population they leave behind) and a "salmon bias" (that less healthy Hispanics return home when they die). A third possible explanation suggested there may be biases in the vital registration data.

In an excellent review on the subject, Markides and Eschbach (2005) compared results from different sources of data used to study this phenomenon: vital statistics, national community surveys linked to the National Death Index, Medicare records linked to applications for social security cards, and regional mortality follow-up studies. They find that studies based on vital statistics, like those shown above, suggest the greatest mortality advantage and that the advantage is greatest for older ages. Indeed there appears to be "agreement that vital statistics death counts linked to census denominators are the least useful source of data to [estimate the size of the Hispanic paradox] because of the inherent uncertainty about the consistency of ethnic classifications in these two sources" (p. 73). Studies that rely on linked records, such as the Medicare-social security linkages, that avoid vital statistics problems suggest there is such an advantage but that it is smaller than what is suggested by vital statistics data.

Despite the lower mortality rates, it is important for public health and aging professionals to keep in mind that those of Hispanic origin face very real disparities in other measures of access to care, in chronic diseases like diabetes and hypertension, and in activity limitations. Examination of cause of death by race/ethnicity underscores this point (NCHS, 2009). The most common causes of death in 2006 for Blacks, Hispanics, and Whites were major cardiovascular disease (including strokes) and cancers. Beyond these, differences begin to emerge. The third most common cause of death for Whites is chronic lower respiratory tract disease, whereas for Blacks and Hispanics it is accidents. Fourth for Whites is accidents, whereas for Blacks and Hispanics, fourth is diabetes. And fifth for Whites is Alzheimer's disease, whereas for Blacks it is assaults, and for those of Hispanic origin it is chronic liver disease and cirrhosis. Understanding the factors—whether they are social, environmental, or biological—that lead a group with greater socioeconomic disadvantage to experience lower than average mortality rates and quite distinct causes of death may hold promise for improving the health and mortality of all groups.

THE HIGH COSTS OF DYING

Medical care in old age is more expensive than medical care for younger age groups because of the greater burden of chronic disease borne by older people. However, as shown earlier, medical management of the chronic diseases of old age is less a burden to Medicare than medical management of dying. Approximately 30% of all Medicare expenditures occur in the year in which people die, that is, the last year of life (Lubitz & Riley, 1993; Miller, 2001). The constancy of this proportion of Medicare spending over a number of decades is impressive, given the huge increases in overall Medicare spending. Between 1976 and 1988, costs in the last year of life increased from $3,488 to $13,316, on average, per decedent. Costs per year for nondecedents rose from $492 to $1,924 in the same period. Thus, both groups saw nearly a fourfold increase over this decade and a half, and accordingly end-of-life care as a proportion of the total Medicare budget changed very little (Lubitz & Riley, 1993). Lubitz and Riley (1993) also note that the proportion of Medicare payments made in the last 60 days of life in 1976 and 1988 was also virtually identical, suggesting no increase in heroic (and perhaps unjustified) efforts to stave off death.

An update of Medicare expenditures in the last year of life shows little change (Hogan, Lunney, Gabel, & Lynn, 2001). Approximately 5% of Medicare enrollees continue to die each year. Not surprisingly, decedents continue to be older, more frail and disabled, and more diseased than survivors. Based on Medicare claims, the typical Medicare decedent has approximately four major disease conditions at the time of death, compared with only one disease condition among survivors. Some three-quarters of decedents have heart disease; one-third have cancer, stroke, chronic obstructive pulmonary disease, or pneumonia/influenza; and more than a fourth have dementia.

Suppose now that we match these decedents to survivors with the same disease profiles. Hogan and colleagues (2001) determined that decedents' costs were approximately 50% higher than those of a survivor cohort matched by age and disease diagnoses, and approximately 30% higher than those of a survivor cohort matched on age, diagnoses, and a hospitalization during the year. This important finding suggests that the high costs of the last year of life are mostly a function of the high disease burden that precedes dying: "Much of what has been labeled the 'high cost of dying' is just the cost of caring for severe illness and functional impairment. Decedents' costs are, roughly speaking, not much different from those of others with similarly complex medical needs" (Hogan et al., 2001, p. 194). This approach also suggests that Medicare data of this sort may be useful in identifying groups at high risk of dying.

Decedents are also more likely to use nursing home care and hence incur high Medicaid costs. Nearly 40% of decedents had some nursing home care in their last year of life. In fact, 22% of decedents were full-time nursing home residents in the year of death, and the remainder had short-term or part-year residence in nursing homes (Hogan et al., 2001).

Hogan and colleagues (2001) also report an important racial difference in Medicare expenditures in the last year of life. End-of-life care costs were higher for minorities and for people living in high-poverty areas. Medicare spending per capita for minority decedents was 28% higher than for nonminorities, and 43% higher in high-poverty areas compared with low-poverty areas. Part of the difference can be attributed to the poorer health of the members of minorities and low-income groups at the end of life. For example, 7% of minority decedents had end-stage renal disease covered in the End-Stage Renal Disease (ESRD) program, a costly death (see the organ failure trajectory described above), compared with only 2% in the remainder of the Medicare decedent population. But costs for minority decedents in the last year of life remained approximately 20% higher even with exclusion of decedents in the ESRD program.

Reasons for the greater expense of dying among minorities remain unclear. Reports also suggest that family members of minority and low-income decedents are more likely to request life-sustaining technologies. A sense of exclusion from medical care earlier in life may be at work here, as well as broader differences in culture and expectations regarding medical care. This question merits further research.

Age also is associated with medical expenditures. Decedents who die at younger ages (age 65–74) are more likely to be male, to die of cancer, and to have higher costs. Older ages at death were associated with a greater prevalence of dementia and nursing home use, with attendant Medicaid expenditures. Women were more prevalent in this group.

Although the relationship between age and medical care costs is well documented, time until death, rather than age, is likely to be the better indicator of health status and biological age (Evans, 2002) and, not surprisingly, a better predictor than age of medical care costs. Miller (2001) has shown that when both time until death and age are considered, Medicare costs are strongly associated with the former and only weakly associated with the latter. For example, using data from 1990, Miller shows that for people aged 75 who were 5 years from death, annual Medicare costs were $3,000. These costs rise to $13,500 for people of the same age in the last year of life. This pattern holds for all age groups and hence "the correlation between age and Medicare costs appears to be explained largely by time until death. Therefore age is a poor measure of health status and cannot reliably be used as a basis for forecasting" (Miller, 2001, p. 217).

Miller also shows that medical care costs decline with older age, especially in the last year of life. Medicare costs in the last year of life in 1990 were $13,500 per enrollee for people aged 75, $10,700 for people aged 85, and $7,000 for people aged 95. In fact, medical care costs in the oldest age groups were lower even 3–4 years before death. For example, 3 years before death, annual medical care costs per enrollee were $4,200 for people aged 75, $4,000 for people aged 85, and $3,200 for people aged 95. This decline is most likely a result of implicit rationing, such as decisions to limit surgery or diagnostic procedures for the very old, but may also reflect greater frailty at older ages. Frailty means that people approach death with less reserve. As a result, their dying is likely to be quicker and hence allow less time or opportunity for expensive interventions.

From these trends, Miller (2001) suggests that increasing longevity may actually result in a decrease in Medicare expenditures. Increasing longevity, if accompanied by delays in late-life morbidity and disability, should postpone the period of high health care costs associated with the end of life. In pushing death to later and later ages, we also push the last year of life to later ages, when frailty and implicit rationing make dying less expensive. Evidence supports indisputable increases in longevity; decreases in disability, although these may have leveled off in recent years (see Chapter 5); and in many cases increases (although perhaps milder and earlier identified forms) of morbidity (see Chapter 4). It is therefore possible, although by no means certain, that progress in keeping people alive to older ages will contribute to lowering medical care costs in the last year of life, the major source of expense to Medicare.

QUALITY OF LIFE NEAR THE END OF LIFE

The mortality statistics above treat death as the event of interest, and are concerned only with the age, cause, and cost of the event. Yet researchers have also been interested in understanding the quality of individuals' lives just before they die. It is very difficult to study end-of-life experiences in community-based studies. Interviewers are considered to be intrusive when a study participant is seriously ill, and family members are often too busy to offer a proxy interview. Researchers instead have relied on samples of individuals who have died, drawn from death certificates or obituaries, and "followed" back these individuals to speak with a surviving relative. This approach is quite different, as we will see, from studying the dying experience, but the studies do provide some window into how family members remember the last year and months of their relative's life.

A key case-control study compared the last year of life in a group of dying elders with an ordinary year of life among surviving elders (Lawton, Moss, & Glicksman, 1993). The study was retrospective and identified dying elders from obituary notices. Next of kin, identified by death certificate, were contacted and interviewed about the dying person's experience 12 months, 3 months, and 1 month before death. Surviving elders were identified in the same neighborhood and matched by age, gender, and source of information. Lawton et al. found that virtually all quality-of-life indicators declined over the 12 months compared with trends in the survivor group, with the exception of visits from family and friends, which increased. Still, they noted that, across the many different indicators of quality, most of these dying elders had good scores on a majority of the measures, suggesting that most experienced relatively good quality of life at the end of life.

Results from the National Mortality Followback Survey suggest that the quality of life among people who are dying may also be improving (Liao, McGee, Cao, & Cooper, 2000). In the Followback Survey a random sample of deaths is drawn from death certificates, with next of kin contacted and interviewed about the decedent's last year of life.

A comparison of results from the 1986 and 1993 surveys shows important gains in quality of life at the end of life. For example, among decedents aged 65–84, the proportion avoiding a hospital admission increased from 21.6% to 25.1% among men and 19.6% to 24.9% among women. Gains were even greater among decedents aged 85 and older. In this group, the proportion avoiding hospitalization increased from 22.3% to 29.1% among men, and 30.7% to 40.6% among women. The proportion without a nursing home admission also increased in all groups, with the exception of younger men. These are welcome findings because they suggest that more people were able to live the last year of life in their own homes, a result consistent with the large increase in hospice use in the same period (see below).

This comparison also revealed better physical and cognitive status in decedents over the decade, a trend especially pronounced among the oldest old. The proportion in the most severely disabled categories declined for all groups. Similarly, a composite measure of quality of life based on time in the hospital or nursing homes, restriction in daily activities, and cognitive status showed improvement for the oldest old. Because the presence of activity limitations in the last year of life declined between 1986 and 1993, the authors conclude that the related decline in hospital and nursing home use was at least partly due to better health even in the last year of life.

ALIGNING PUBLIC HEALTH AND END-OF-LIFE GOALS

These studies provide a glimpse into the last year of life, but what about the actual dying experience? A 1997 Report by the Institute of Medicine, "Approaching Death: Improving Care at the End of Life," explored several interrelated themes along these lines. The report stressed that too many dying people have pain and distress that could be prevented or relieved and identified remediable impediments to a good death (including organizational, economic, legal, and educational barriers). They also identified gaps in scientific knowledge about how to improve end-of-life care and the need to develop tools for evaluating end-of-life outcomes to improve accountability for the quality of end-of-life care delivered.

End-of-Life Goals

Much of what we know about end-of-life experiences comes from The Study to Understand Prognoses and Preferences for Outcomes and

Risks of Treatments (SUPPORT) and ancillary study on the Hospitalized Elderly Longitudinal Project (HELP). SUPPORT monitored 9,105 seriously ill hospital patients at five sites, 4,274 of whom died within 6 months. HELP monitored 1,286 persons ages 80 and older in four of the five SUPPORT hospitals, 25% of whom died within 6 months. These studies aimed to describe the decision-making that affected seriously ill patients, but also provided important insights into the course of death. For example, analyses of the study data suggested high levels of untreated symptoms, minimal advance planning, site of death and treatments were in conflict with patient preferences, and a high burden was placed on family members. Lynn et al. (1997), for example, found that most study participants died in acute care hospitals and that pain was commonplace in the last few days. Family members who were interviewed most often reported (59%) that the patient preferred comfort care, but life-sustaining treatments were not uncommon (11% had a final resuscitation attempt; 25% had a ventilator; and 4% had a feeding tube in place).

The IOM report also put forth a definition of a good death as "one that is free from avoidable distress and suffering for patients, families, and caregivers; in general accord with patients' and families' wishes; and reasonably consistent with clinical, cultural, and ethical standards." The committee who wrote the report asserted that every person dying in the United States should be able to achieve a good death. Nevertheless, current public policy goals have not been explicitly aligned with such an end-of-life goal. In fact, in some cases, the current policy environment may actually hinder a good death.

The End-of-Life System: Hospice

As we discussed in Chapter 4, Medicare covers acute health care costs for older adults in the United States. A hospice benefit to cover end-of-life costs was first added to the menu of benefits in 1982. The benefit provides care to a patient under two conditions: first, a physician must certify that he or she is within 6 months of death, if the disease follows its "usual" course, and second, that the patient is willing to forego coverage for life-prolonging treatment.

The hospice model sets up as an either/or choice "curative" and "end-of-life" care: a patient receives curative care until he or she decides it is time to stop curative care and begin hospice care. Once on the hospice care benefit, a patient is eligible for a variety of services, including physician services, nursing care, medical appliances and supplies, drugs for symptom management and pain relief, short-term inpatient and respite care, homemaker and home health aide services, counseling and social work services, and spiritual care and bereavement services. Medicare's hospice benefit pays a per diem rate intended to cover all expenses related to the terminal illness ($120 per day). Beneficiary copays for these services are minimal.

Hogan et al. (2001) report an increase in hospice use from 11% in 1994 to 19% in 1998. This percentage grew again to 25% in fee-for-service and 34% in managed care in 1998 (MedPac, 2004). A majority of people who die of cancer now use hospice, but growth in hospice use has been substantial among patients with noncancer diagnoses and among patients in nursing homes.

Studies that have examined the benefits of hospice have provided evidence that patients on hospice receive more support than other patients and are more likely to receive pain management (Miller, Gozalo, & Mor, 2000). However, studies of cost savings have suggested only minimal savings from the hospice benefit. For example, one study (Campbell, Lynn, Louis, & Shugarman, 2004) suggested that beneficiaries who used the hospice benefit had Medicare spending that was 4% higher, on average, than beneficiaries who did not elect hospice care. However, this finding masks important differences by trajectory. Among decedents with cancer, Medicare spending was 10% less for those who elect hospice care in the last year of life compared with those who did not. Among those with all other diagnoses, hospice use was associated with higher Medicare spending, in particular, for those with dementia.

At the same time, the choice between life prolongation and attention to quality of life that is at the heart of the hospice benefit results in both ineffective life-prolonging treatment and preventable suffering among those who do not choose the hospice benefit in a timely manner. Indeed, timely referral to hospice has been a problem with the benefit, which is linked to the uncertainty of prognosis among older adults. Christakas and Lamont (2000), for example, demonstrate that physicians are inaccurate in their prognoses for terminally ill patients, and more often than not are too optimistic in their predictions.

Aligning Goals With End-of-Life Trajectories

The hospice model grew out of and appears to work best for patients that die of cancer. But this is only one of several typical pathways to death that are experienced in later life. Lynn (2001) has distinguished three trajectories of dying: a relatively compressed period of disability followed by death from cancer; a longer period of declines, recoveries, and relapses in function that ends with death from organ failure; and a much longer period of slow dwindling and decline typical of increasing physical and cognitive frailty (i.e., dementia). In an attempt to quantify these trajectories, Lunney and colleagues (2002) have proposed a slightly different typology based on Medicare claims for decedents. They identified four trajectories based on three criteria: medical expenditures, length of illness, and diagnostic category. They identified one trajectory characterized by a short but expensive death; this kind of dying is typical of deaths from cancer, accounts for about a quarter of American deaths, and entails a mean cost of $31,000 in the last year a life. A second trajectory summarizes dying of dementia and physical frailty; this trajectory of dying accounts for about half the deaths of older people and carries a mean cost of $25,000 in the last year of life. The third trajectory is typical of deaths due to organ failure; approximately 20% of deaths follow this pattern, which carries a cost of $37,000 in the last year of life. Finally, a fourth trajectory summarizes the experience of people who die suddenly and with little contact with medical care in the last year of life. This trajectory accounts for the smallest proportion of deaths, some 7%, and is the least expensive; Medicare costs for this kind of dying run about $2,000 in the last year of life.

Lynn and Adamson (2003) have proposed a way to better align the health care system's delivery of care with end-of-life needs by drawing on the illness trajectories approach. They argue that much of the health care system has been built to meet the needs of individuals early in their trajectories who have not yet faced chronic care needs. They suggest that during the healthy period, before the onset of chronic illness, that managed care, preventive care, and acute care when needed are the appropriate benefits. However, for each of the other three trajectories— cancer, organ failure, and dementia/frailty—they suggest a unique bundle of services. For those on the cancer trajectory, for example, they suggest building advance-care planning into early treatment, providing palliation for symptoms and rehabilitation for disabilities, providing some aggressive treatments when they work to enhance life, providing smooth transitions across settings and attending to the family's needs and spiritual/emotional needs of the patient. For patients experiencing organ failure, a different package is in order: teaching the essentials of disease management, including how to recognize symptoms that need medical care; ensuring the availability of medications; planning for sudden death; providing early interventions in the patient's home; offering in-home adaptations and equipment to ensure comfort and maximize functioning; and individualizing care planning to meet the family's and patient's needs. Finally, for those patients with dementia and/or frailty, Lynn and Adamson propose attention to training, support, benefits, and respite for family caregivers; ensuring the quality of care in long-term care facilities and the availability of quality home health aides and home- and community-based services, flexible end-of-life planning, and attention to palliative care.

The last service deserves expansion, because it is a term we have not previously used. Palliative care is an alternative model of care that has received much attention of late, but it is not a benefit in the Medicare program. Palliative care focuses on prevention and relief of suffering through symptom management, as well as on the spiritual and emotional needs of the patient and family. Such care ideally is delivered to the patient early in the disease and sustained throughout the final stages of an illness. Unlike an "either/or" choice associated with hospice care, palliative care may be combined with curative and life-prolonging care, if it is beneficial, and may be increased over time as curative attempts are gradually diminished. Studies evaluating the benefits of palliative care suggest modest benefits in terms of the quality of the end of life, but thus far the research has been hampered by poor research designs, including small sample sizes and the lack of large, randomized trials. Further research is needed to understand whether the palliative care philosophy can be integrated into the Medicare program to achieve the experience of a good death for more adults dying in the United States.

TERMINAL DROP

What sorts of changes mark the point when people begin to die? If we start with a group that has died and work backward to examine changes in health before the death, can we identify a point when decline begins? Finally, how much of the negative changes in health that we see in late life can be attributed to predeath decline?

Inquiry in this area has led to the suggestion of a period of "terminal drop" before death (Kleinmeier, 1962). However, in practice it is hard to date the start of this period of terminal decline, because this inquiry requires prospective follow-up in a cohort of people who have died. Wilson and colleagues (2002) reported the results of such a study and determined that cognitive decline began, on average, about 4 years before death. This cohort involved the Religious Orders cohort, a group of highly educated nuns and priests. People in the cohort who did not die showed almost no change in cognitive performance over the same period.

More generally, little research has been conducted on changes prior to the last year of life. This is an important and neglected area of research.

SUMMARY

Causes of Death. Death certificates distinguish between "underlying" or "primary" causes of death and "contributory" causes. "Underlying causes" indicate proximal or immediate conditions that led to the death, whereas "contributory causes" indicate more distal or remote causes, that is, longstanding chronic conditions that may have played a role in the death. Heart disease (25% of deaths), cancer (24%), and stroke (6%) were the leading causes of death, together accounting for 55% of all deaths. For older adults who often have many chronic conditions and symptoms, the cause of death is not always obvious.

Death Rates. Both age-adjusted and crude death rates have declined over the past 50 years as have age-specific death rates. The age-specific mortality curve is shaped like a "check-mark" or "j" shape and many of the most common causes of death follow this pattern. Over the past hundred years, deaths from acute conditions have been replaced gradually by deaths from chronic conditions. Over the past 25 years we have seen Alzheimer's disease and septicemia take the place of atherosclerosis and liver disease in top 10 causes of death. The latter changes are likely due to a combination of medical (treatment-related) and nonmedical (changes in coding) reasons.

Disparities in Mortality Risks. The risks of dying for someone with more than a high school education are one-third the risks of someone with less than a high school education, down from one-half just 10 years ago. This relationship holds for late life, although it is attenuated somewhat. Mortality rates have declined consistently across racial/ethnic groups; however, mortality rates for Blacks continue to be higher than for Whites, and Hispanics continue to experience lower than average mortality rates than Whites, despite having socioeconomic profiles similar to Blacks (the so-called "Hispanic paradox").

Costs and Quality of Life at the End of Life. Approximately 30% of all Medicare expenditures occur in the year in which people die, that is, the last year of life. These costs are mostly a function of the high care needs that precede dying and not the costs of dying itself. Although time to death is a better predictor of medical expenditures than age, people who die at older ages have, on average, lower medical costs in the last year of life than people who die at younger ages. This finding suggests that increasing longevity may lower medical care costs in the last year of life in the future. Studies of the quality of life in the last year suggest quality of life does decline as individuals approach death; however, there is some evidence that recently individuals have experienced some gains in quality of life at the end of life.

Aligning Public Health and End-of-Life Goals. Current public health systems are not aligned with the goal of ensuring that all persons who die in the United States experience a good death. Instead, many patients die in avoidable pain with life-sustaining treatments rather than in comfort care. The current Medicare hospice care benefit provides comfort care to those who have a physician's certification of being within 6 months of death and who are willing to forego coverage for life-prolonging treatment. The benefit has been used increasingly, but the choice between life prolongation and attention to quality of life continues to facilitate ineffective life-prolonging treatments and preventable suffering. Alignment of the health care system with end-of-life goals would benefit from attention to the different trajectories that older adults follow at the end of life. Attention to palliative care, which focuses on prevention and relief of suffering through symptom management, and on the spiritual and emotional needs of the patient and family, irrespective of the stage of illness, may also be a fruitful avenue for improving end-of-life care, but more research is needed in this arena.

11 Ethical Issues in Public Health and Aging

Headlines in popular magazines suggest a new interest in global aging. However, when it is mentioned, it is usually as a problem with dire consequences. *Business Week* reminds us that "it's not just Europe—China and other emerging-market economies are aging fast, too. There are solutions, but it's time to act" (Engardio & Matlack, 2005). The foreign policy establishment is also interested and equally concerned (Department of State, 2007). These sources sound the alarm of the "graying of the great powers" (Jackson & Howe, 2007). What will happen in 2050, they ask, when 20% of the population of the developed world, and nearly a third in Japan, are over age 60? Will these societies be able to afford the burden of care? Will there be enough younger people to provide for elders? And will aged countries be able to compete against newly emerging countries with younger populations and presumably more dynamic economies?

The aging of populations is undeniable, but it is worth stepping back a minute to ask whether global aging really is a problem. Is it? Greater survival, with greater function until increasingly later ages, seems like the crowning achievement of human science and technology. Who would quibble with greater opportunity to flourish longer over the life span? Nations seek to jump from low-life-expectancy "mortality traps" (where life expectancy hovers between 40 and 50) to high-life-expectancy

353

demographic regimes (Bloom & Canning, 2007). And at least one strand of research suggests that nations with older populations are more likely to produce wealth and achieve higher standards of living than younger populations (Bloom & Canning, 2007). Why then is an increasingly older world a source of concern? The economists and foreign policy theorists who fear this latest version of the "population bomb" are not swayed by the benefits offered by an aging world.

Despite declines in disability in old age approaching 2.2% per year between 1999 and 2004 (see Chapter 5), continuing increases in longevity (Chapter 2), and greater civic involvement and employment at older ages than ever before, aging is still feared and unwelcome. And despite the great promise of longer, richer lifetimes available to more and more people, old age is still inescapably stamped by decline and the end of life, with "voice broken, mind short, chin double, every part about you blasted with antiquity" (Shakespeare, *Henry IV*). Against the greater potential of longer life and more opportunity to flourish, the critic can still point to failing faculties and corresponding loss of acuity, flexibility, fecundity, strength, and speed, the wonderful qualities of younger ages.

Moreover, one might argue that loss of these qualities in old age after a well-lived life is reasonable. As one has noted, "I have never heard anyone remember with bitterness, or sharp regret, the death of an elderly person who lived a full and long life" (Callahan, 2001, p. 71). Behind the fear of our increasingly grayer world is the concern that we have gone too far in using science and medicine to extend life. Have we reached a point where we can say we have too much of a good thing? This was an early fear of epidemiologists of aging, who pointed out that reducing case fatality rates and providing better chronic care inexorably leads to more cases of people living with disease and thus "rising pandemics of mental disorders, associated chronic diseases, and disability" (Kramer, 1980). Could public health successes have created a new species of problem, in which care for older people now competes with other equally or more pressing needs?

Thus, a first ethical challenge for public health and aging is whether "old age is a reason in itself to think about medical care in a different way" (Callahan, 2001). Callahan suggests that age is a reasonable criterion for limiting medical care. We take up this challenge first. But we can also turn this question around and ask whether old age is reason enough for thinking about the life span in a different way. We take an anthropological digression to see how the ethics of care at older ages may differ in cultures that think of the life span in different ways. This may suggest alternative ways to think about the connection between generations, and between parents and children, that might inform ethics.

Declining health and, in particular, loss of cognitive function, poses additional ethical challenges (Ravitsky, Fiester, & Caplan, 2009). The President's Council on Bioethics suggests that the goal of care for the elder with dementia is to maximize care and not just minimize suffering. We examine how the distinction might be useful and what it implies. Loss of cognitive ability also implies a need to rethink autonomy and perhaps recognize that our model of competent, fully informed patients dealing with physicians who fully include them as partners in care may be more ideal than fact. Finally, we conclude with different visions of medical care in late life, regenerative versus "spare parts" medicine, and how differences between the two may affect efforts in public health and aging.

AGE AS A CRITERION TO RATION MEDICAL CARE

As earlier chapters have shown, life expectancy has increased dramatically in the United States and continues to increase. Most commentators note the greater number of years lived by successive birth cohorts and hence the additional years of life expectancy they accrue, 78.5, for example, compared with 76. But an alternative rendering is given in Table 11.1. The table again shows how life expectancy has increased in the United States over the past 50 years, but instead displays the proportion of Americans who can expect to reach the oldest ages according to birth cohort. Of people born in 1959–1961, for example, approximately 7% were projected to reach age 90. For the most recent birth cohort (2004), by contrast, 22% can expect to reach this age. In less than 50 years, the proportion who will reach age 90 has tripled.

Many people think that the increasing proportion of very old people means an increasing prevalence of chronic conditions, physical and cognitive limitations, and need for medical and supportive care. As analyses of trends in active life expectancy show us (see Chapter 6), this conclusion is not necessarily the case. But certainly within the oldest age group care needs are extraordinarily high. The prevalence of dementia among people aged 85 and older is more than a third, and the proportion with mobility and ADL limitation is even higher, reaching perhaps 50%. In *Setting Limits,* Daniel Callahan asks whether providing intensive medical care to people who have reached these ages is morally justified. He argues no, not because of the costs nor because of inadequacies of medical science,

Table 11.1

LIFE TABLES, UNITED STATES, SELECTED PERIODS

	2004	1989–1991	1979–1981	1969–1971	1959–1961
0	100,000	100,000	100,000	100,000	100,000
1	99,320	99,064	98,740	97,998	97,407
5	99,202	98,877	98,495	97,668	96,998
10	99,129	98,766	98,347	97,460	96,765
15	99,036	98,635	98,196	97,261	96,551
20	98,709	98,215	97,741	96,716	96,111
25	98,246	97,671	97,110	96,000	95,517
30	97,776	97,070	96,477	95,307	94,905
35	97,250	96,322	95,808	94,482	94,144
40	96,517	95,373	94,926	93,322	93,064
45	95,406	94,154	93,599	91,587	91,378
50	93,735	92,370	91,526	88,972	88,756
55	91,357	89,658	88,348	85,110	84,711
60	88,038	85,537	83,726	79,529	79,067
65	83,114	79,519	77,107	71,933	71,147
70	76,191	71,357	68,248	61,984	60,857
75	66,605	60,449	56,799	49,705	48,170
80	53,925	47,084	43,180	35,285	33,576
85	38,329	31,770	27,960	20,908	18,542
90	22,219	17,046	14,154	9,297	7,080
95	9,419	6,282	5,043	2,786	1,524
100	2,510	1,424	1,150	542	183

but because people reaching advanced age have already lived (or had an opportunity to live) a complete life. His argument, reduced to syllogism, runs something like this:

1. There is a natural and fitting life span for people, a time over which people develop a career, have families, travel, learn, and generally flourish. By approximately age 80, this "biographical life

span" is complete; no really new career or life span accomplishments remain unrealized.

2. Modern biomedicine and its ethos of aggressive medical care have allowed people to live beyond this biographical life span.
3. Therefore, limits on medical care for the oldest old are appropriate; we should not attempt to treat or cure older people in ways we might treat younger people who have not yet lived a full life.

Students of public health and aging (along with researchers who study aging and clinicians who treat seniors) typically find this argument very disturbing. It is difficult to find students willing to defend this viewpoint in class presentations. Students usually begin by saying that the older people important in their lives deserve medical treatment if they need it just like anyone else, and that they themselves would not want to be excluded from medical care simply by virtue of age. After examining the argument more carefully, they quickly learn that it is difficult to challenge the minor premise (2). As we have seen, geriatric medicine has added years of life even to people who have already reached very old ages. And a visit to any intensive care unit or emergency room shows that preventing aggressive care, even in the case of people very near the end of life, is often a great challenge to families (who are themselves in many cases unsure of what limits to place on medical intervention [Kaufman, 2005]). The "slow medicine" movement is a response to this orientation in medicine (McCullough, 2008).

Callahan is on weaker ground with the major premise (1). After all, people who have reached advanced age may still flourish, travel, and learn. Although they have completed some careers, such as work, marriage, or child-rearing, why should we assume their biography is complete? With reasonable health, their contribution to families, communities, and society need not come to an end. Callahan is ageist to the extent that he only uses criteria from earlier stages of the life span to define a completed biography. Callahan also does not draw out the full implications of his argument. If where you are in a "biographical life span" determines access to medical care, should people unable to have such a biography (because of developmental disorders, early onset disease, or brain injury, for example) also be denied full access to medical care? This is a conclusion he does not want to draw, but the argument leads to such morally unpalatable conclusions.

The weakness of using age as a criterion for rationing medical care becomes even clearer when Callahan tries to state who should and should not receive particular kinds of medical treatments. What he thinks is morally justified, given that a person has reached old age in a particular health state, is shown in Table 11.2.

Curiously, Callahan retreats from the strong claim of limiting care according to age. Instead, health status drives moral claims to medical care, with elders in the best health (the physically vigorous and mentally alert) receiving unlimited medical access (including emergency life-saving technology and advanced life support care). With failing health, especially dementia, the claims of older people on medical care become more and more limited and finally narrow to nursing care and palliation. Some of these suggestions seem quite arbitrary, such as tube feeding for people with dementia, which in fact has not been shown to offer benefit (Casarett et al., 2005).. Likewise, physical illness trumps cognitive

Table 11.2

CALLAHAN'S LIMITATION OF CARE (*SETTING LIMITS*)

	EMERGENCY LIFE-SAVING TECHNOLOGY	ICU & ADVANCED LIFE SUPPORT	GENERAL MEDICAL CARE	NURSING CARE, PALLIATION
Physically vigorous, mentally alert	X	X	X	X
Physically frail, mentally alert	X		X	X
Severely ill, mentally alert			Only to relieve suffering	X
Mild–moderate cognitive deficit			X	X
Severe dementia			Artificial hydration & nutrition only	X
Persistent vegetative state				X
Brain death				

From *Setting the Limits: Medical Goals in an Aging Society* (pp. 181ff), by D. Callahan, 2001, Washington, DC: Georgetown University Press.

disorders, with the physically frail-mentally alert elder entitled to greater access to care than elders with mild to moderate cognitive deficit.

Callahan recognizes his retreat from a strict age-based criterion. "But is it not a contradiction to my age criteria—if a person has lived out a natural life span—to say that all forms of treatment are appropriate? Yes, but public consensus might allow no other course in such cases" (2001, p. 184). He adds in a footnote that "my arguments for this category of persons have been revised from the original edition."

Callahan's arguments have been the subject of much spirited debate, which we cannot recapitulate here. Still, the retreat from an age-based criterion and attempt to specify a basis for rationing based on health status suggest that Callahan himself recognizes the inadequacy of age as a standard and falls back on it only as a stopgap to limit what he sees as irrational attempts to prolong life with technology. He does not believe that physicians can make reasonable judgments in this area under the pressure of available technology (and society-wide denial of the "fittingness" of death in late life). Indeed, he states that "'medical need' is too indeterminate and elastic a concept to be used by itself [in limiting care]," and therefore "some use of age will be necessary to make a judgment about terminating care of the elderly" (2001, p. 170).

Here, Callahan could profit from the kinds of analyses presented in earlier chapters. Why not base access to advanced medical care or technology on the criterion of what works and what a society can afford—in short, on potential to maximize functioning and well-being? This approach is more reasonable for many reasons: it provides benefit to people likely to benefit, allows limitation in care for people near the end of life, makes a rational case for palliation when appropriate, and can be uniformly implemented. This is the approach we advocated earlier when examining the end of life as a public health problem (Chapter 10). Here, research and evidence-based approaches to interventions in aging provide the best guidance.

OTHER CONCEPTIONS OF THE LIFE COURSE AND THE ETHICS OF CARE AT THE END OF LIFE

Callahan raised the question of a "biographical life span," a completed life course, which might be relevant for thinking about the limits to care in late life. We are all familiar with the Western model of the life course, nicely articulated by Shakespeare: (a) infancy, (b) "whining school-boy . . . creeping unwillingly to school," (c) lover, (d) soldier ("seeking the bubble reputation even in the cannon's mouth"), (e) judge or administrator, (f) retirement based on frailty ("his big manly voice, turning again towards childish treble"), and finally (g) "second childishness and mere oblivion . . . sans teeth, sans eyes, sans taste, sans everything" (*As You Like It* II, 7). But imagine a society in which decline is not the primary motif for the second half of life. In some societies transformation or transcendence is at least as important as decline when thinking about the second half of the life span.

In a number of African societies powerful seniors who decline into frailty and death travel a parallel course to spiritual power and activity as ancestors (Cattell & Albert, 2009). The boundary between very old person and ancestor may be porous, as in the case of Sukuma agropastoralists in Tanzania, among whom the very old live in an ambiguous zone between life and death, elderhood and ancestorhood. In this situation, death is not a sharp dividing line and elders fade into an ancestral state in a gradual process that imbues those still living with the qualities and powers of ancestral spirits (Stroeken, 2002). In the worldview of sub-Saharan African societies, decline and death open the door to ancestorhood, where ancestors may play an active role in the lives of their descendants.

For example, among mid-twentieth century Tallensi in Ghana, dead lineage elders were transformed into ancestor spirits with great power and authority, both mystical and worldly (Fortes, 1961). Ancestors were fed at gravesites and crossroads and regularly consulted by their descendants. They were petitioned when crops failed or someone was sick, or when a lineage's fortunes declined. An ancestor's response could be to curse or to bless, to bring further disaster or good fortune. Junior lineage members were linked to clan ancestors through living elders who represented the ancestors. The living elders communicated with ancestors, spoke for them, and drew on ancestors' authority to enhance their own.

While Meyer Fortes was working with the Tallensi, a man named Teezien gave him a vivid account of the immediate, direct connection Tallensi saw between themselves and their ancestors: "We provide for them . . . and beg crops. . . . If we deny him [ancestor], he will not provide for us, he will not give to us, neither wife nor child. It is he who rules over us so that we may live. . . . If you gave him nothing, will he give you anything? He is the master of everything. We brew beer for him and sacrifice fowls so that he may eat to satisfaction and then he will secure guinea corn and millet for us" (Fortes, 1961, p. 186). Fortes challenged Teezien: "Ancestors . . . are dead; how can they eat and do such material things as making crops thrive?" Imperturbable, Teezien responded: "It is exactly as with living people."

This kind of status for the declining (or even dead) elder may invest old age with an entirely different meaning. For example, the Samia of Kenya view it as a time to sit around the fire and be fed, not an unwelcome prospect at all (Albert & Cattell, 1994). The Ju'hoansi of Namibia defend the right of older people to complain even when they are well taken care of; it is the reward of very old age (Rosenberg, 2009). The centrality of the frail declining elder in these villages, who is cared by the whole community and the first stop for any visitor to the village, is striking. This connectedness of elders to families and communities may be more pronounced in other societies with different approaches to aging. Thus, South Asian elderly must work hard to *separate* themselves from adult children as they approach very old age and mark this separation with an elaborate ritual cycle (Lamb, 2009).

The conclusion to draw from this brief excursion is only that the life course, and the position of people approaching the end of life, varies across cultures. We may learn something about the ethics of care at older ages by examining cultural variation in approaches to the life course.

MINIMIZE SUFFERING OR MAXIMIZE CARE?

In striking contrast to Callahan's use of age to limit care, the President's Council on Bioethics (2005) has proposed a vision of ethical caregiving and access to medical care that is completely age neutral. For the Council, age and its infirmities offer "hard cases" that help define moral clarity in medical care. The Council emphasized best care guided by "loving prudence." The lodestar for such care is "the obligation never to seek a person's death in making decisions about a person's care" (2005, p. 151). This injunction follows from the need to recognize the humanity of even the most frail elder with dementia, who is entitled as a result of this humanity to reasonable access to care. The Council applied this framework to a series of progressively more challenging hypothetical cases involving elders with cognitive impairment. Summaries of the cases and proposed ethical analyses are shown in Table 11.3.

As the cases show, "the obligation to serve the patient now living among us, by always seeking the best care possible under the circumstances" (2005, p. 196) makes the decision not to treat morally suspect in most cases. In only one of the four cases shown in the table, the case of

Table 11.3

HARD CASES FROM THE PRESIDENT'S COUNCIL ON BIOETHICS

MEDICAL CONDITION	TREATMENT DILEMMA	ETHICAL RECOMMENDATION
Mild cognitive impairment; patient aware of impending Alzheimer's	Candidate for bypass surgery due to vessel blockage; patient declines and decides to stop heart medication. Decision not coerced and patient reasonably informed about benefits and risks of treatment; patient not depressed.	Because patient may (i) face subtle self-imposed coercion based on fear of being burden; (ii) not appreciate burden posed by untreated heart disease; (iii) not appreciate effect on family of hastened death; (iv) not recognize likelihood of some years of reasonable health even with AD, *no compelling reason to stop medication or avoid procedure*
Severe dementia; severe dependency in ADL; little recognition of others; calm and compliant; some pleasure in daily contacts	Decision whether to treat bacterial pneumonia in hands of family members	Because (i) she is not irreversibly dying, (ii) the treatment is not overly burdensome, and (iii) the treatment is best care for the person as she now exists (and denying it would violate principle of equal access to such care), *no compelling reason not to treat*
Middle-stage dementia; aggressive and violent, treated with sedatives; occasionally needs physical restraints	Decision regarding pacemaker implant for transient loss of consciousness due to heart disease Psychiatric symptoms resistant to number of medication regimens	Because (i) nontreatment is also risky (e.g., hip fracture), (ii) death is not imminent; and (iii) nontreatment indicates that the impairments of AD are, by themselves, a legitimate reason to aim at death, *no compelling reason not to install pacemaker*
Middle-stage dementia; severe ADL dependency, bathing a struggle; reasonable daily routine	Kidney failure, dialysis; patient resists going to dialysis center, family burned out Decision whether to end dialysis	Because (i) treatment is severe burden, and (ii) after determining that other alternatives (i.e., home dialysis) do not improve situation, *decision to cease treatment morally permissible*

dialysis in a highly resistant patient, is it permissible to cease treatment; and even this decision depends heavily on first considering treatment alternatives. Here, the invasiveness of the treatment, the active approach of death represented by kidney failure, and the burden to patient and family make the decision to stop treatment ethically acceptable. But the other decisions do not pass this test, because they all imply that death due to nontreatment is superior to lives lived with disability or distress, and the Council begins with the fundamental principle that human worth does not depend on possession of particular capacities.

One implication of this principle is that minimizing suffering and maximizing care for vulnerable elders may conflict. Treating pneumonia and implanting a pacemaker maximize care but may increase patient suffering to the extent that patients live longer and suffer increasing loss of function with the progression of dementia. The Council asks that we err on the side of maximizing care because it demonstrates our commitment to the worth of the person as a person. But the cost of such care must also be recognized. "Often, with regret and anguish, we must opt for affirming what seems to be miserable or undignified life over death" (2005, p. 182).

The public health implications of this position are also worth comment. Certainly, this approach strengthens the claim of people who have dementia and their families to adequate respite, aging services, and long-term care. The Council's position also draws attention to a certain humility and realism to end-of-life care and the infirmities of very late life. There is suffering that we cannot remediate, but instead must simply bear and witness.

RETHINKING AUTONOMY

Research in psychology and aging suggests important changes over the life span in novelty seeking (less), altruism (more), social selectivity (more), deliberation in decision making (more), risk aversion (more), emotional range (less), emotional regulation (more), and many other domains. These kinds of changes may be relevant to a key element in moral theory, namely autonomy.

Older adults prefer fewer choices or options than younger people. When asked the optimal number of options for a decision involving choice of drug plans and physicians, for example, or purchases of cars or jams, older people prefer about half the number of options mentioned by college students (Reed, Mikels, & Simon, 2008). Even among older people, increasingly late age is associated with preferences for fewer choices. Why should this be? Restricting the range of choices offers a number of benefits in old age. For example, reducing the amount of information in a decision may make the decision easier, important if one is aware of reduced competence in complex decision making. Also, fewer decision choices may mean less regret or self-blame if a decision proves to be wrong, because having many choices may increase expectations for better decisions. Finally, seeking fewer choices is consistent with broader self-regulation strategies in older age. Older adults are more likely to aim for satisfaction and avoidance of negative affect than younger people, and more choice may mean more opportunity for negative outcomes.

Thus, it is not surprising that older adults are less likely than younger people to seek second opinions in medical care (Zwahr, Park, & Shifren, 1999), or that they are more deferential to physicians and desire less responsibility for decisions (Finucane et al., 2002). Is autonomy, as currently construed, an appropriate standard, then, for thinking about medical decision making in later life?

Some doubt comes from empirical studies that document how older people seek medical care. Among the very old, the doctor-patient relationship is usually set within a triad of doctor-patient-caregiving spouse or adult child (Silliman, 2000). Physicians need to attend to this family setting of care and decision making. By their mid-sixties, about a third of patients with chronic disease are already accompanied by family when they make doctor visits (Silliman, Bhatti, Khan, Dukes, & Sullivan, 1996).

Questions about the focus on autonomy come to the fore when elders begin to lose the cognitive capacity required for complex medical decisions. The capacity to consent for treatment, and especially research, is an active research area. A series of studies have applied the MacArthur Competency Assessment Tool for Clinical Research, MacCAT-CR (Appelbaum & Grisso, 2000) to people with cognitive impairment (along with family proxies) in the setting of clinical trials to determine what proportion are capable of understanding consent. The MacCAT-CR assesses the ability to express a choice, comprehend information, appreciate facts relevant to a decision, and reason about the consequences of an action. In one clinical trial on Alzheimer's disease, consent forms were read to participants and proxies and coupled with MacCAT-CR indicators, so that participants could be assessed on choice, understanding, reasoning, and appreciation of information. Audiotapes of the sessions were reviewed by experienced clinicians with experience in determining capacity. In this sample of people with Mini-Mental State Examination scores of 12–26, and thus mild to moderate dementia, clinicians found that approximately half were capable of providing informed consent. It is noteworthy that among caregivers without dementia, more than 85% received maximum scores on the four dimensions of competency (Karlawish et al., 2008).

Clearly, capacity to provide informed consent for medical treatment or research cannot be assumed in older people with cognitive disorders (and a larger literature also suggests that even when consent is obtained, people often do not understand that they have been enrolled in research studies). Should people with cognitive disorders be barred from participation in clinical research because of this inability to provide consent? This is an unwelcome conclusion, because it excludes a large class of people from any benefits associated with participation (including the more extensive care and medical attention typical of such trials) and makes it hard to test therapies to treat disease. The alternative is surrogate consent. Americans, on the whole, support such consent for research involving older people (Kim et al., 2009). But who should serve as surrogate? The family member with power of attorney, as has been suggested by legal authorities? The family member in the best position to judge what the person may have wanted or what is in his or her best interest? No firm guidelines are available.

These issues rear their head again in advanced directives for end-of-life care. Advanced directives can be absent, completed, but not available to intensive care unit staff or emergency medical services (EMS), completed but underspecified, or completed but overridden by family members. Elders and others near the end of life rely on these instruction directives to ensure that their preferences are respected when they can no longer communicate them. But a steady stream of research has demonstrated that these documents are not always available when patients are admitted for emergency care and are no match for the treatment-centric setting of the modern hospital.

At least for the nursing home and hospice setting, and more recently for EMS, a new paradigm for such instructions is now available in certain states, the Physician Orders for Life-Sustaining Treatment (POLST). The POLST differs from the advanced directive or living will in its standardization of key end-of-life treatment choices and, most importantly, its requirement that it be signed by a physician and placed in patient medical charts (Schmidt, Hickman, Tolle, & Brooks, 2004b). Already, evidence suggests that patient preferences, as expressed in the POLST, are more likely to be followed than the standard advanced directive in the nursing home setting. On the other hand, first reports of its use in nursing homes raise some question about who is completing it (family member, physician, social worker?), whether it is ever updated, and whether residents or families comprehend its features. The POLST paradigm of training and implementation attempts to overcome challenges to end-of-life advanced directives by limiting its use to people highly likely to die in a year (so that preferences would not be expected to change in people who already have severe debility and chronic disease), standardizing elicitation of end-of-life preferences and completion of the form, and training nursing home staff in conducting POLST conversations with residents and families.

The POLST may indeed be an improvement over current practice and seems to be on its way to adoption across the United States. Still, caution is probably appropriate in its extension beyond the nursing home or hospice. Palliative care physicians and more experienced clinicians insist that what is important in an advanced directive or POLST is not the signed document, but rather the discussion that allows patient and physician to figure out what a patient's preferences really are. Such a discussion is obviously critical but probably needs to be supplemented with a document like the POLST that will guide care when that physician is unavailable to advocate for the patient.

BEYOND SPARE-PARTS MEDICINE

> *It is grossly unfair to blame people for the health consequences of inheriting a body that lacks perfect maintenance and repair systems and was not built for extended use or perpetual health.*
> —Olshansky, Carnes, & Butler

It is hard to know whether the authors meant it as a tongue-and-cheek exercise, but Olshansky and colleagues offer a redesigned human body consistent with our wishes to live long and age well. Table 11.4 shows some of the flaws our current bodies present for this effort (driven largely by evolutionary pressures that benefit survival only through the reproductive period) and some fixes. The table shows how we might redesign bones, joints, and musculature for optimal long life. Thus, shorter stature is advantageous because we face bone mineral loss in old age. The authors also present fixes for other aspects of human bodies, which are clearly poorly designed for function in very late age.

The redesigned body is a caricature. Clearly, we cannot expect to reduce stature, change neck curvature, or redesign leg vasculature. This replacement of defective organs, which Butler (2008) has called spare parts medicine, can only go so far, although joint replacement is far advanced and nerve and muscle regeneration may be on the horizon. Butler and his colleagues think the real payoff for securing better aging lies in basic science to determine how genetic mutations influence the rate at which we age. The goal is to design therapies that slow aging. The gains from such therapy would be immense. Slowing the rate of aging would reduce the age-specific risk of mortality and disabilities at all ages and transform the face of very old age.

Advocates of a limited natural life span, such as Daniel Callahan, do not want to hear such speculation and certainly do not think it is appropriate for research funding. Yet, it seems likely that knowledge of genetic mechanisms involved in aging will help us reduce the prevalence of age-related diseases, such as diabetes, osteoporosis, heart and kidney failure, and Parkinson's and Alzheimer's disease. The effort will likely spin off medical advances welcome for health at any age.

So, public health and aging is left with many large questions, all with ethical consequences. For the largest question of control over the aging process itself, it may be useful to look back to the humble *Caenorhabditis elegans,* the nematode that has taught us so much about aging.

Table 11.4

FLAWS AND FIXES FOR THE HUMAN BODY: BONE AND MUSCULATURE

FLAW	FIX
Bone mineral loss	Shorter stature
Fallible spinal disks	Forward-tilting upper torso; curved neck with enlarged vertebrae; thicker disks
Muscle loss	Extra muscle and fat
Vein varicosity	Leg veins with check veins
Short rib cage	Additional ribs
Joint degeneration	Knee able to bend backward; larger hamstrings and tendons

Figure 11.1 shows mobility trajectories for this worm as it enters old age at day 12 of its short life span. Herndon and colleagues (2002) exquisitely measured locomotor phenotypes in the worms and defined three states of mobility (very fast and active in response to stimulation and a food source; somewhat fast; and slow). Half the worms entered old age at day 12 with excellent mobility, but the other half were already slower. With each additional day, the number with better locomotor status declined. A few worms maintained superior locomotor ability up to day 22, but the trend with time was toward the poorest mobility state, which is highly correlated with time to death. All worms were dead by day 38. No worms reversed the downward locomotor trajectory; but the results show that the longer one maintains high-level mobility, the less the proportion of life span lived with disability and the longer the life span.

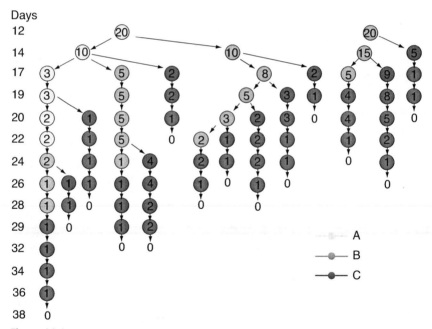

Figure 11.1 Mobility trajectories in *C. elegans*.

Note: Three locomotor phenotypes for *C. elegans* based on speed and amplitude of movement: A, fastest; B, middle state; C, slowest.

Source: Reprinted by permission from Macmillan Publishers Ltd: Herndon, L. A., Schmeissner, P. J., Dudaronek, J. M., Brown, P. A., Listner, K. M., Sakano, Y., et al. Stochastic and genetic factors influence tissue-specific decline in ageing *C. elegans*. *Nature, 419*, 808–814. Copyright 2002.

This should sound familiar because it is also our condition, with perhaps one exception. Medical and public health and aging efforts have allowed people to reverse these trajectories, at least to some extent, as people regain function through treatment and draw on physiological reserve banked over the life span. How far can we push the delay of locomotor decline? For how long and for how many can we reverse it? Perhaps the central question raised by public health and aging is simply to determine how far we differ from this simple organism in its old age trajectories of function and well-being.

SUMMARY

Age as a Criterion to Ration Medical Care. People are not overly sad when a person who has lived a long and full life dies. Starting from this important insight, Daniel Callahan builds a case for rationing medical care based on age. This criterion is inadequate in many ways and leads to a number of ethically unpalatable conclusions. If a principle for rationing is required, a much simpler and fairer criterion is what works and what a society can afford—in short, evidence-based medical effectiveness.

Other Conceptions of the Life Course and the Ethics of Care at the End of Life. In some societies, transformation or transcendence is at least as important as decline when thinking about the second half of the life span. This kind of status for the declining (or even dead) elder may invest old age with an entirely different meaning. We may learn something about the ethics of care at older ages by examining cultural variation in approaches to the life course.

Minimize Suffering or Maximize Care? In striking contrast to Callahan's use of age to limit care, the President's Council on Bioethics (2005) proposed a vision of ethical caregiving and access to medical care that is completely age neutral. Their approach begins with the fundamental principle that human worth does not depend on possession of particular capacities. This principle leads to severe limitation on restrictions of care because such limitations in care often imply that death due to nontreatment is superior to lives lived with disability or distress. The Council suggests we err on the side of maximizing care rather than minimizing suffering.

Rethinking Autonomy. Older adults desire fewer choices than younger people, seek less information in health decisions, and desire less responsibility for decisions. Is autonomy, as currently construed, an appropriate standard, then, for thinking about medical decision making in later life? In practice, autonomy in decision making in old age is diffused among other family members, and adequate guidelines for specifying surrogacy are still unavailable.

Beyond Spare-Parts Medicine. Knowledge of genetic mechanisms involved in aging will help us reduce the prevalence of age-related diseases, such as diabetes, osteoporosis, heart and kidney failure, and Parkinson's and Alzheimer's disease. The effort will likely spin off medical advances welcome for health at any age. Public health opportunities for aging will shift when we move from spare parts medicine to greater control of the rate of aging.

References

AARP. (2006). Valuing the invaluable: A new look at the economic value of family caregiving (Issue Brief). Retrieved September 29, 2009, from http://assets.aarp.org/rg center/il/ib82_caregiving.pdf

Abrams, R. C., Lachs, M., McAvay, G., Keohane, D. J., & Bruce, M. L. (2002). Predictors of self-neglect in community-dwelling elders. *American Journal of Psychiatry,159*, 1724–1730.

Ackermann, R. T., Cheadle, A., Sandhu, N., Madsen, L., Wagner, E. H., & LoGerfo, J. P. (2003). Community exercise program use and changes in healthcare costs for older adults. *American Journal of Preventive Medicine, 25*(3), 232–237.

Agency for Healthcare Research and Quality (AHRQ). (2002). Preventing disability in the elderly with chronic disease. *Research in action*, Issue 3. Retrieved May 15, 2009, from http://www.ahrq.gov/research/elderis.htm

Agency for Healthcare Research and Quality (AHRQ). (2008). *Recommendations of the U.S. Preventive Services Task Force*. Guide to Clinical Preventive Services. AHRQ Publication No. 08-05122, September. Rockville, MD: Author. Retrieved May 15, 2009, from http://www.ahrq.gov/clinic/pocketgd08/

Agree, E. M., & Freedman, V. A. (2003). A comparison of assistive technology and personal care in alleviating disability and unmet need. *Gerontologist, 43*(3), 335–344.

Agree, E. M., Freedman, V. A., Cornman, J. C., Wolf, D. A., & Marcotte, J. E. (2005). Reconsidering substitution in long-term care: When does assistive technology take the place of personal care? *The Journals of Gerontology. Series B, Psychological Sciences and Social Sciences, 60*(5), S272–S280.

Ahronheim, J. C., Morrison, R. S., Baskin, S. A., Morris, J., & Meier, D. E. (1996). Treatment of the dying in the acute care hospital. Advanced dementia and metastatic cancer. *Archives of Internal Medicine, 156*(18), 2094–2100.

Aizenstein, H. J., Nebes, R. D., Saxton, J. A., Price, J. C., Mathis, C. A., Tsopelas, N. D., et al. (2008). Frequent amyloid deposition without significant cognitive impairment among the elderly. *Archives of Neurology, 65*(11), 1509–1517.

Albert, S. M. (1997). Assessing health-related quality of life in elderly chronic care populations. In J. A. Teresi, M. P. Lawton, D. Holmes, & M. Ory (Eds.), *Measurement in elderly chronic care populations* (pp. 210–227). New York: Springer.

Albert, S. M. (1998). Defining and measuring quality of life in medicine. *Journal of the American Medical Association, 279*(6), 429.

Albert, S. M. (2002). *Speaking from experience: Home attendants speak about home care*. New York, Fan Fox & Leslie R. Samuels Foundation.

371

Albert, S. M. (2004). Beyond ADL-IADL: "Recognizing the full scope of family caregiving." In C. Levine (Ed.), *Family caregivers on the job: Moving beyond ADLs and IADLs.* New York, United Hospital Fund.

Albert, S. M., Bear-Lehman, J., & Burkhardt, A. (2009, in press). Lifestyle-adjusted function: Variation beyond BADL and IADL competencies. *The Gerontologist.*

Albert, S. M., Bear-Lehman, J., Burkhardt, A., Merete-Roa, B., & Noboa-Lemonier, R. (2006). Variation in sources of clinician- and self-rated IADL disability. *Journal of Gerontology: Medical Sciences, 61A,* 826–831.

Albert, S. M., & Brody, E. M. (1996). When elder care is viewed as child care. Significance of elder's cognitive impairment and caregiver burden. *American Journal of Geriatric Psychiatry, 4,* 121–130.

Albert, S. M., Castillo-Castaneda, C., Jacobs, D. M., Sano, M., Bell, K., Merchant, C., et al. (1999a). Proxy-reported quality of life in Alzheimer's patients: Comparison of clinical and population-based samples. *Journal of Mental Health and Aging, 5*(1), 49–58.

Albert, S. M., & Cattell, M. G. (1994). *Old age in global perspective.* New York: GK Hall/ McMillan.

Albert, S. M., Colombi, A., & Hanlon, J. (in press). Potentially inappropriate medications and risk of hospitalization in retirees. *Drugs and Aging.*

Albert, S. M., Costa, R., Merchant, C., Small, S., Jenders, R. A., Stern, Y. (1999b). Hospitalization and Alzheimer's disease: Results from a community-based study. *The Journals of Gerontology. Series A, Biological Sciences and Medical Sciences, 54A,* M267–M271.

Albert, S. M., Dienstag, A., Tabert, M. H., Pelton, G., & Devanand, D. P. (2002a). The impact of mild cognitive impairment on functional abilities in the elderly. *Current Psychiatry Reports, 4*(1), 64–68.

Albert, S. M., Glied, S., Andrews, H., Stern, Y., & Mayeux, R. (2002b). Primary care expenditures before the onset of Alzheimer's disease. *Neurology, 59*(4), 573–578.

Albert, S. M., Im, A., & Raveis, V. (2002c). Public health and the second 50 years of life. *American Journal of Public Health, 92,* 1214–1216.

Albert, S. M., & Logsdon, R. G., Eds. (2001). *Assessing quality of life in Alzheimer's disease.* New York: Springer Publishing.

Albert, S. M., Michaels, K., Padilla, M., Pelton, G., Bell, K., Marder, K., et al. (1999c). Functional significance of mild cognitive impairment in elderly patients without a dementia diagnosis. *American Journal of Geriatric Psychiatry, 7,* 213–220.

Albert, S. M., Musa, D., Kwoh, K., & Silverman, M. (2008). Defining optimal self-management in osteoarthritis: Racial differences in a population-based sample. *Journal of Cross-Cultural Gerontology, 23,* 349–360.

Albert, S. M., O'Neil, M., Muller, C., & Butler, R. (2002d). *When does old age begin? Results from a national survey.* New York, International Longevity Center.

Albert, S. M., Rabkin, J. G., Del Bene, M. L., Tider, T., O'Sullivan, I., Rowland, L. P., et al. (2005a). Wish to die in end-stage ALS. *Neurology, 65*(1), 68–74.

Albert, S. M., Sano, M., Bell, K., Merchant, C., Small, S., & Stern, Y. (1998). Hourly care received by people with Alzheimer's disease: Results from an urban, community-based survey. *The Gerontologist, 38*(6), 704–714.

Albert, S. M., Simone, B., Brassard, A., Stern, Y., & Mayeux, R. (2005b). Medicaid home care services and survival in New York City. *The Gerontologist, 45*(5), 609–616.

Albert, S. M., & Teresi, J. A. (1999). Reading ability, education, and cognitive status assessment among older adults in Harlem, New York City, *American Journal of Public Health, 89*, 95–97.

Albert, S. M., & Teresi, J. A. (2002). Quality of life, definition and measurement. In D. J. Eckert (Ed.), *Encyclopedia of aging* (Vol. 4, pp. 1158–1161). New York: MacMillian.

Alecxih, L. (2006). *Long term care financing in the U.S.* The Lewin Group. Retrieved June 1, 2009, from http://www.allhealth.org/BriefingMaterials/Alecxih-443.pdf

Alecxih, L. M. B., Zeruld, S., & Olearczyk, B. (2000). *Characteristics of caregivers based on the survey of income and program participation.* Washignton, D.C., The Lewin Group.

Alexopoulos, G. S., Borson, S., Cuthbert, B. N., Devanand, D. P., Mulsant, B. H., Olin, J. T., et al. (2002). Assessment of late life depression. *Biological Psychiatry, 52*(3), 164–174.

Alexopoulos, G. S., Katz, I. R., Bruce, M. L., Heo, M., Ten Have, T., Raue, P., et al. (2005). Remission in depressed geriatric primary care patients: A report from the PROSPECT Study. *American Journal of Psychiatry, 162*(4), 718–724.

Allen, S., & Mor, V. (1998). Unmet need and its consequences: Contrasts between older and younger adults with disability. *Medical Care, 35*(11), 1132–1148.

Alzheimer's Association. (2009). Alzheimer's disease facts and figures. *Alzheimers & Dementia: The Journal of the Alzheimer's Association, 5*(3), 234–270.

American Psychiatric Association. (2000). *Diagnostic and statistical manual of mental disorders* (4th ed.). Washington, DC: Author.

Amirkhanyan, A. A., & Wolf, D. A. (2006). Parent care and the stress process: Findings from panel data. *The Journals of Gerontology. Series B, Psychological Sciences and Social Sciences, 61*(5), S248–S255.

Anderson, R. N., & Smith, B. L. (2005). Deaths: Leading causes for 2002. *National Vital Statistics Reports, 53*(17), 1–89.

Appelbaum, P. S., & Grisso, T. (2000). *The MacArthur competence assessment tool—Clinical research.* Sarasota, FL: Professional Resources.

Arias, E. (2007). United States life tables, 2004. *National Vital Statistics Reports* (Vol. 56). Hyattsville, MD: National Center for Health Statistics. Retrieved May 15, 2009, from http://www.cdc.gov/nchs/data/nvsr/nvsr56/nvsr56_09.pdf

Arno, P. S., Levine, C., & Memmott, M. M. (1999). The economic value of informal caregiving. *Health Affairs (Project Hope), 18*, 182–188.

Asthana, S., Brinton, R. D., Henderson, V. W., McEwen, B. S., Morrison, J. H., & Schmidt, P. J. (2009). Frontiers proposal. National Institute on Aging "bench to bedside: Estrogen as a case study." *Age (Dordr)* 31, 199–210.

Balfour, J. L., & Kaplan, G. A. (2002). Neighborhood environment and loss of physical function in older adults: Evidence from the Alameda County Study. *American Journal of Epidemiology, 155*(6), 507–515.

Ball, K., Berch, D. B., Helmers, K. F., Jobe, J. B., Leveck, M. D., Marsiske, M., et al. (2002). Effects of cognitive training interventions with older adults: A randomized controlled trial. *Journal of the American Medical Association, 288*(18), 2271–2281.

Baltes, M., & Carstensen, L. (1996). The process of successful ageing. *Ageing and Society, 16*, 397–422.

Baltes, P. B., & Baltes, M. M. (1990). *Successful aging: Perspective from the behavioral sciences* (pp. 1–34). New York: Cambridge University Press.

Baltes, P. B., & Smith, J. (2003). New frontiers in the future of aging: From successful aging of the young old to the dilemmas of the fourth age. *Gerontology, 49*(2), 123–135.

Bayles, C. N., Milas, C. N., Kuller, L. H., Newman, A. B., McTigue, K., & Williams, K. (2008). *The 10 keys to healthy aging.* Pittsburgh, PA: Center for Healthy Aging, University of Pittsburgh.

Beekman, A. T., Geerlings, S. W., Deeg, D. J., Smit, J. H., Schoevers, R. S., de Beurs, E., et al. (2002). The natural history of late-life depression: a 6-year prospective study in the community. *Archives of General Psychiatry, 59*(7), 605–611.

Beers, M. H., Ouslander, J. G., Fingold, S. F., Morgenstern, H., Reuben, D. B., Rogers, W., et al. (1992). Inappropriate medication prescribing in skilled-nursing facilities. *Annals of Internal Medicine, 117*(8), 684–689.

Belle, S. H., Burgio, L., Burns, R., Coon, D., Czaja, S. J., Gallagher-Thompson, D., et al. (2006). Enhancing the quality of life of dementia caregivers from different ethnic or racial groups: A randomized, controlled trial. *Annals of Internal Medicine, 145*(10), 727–738.

Benton, A. L. (1955). *The Benton visual retention test.* New York: The Psychological Corporation.

Benton, A. L. (1967). *FAS Test.* Victoria, BC, Canada: University of Victoria.

Bergner, M., Bobbitt, R. A., Pollard, W. E., Martin, D. P., & Gilson, B. S. (1976). The sickness impact profile: Validation of a health status measure. *Medical Care, 14*(1), 57–67.

Berzon, R. A., Leplege, A. P., Lohr, K. N., Lenderking, W. R., & Wu, A. (1997). Summary and recommendations for future research. *Quality of Life Research: An International Journal of Quality of Life Aspects of Treatment, Care and Rehabilitation, 6,* 601–605.

Beswick, A. D., Rees, K., Dieppe, P., Ayis, S., Gooberman-Hill, R., Horwood, J., et al. (2008). Complex interventions to improve physical function and maintain independent living in elderly people: A systematic review and meta-analysis. *Lancet, 371*(9614), 725–735.

Bhalla, R. K., Butters, M. A., Becker, J. T., Houck, P. R., Snitz, B. E., Lopez, O. L., et al. (2009). Patterns of mild cognitive impairment after treatment of depression in the elderly. *American Journal of Geriatric Psychiatry, 17*(4), 308–316.

Bhattacharya, J., & Bundorf, M. K. (2009). The incidence of the healthcare costs of obesity. *Journal of Health Economics, 28,* 649–658.

Bhattacharya, J., Choudhry, K., & Lakdawalla, D. (2006). Appendix F: Chronic disease and trends in severe disability in working-age populations. In M. J. Field, A. Jette, & L. M. Martin (Eds.), *Workshop on disability in America.* Washington, DC: National Academies Press.

Blazer, D. G. (2002). The prevalence of depressive symptoms. *The Journals of Gerontology. Series A, Biological Sciences and Medical Sciences, 57*(3), M150–M151.

Bloom, D. E., & Canning, D. (2007). Mortality traps and the dynamics of health transitions. *Proceedings of the National Academy of Sciences of the United States of America, 104*(41), 16044–16049.

Bloom, D. E., Canning, D., & Fink, G. (2008). Urbanization and the wealth of nations. *Science, 319*(5864), 772–775.

The Boards of Trustees, Federal Hospital Insurance and Federal Supplementary Medical Insurance Trust Funds. (2009). *Annual report of the Boards of Trustees of the*

Federal Hospital Insurance and Federal Supplementary Medical Insurance Trust Funds Communication. Available at http://www.ssa.gov/OACT/TR/2009/index.html

Borson, S., Barnes, R. A., Kukull, W. A., Okimoto, J. T., Veith, R. C., Inui, T. S., et al. (1986). Symptomatic depression in elderly medical outpatients. I. Prevalence, demography, and health service utilization. *Journal of the American Geriatrics Society,* 34(5), 341–347.

Boult, C., & Pacala, J. T. (1999). Care of older people at risk. In E. Calkins, C. Boult, E. H. Wagner, & J. T. Pacala (Eds.), *New ways to care for older people: Building systems based on evidence* (pp. 65–81). New York: Springer Press.

Breitner, J. C., Haneuse, S. J., Walker, R., Dublin, S., Crane, P. K., Gray, S. L., et al. (2009). Risk of dementia and AD with prior exposure to NSAIDs in an elderly community-based cohort. *Neurology, 72,* 1899–1905.

Brod, M., Stewart, A. L., & Sands, L. (2001). Conceptualization of quality of life in dementia. In S. M. Albert, & R. G. Logsdon (Eds.), *Assessing quality of life in Alzheimer's disease* (pp. 3–16). New York: Springer Publishing.

Brookmeyer, R., Corrada, N. M., Curriero, F. C., & Kawas, C. (2002). Survival following diagnosis of Alzheimer's disease. *Archives of Neurology, 59*(11), 1764–1767.

Brookmeyer, R., Gray, S., & Kawas, C. (1998). Projections of Alzheimer's disease in the United States and the public health impact of delaying disease onset. *American Journal of Public Health, 88*(9), 1337–1342.

Bruce, M. L., Seeman, T. E., Merrill, S. S., & Blazer, D. G. (1994). The impact of depressive symptomatology on physical disability: MacArthur Studies of Successful Aging. *American Journal of Public Health, 84,* 1796–1799.

Bruce, M. L., Ten Have, T. R., Reynolds, C. F., III, Katz, I. I., Schulberg, H. C., Mulsant, B. H., et al. (2004). Reducing suicidal ideation and depressive symptoms in depressed older primary care patients: A randomized controlled trial. *Journal of the American Medical Association, 291*(9), 1081–1091.

Buchner, D. M. (1999). Prevention of frailty. In E. Calkins, C. Boult, E. H. Wagner, & J. T. Pacala (Eds.), *New ways to care for older people: Building systems based on evidence* (pp. 3–19). New York: Springer Publishing.

Buchner, D. M., Cress, E., de LaTour, B. J., Essleman, P. C., et al. (1997). The effect of strength and endurance training on gait, balance, fall risk, and health services use in community-living older adults. *The Journals of Gerontology. Series A, Biological Sciences and Medical Sciences, 52A,* M218–M224.

Buchner, D. M., Larson, E. B., Wagner, E. H., Koepsell, T. D., & de Lateur, B. J. (1996). Evidence for a non-linear relationship between leg strength and gait speed. *Age and Aging, 25,* 386–391.

Burgio, L. D., Stevens, A., Burgio, K. L., Roth, D. L., Paul, P., & Gerstle, J. (2002). Teaching and maintaining behavior management skills in the nursing home. *Gerontologist, 42*(4), 487–496.

Bureau of Labor Statistics 2007. (2008). *Volunteering in the United States,* USDL 09–0078. Retrieved October 15, 2009, from http://www.bls.gov/news.release/pdf/volun.pdf

Buschke, H., & Fuld, P. A. (1974). Evaluating storage, retention, and retrieval in disordered memory and learning. *Neurology, 24,* 1019–1025.

Buszewicz, M., Rait, G., Griffin, M., Nazareth, I., Patel, A., Atkinson, A., et al. (2006). Self management of arthritis in primary care: Randomised controlled trial. *British Medical Journal, 333*(7574), 879.

Butler, R. (2008). The careers of people with dementia. *British Medical Journal,* *336*(7656), 1260–1261.

Butler, R. N. (1969). Age-ism: Another form of bigotry. *Gerontologist, 9,* 243–246.

Cadogan, M. P., Schnelle, J. F., Yamamoto-Mitani, N., et al. (2004). A minimum data set prevalence of pain quality indicator: Is it accurate and does it reflect differences in care processes? *The Journals of Gerontology. Series A, Biological Sciences and Medical Sciences, 59,* 281–285.

Cai, L., & Lubitz, J. (2007). Was there compression of disability for older Americans from 1992 to 2003? *Demography, 44*(3), 479–495.

Callahan, D. (2001). *Setting limits: Medical goals in an aging society.* Washington, DC: Georgetown University Press.

Campbell, D. E., Lynn, J., Louis, T. A., & Shugarman, L. R. (2004). Medicare program expenditures associated with hospice use. *Annals of Internal Medicine, 140*(4), 269–277.

Cannuscio, C. C., Jones, C., Kawachi, I., Colditz, G. A., Berkman, L., & Rimm, E. (2002). Reverberations of family illness: A longitudinal assessment of informal caregiving and mental health status in the Nurses' Health Study. *American Journal of Public Health, 92*(8), 1305–1311.

Carpenter, B. D., Van Haitsma, K., Ruckdeschel, K., & Lawton, M. P. (2000). The psychosocial preferences of older adults: A pilot examination of content and structure. *Gerontologist, 40*(3), 335–348.

Carstensen, L. L. (1992). Social and emotional patterns in adulthood: Support for socioemotional selectivity theory. *Psychology of Aging, 7*(3), 331–338.

Casarett, D., Karlawish, J., Morales, K., Crowley, R., Mirsch, T., & Asch, D. A. (2005). Improving the use of hospice services in nursing homes. A randomized controlled trial. *Journal of the American Medical Association, 294,* 211–217.

Cattell, M. G., & Albert, S. M. (2009). Elders, ancients, ancestors and the modern life course. In J. Sokolovsky (Ed.), *The cultural context of aging: Worldwide perspectives* (3rd ed., pp. 115–133). New York; Garvey.

Cella, D. F., & Bonomi, A. E. (1996). The functional assessment of cancer therapy (FACT) and functional assessment of HIV infection (FAHI) quality of life measurement system. In B. Spilker (Ed.), *Quality of life and pharmacoeconomics in clinical trials* (pp. 203–225). Philadelphia: Lippincott-Raven.

Centers for Disease Control and Prevention. (2000a, July 24). Deaths, United States, 2000. *National Vital Statistics Reports, 48*(11). Hyattsville, MD: National Center for Health Statistics.

Centers for Disease Control and Prevention. (2000b). *Measuring healthy days. Population assessment of health-related quality of life.* National Center for Chronic Disease Prevention and Health Promotion. Division of Adult and Community Health. Retrieved May 15, 2009, from www.cdc.gov/hrqol/pdfs/mhd.pdf

Centers for Disease Control and Prevention. (2003). Trends in aging—United States and worldwide. *Morbidity and Mortality Weekly Report, 53,* 102–106.

Centers for Disease Control and Prevention. (2007). *State of health and aging in America 2003.* Testimony, U.S. Senate. J. S. Marks, May 19, 2003. Retrieved April 20, 2006, from http://www.cdc.gov/aging/saha.htm

Centers for Disease Control and Prevention. (2009). *Healthy People 2010. Midcourse Review, Goal 1.* Retrieved May 15, 2009, from http://www.healthypeople.gov/data/midcourse/html/

Centers for Medicare and Medicaid Services. (2007). *Medicare hospice data: 1998–2005.* Retrieved September 26, 2009, from http://www.cms.hhs.gov/ProspMedicareFee SvcPmtGen/downloads/HospiceData1998-2005.pdf

Centers for Medicare and Medicaid Services/Office of Research, Development, and Information (ORDI). (2008). *Key milestones in the Medicare programs.* Retrieved August 11, 2008, from http://www.cms.hhs.gov/History/Downloads/CMSProgram KeyMilestones.pdf

Centers for Medicare and Medicaid Services. (2009). *Trustees report.* Retrieved April 15, 2009, from http://www.cms.hhs.gov/ReportsTrustFunds/

CESSI. (2003). *Federal statutory definitions of disability*: Prepared for the Interagency Committee on Disability Research. Retrieved March 15, 2009, from http://www.icdr.us/documents/definitions.htm

Chang, J.T., Morton, S.C., Rubenstein, L.Z., Mojica, W.A., Maglione, M., Suttorp, M.J., et al. (2004). Interventions for the prevention of falls in older adults: Systematic review and meta-analysis of randomised clinical trials. *British Medical Journal, 328,* 680.

Christakis, N. A., & Lamont, E. B. (2000). Extent and determinants of error in doctors' prognoses in terminally ill patients: Prospective cohort study. *British Medical Journal, 320,* 469–472.

Chronic Disease Directors, National Association of State Units on Aging. (2003). *The Aging States Project: Promoting Opportunities for Collaboration Between the Public Health and Aging Services Network.* Centers for Disease Control and Prevention.

Ciechanowski, P., Wagner, E., Schmaling, K., Schwartz, S., Williams, B., Diehr, P., et al. (2004). Community-integrated home-based depression treatment in older adults: A randomized controlled trial. *Journal of the American Medical Association, 291*(13), 1569–1577.

Clark, F., Azen, S. P., Zemke, R., Jackson, J., Carlson, M., Mandel, D., et al. (1997). Occupational therapy for independent-living older adults. *Journal of the American Medical Association, 278*(16), 1321–1325.

Clarke, P., & George, L. K. (2005). The role of the built environment in the disablement process. *American Journal of Public Health, 95*(11), 1933–1939.

Cohen, J. T., Neumann, P. J., & Weinstein, M. C. (2008). Does preventive care save money? Health economics and the presidential candidates. *New England Journal of Medicine, 358*(7), 661–663.

Congressional Budget Office. (2007a). *Restrict Medigap coverage of Medicare's cost sharing, budget options* (February). Washington: Author.

Congressional Budget Office. (2007b). Statement of Peter R. Orszag. *The Medicare Advantage Program: Trends and options before the Subcommittee on Health Committee on Ways and Means U.S. House of Representatives.* Retrieved March 21, 2007 from http://www.cbo.gov/ftpdocs/78xx/doc7879/03-21-Medicare.pdf

Cooper, C., Selwood, A., Blanchard, M., Walker, Z., Blizard, R., & Livingston, G. (2009). Abuse of people with dementia by family carers: Representative cross sectional survey. *British Medical Journal, 338,* b155.

Corder, E. H., Saunders, A. M., Risch, N. J., Strittmatter, W. J., Schmechel, D. E., Gaskell, P. C., Jr., et al. (1994). Protective effect of apolipoprotein E type 2 allele for late onset Alzheimer disease. *Nature Genetics, 7,* 180–184.

Corder, E. H., Saunders, A. M., Strittmatter, W. J., Schmechel, D. E., Gaskell, P. C., Small, G. W., et al. (1993). Gene dose of apolipoprotein E type 4 allele and the risk of Alzheimer's disease in late onset families. *Science, 261,*(5123), 921–923.

Cornman, J. C., Freedman, V. A., & Agree, E. M. (2005). Measurement of assistive device use: Implications for estimates of device use and disability in late life. *Gerontologist, 45*(3), 347–358.

Corporation for National and Community Service. (2007). *Volunteering in Pittsburgh, PA, Volunteering in America, Cities 2007.* Available at http://www.volunteeringinamerica. gov/PA/Pittsburgh.

Costa, D. (2000). Understanding the twentieth century decline in chronic conditions among older men. *Demography, 37*(1), 53–72.

Covinsky, K. E., Hilton, J., Lindquist, K., & Dudley, R. A. (2006). Development and validation of an index to predict activity of daily living dependence in community-dwelling elders. *Medical Care, 44*(2), 149–157.

Crews, D. E. (1990). *Anthropological issues in biological anthropology.* In R. Rubenstein (Ed.), *Anthropology and aging: Comprehensive reviews* (pp. 11–39). Dordrecht: Kluwer Academic Publishers.

Crimmins, E. M., Hayward, M. D., Hagedorn, A., Saito, Y., & Brouard, N. (2009). Change in disability-free life expectancy for Americans aged 70+. *Demography, 46*(3), 627–646.

Crimmins, E. M., & Saito, Y. (2001). Trends in healthy life expectancy in the United States, 1970–1990: Gender, racial, and educational differences. *Social Science and Medicine, 52,* 1629–1641.

Crimmins, E. M., Saito, Y., & Ingegneri, D. (1997a). Trends in disability-free life expectancy in the United States, 1970–1990. *Population and Development Review, 23*(3), 555–572.

Crimmins, E. M., Saito, Y., & Reynolds, S. L. (1997b). Further evidence on recent trends in the prevalence and incidence of disability among older Americans from two sources: The LSOA and the NHIS. *The Journal of Gerontology, Psychological Science and Social Sciences, 52B*(2), S59–S71.

Crook, T., Bartus, R. T., Ferrish, S. H., et al. (1986). Age-associated memory impairment: Proposed diagnostic criteria and measures of clinical change. Report of a National Institute of Mental Health Work Group. *Developmental Neuropsychology, 2,* 261–276.

Crum, R. M., Anthony, J. C., Bassett, S. S., & Folstein, M. F. (1993). Population-based norms for the Mini-Mental State Examination by age and educational level. *Journal of the American Medical Association, 269*(18), 2386–2391.

Cummings, J. L. (1997). The neuropsychiatric inventory: Assessing psychopathology in dementia patients. *Neurology, 48,* 10S–16S.

Current trends. (1994, May 27). Quality of life as a new public health measure: Behavioral Risk Factor Surveillance System, 1993, *Morbidity and Mortality Weekly Report,* pp. 375–380.

Czaja, S. J., Gitlin, L. N., Schulz, R., Zhang, S., Burgio, L. D., Stevens, A. B., et al. (2009). Development of the risk appraisal measure: A brief screen to identify risk areas and guide interventions for dementia caregivers. *Journal of the American Geriatrics Society, 57*(6), 1064–1072.

DeFries, E. L., McGuire, L. C., Andresen, E. M., Brumback, B. A., & Anderson, L. A. (2009). Caregivers of older adults with cognitive impairment. *Preventing Chronic Disease, 6*(2). http://www.cdc.gov/pcd/issues/2009/ apr/08_0088.htm

Department of State, Department of Health and Human Services, National Institute on Aging, & National Institutes of Health. (2007). *Why population aging matters: A global perspective.* Washington, DC: Author. Retrieved March 13, 2009, from http://www.nia.nih.gov/ResearchInformation/ExtramuralPrograms/BehavioralAndSocial Research/GlobalAging.htm

Derogatis, L. R., Lipman, R. S., Rickels, K., Uhlenhuth, E. H., & Covi, L. (1974). The Hopkins Symptom Checklist (HSCL): A self-report symptom inventory. *Behavioral Science, 19*(1), 1–15.

Devanand, D. P., Sano, M., Tang, M. X., Taylor, S., Gurland, B. J., Wilder, D., et al. (1996). Depressed mood and the incidence of Alzheimer's disease in the elderly living in the community. *Archives of General Psychiatry, 53*(2), 175–182.

Dolan, P., Gudex, C., Kind, P., & Williams, A. (1996). Valuing health states: A comparison of methods. *Journal of Health Economics, 15*, 209–231.

Dong, X., Mendes de Leon, C. F., & Evans, D. A. (2009). Is greater self-neglect severity associated with lower levels of physical function? *Journal of Aging Health, 21*(4), 596–610.

Dooneief, G., Marder, K., Tang, M.-X., & Stern, Y. (1996). The Clinical Dementia Rating scale: Community-based validation of "profound" and "terminal" stages. *Neurology, 46*, 1746–1749.

Draper, P., & Harpending, H. (1990). Work and aging in two African societies: Kung and Herero. In B. R. Bonder (Ed.), *Occupational performance in the elderly.* Philadelphia: FA Davis.

Dubois, B., Feldman, H. H., Jacova, C., Dekosky, S. T., Barberger-Gateau, P., Cummings, J., et al. (2007). Research criteria for the diagnosis of Alzheimer's disease: Revising the NINCDS-ADRDA criteria. *Lancet Neurology, 6*(8), 734–746.

Dyer, C. B., Goodwin, J. S., Pickens-Pace, S., Burnett, J., & Kelly, P. A. (2007). Self-neglect among the elderly: A model based on more than 500 patients seen by a geriatric medicine team. *American Journal of Public Health, 97*(9), 1671–1676.

Edelman, P., Fulton, B. R., Kuhn, D., & Chang, C. H. (2005). A comparison of three methods of measuring dementia-specific quality of life: Perspectives of residents, staff, and observers. *Gerontologist, 45 Spec No 1*(1), 27–36.

Elo, I. T., & Preston, S. H. (1996). Educational differentials in mortality: United States, 1979–85. *Social Science and Medicine, 42*(1), 47–57.

Engardio, P., & Matlack, C. (2005, January 31). Global aging. *Business Week.*

Erickson, P., Wilson, R., & Shannon, I. (1995). *Years of healthy life.* Healthy People 2000, Statistical Notes, No. 7. Atlanta, GA: Centers for Disease Control and Prevention.

Etkin, C. D., Prohaska, T. R., Harris, B. A., Latham, N., & Jette, A. (2006). Feasibility of implementing the strong for life program in community settings. *The Gerontologist, 46*, 284–292.

Evans, J. E. (2002). *What does the epidemiology of ageing tell us now?* Valencia Forum. Retrieved March 15, 2009, from http://www.valenciaforum.com/Keynotes/ge.html

Evers, M. M., Purohit, D., Perl, D., Khan, K., & Marin, D. B. (2002). Palliative and aggressive end-of-life care for patients with dementia. *Psychiatric Services, 53*, 609–613.

Fabiszewski, K. J., Volicer, B., & Volicer, L. (1990). Effect of antibiotic treatment on outcome of fevers in institutionalized Alzheimer patients. *Journal of the American Medical Association, 263*(23), 3168–3172.

Farrer, L., & American College of Medical Genetics/American Society of Human Genetics Working Group on ApoE and Alzheimer Disease. (1995). Statement on use of apolipoprotein E testing for Alzheimer disease. *Journal of the American Medical Association, 274,* 1627–1629.

Feder, J., Komisar, H. L., & Niefeld, M. (2001). Long-term care in the United States: An overview. *Health Affairs, 19*(3), 40–56.

Federal Interagency Forum on Aging-Related Statistics. (2008). *Older Americans 2008: Key indicators of well-being.* Retrieved September 15, 2009, from http://www.aging stats.gov/chartbook2008/default.htm

Feeney, D., Furlong, W., Boyle, M., & Torrance, G. W. (1995). Multi-attribute health status classification systems. Health Utilities Index. *Pharmacoeconomics, 7,* 490–502.

Feher, E. P., Larrabee, G. J., Sudilovsky, A., & Crook, T. H. (1994). Memory self-report in Alzheimer's disease and in age-associated memory impairment. *Journal of Geriatric Psychiatry Neurology, 6,* 58–65.

Feinstein, A. R., Josephy, B. R., & Wells, C. K. (1986). Scientific and clinical problems in indexes of functional disability. *Annals of Internal Medicine, 105*(3), 413–420.

Feldman, P. H., & Oberlink, M. (2003). Developing community indicators to promote the health and well-being of older people. *Family and Community Health Journal, 26*(4), 268–274.

Feldman, P. H., Oberlink, M. R., Simantov, E., & Gursen, M. D. (2004). *A tale of two older Americas: Community opportunities and challenges.* The AdvantAge Initiative 2003 National Survey of Adults Aged 65 and Older. New York: The Center for Home Care Policy and Research, Visiting Nurse Service of New York.

Ferrucci, L., Harris, T. B., Guralnik, J. M., Tracy, R. P., Corti, M. C., & Cohen, H. (1999). Serum IL-6 level and the development of disability in older persons. *Journal of the American Geriatrics Society, 47,* 639–646.

Ferrucci, L., Penninx, B. W., Volpato, S., Harris, T. B., Bendeen-Roche, K., Balfour, J., et al. (2002). Change in muscle strength explains accelerated decline of physical function in older women with high interleukin-6 serum levels. *Journal of the American Geriatrics Society, 50,* 1947–1954.

Fialová, D., Topinková, E., Gambassi, G., Finne-Soveri, H., Jónsson, P. V., Carpenter, I., et al. (2005). AdHOC Project Research Group. Potentially inappropriate medication use among elderly home care patients in Europe. *Journal of the American Medical Association, 293*(11), 1348–1358.

Fiatarone, M. A., Marks, E. C., Ryan, N. D., Meredith, C. N., Lipsitz, L. A., & Evans, W. J. (1990). High-intensity strength training in nonagenarians: Effects on skeletal muscle. *Journal of the American Medical Association, 263,* 3029–3034.

Fillenbaum, G., Heyman, A., Peterson, B., Pieper, C., & Weiman, A. L. (2000). Frequency and duration of hospitalization of patients with AD based on Medicare data: CERAD XX. *Neurology, 54*(8), 740–743.

Finucane, M. L., Slovic, P., Hibbard, J. H., Peters, E., Mertz, C. K., & McGregor, D. G. (2002). Aging and decision-making competence: An analysis of comprehension and consistency skills in older versus younger adults considering health-plan options. *Journal of Behavioral Decision Making, 15,* 141–164.

Fisher, A. G. (2006a). *Assessment of motor and process skills, Vol. 1: Development, standardization, and administration manual* (6th ed.). Fort Collins, CO: Three Star Press.

Fisher, A. G. (2006b). *Assessment of motor and process skills, Vol. 2: User manual* (6th ed.). Fort Collins, CO: Three Star Press.

Fitzpatrick, A. L., Kuller, L. H., Lopez, O. L., Diehr, P., O'Meara, E. S., Longstreth, W. T., Jr., et al. (2009). Midlife and late-life obesity and the risk of dementia: Cardiovascular health study. *Archives of Neurology, 66*(3), 336–342.

Fleming, M. F., Manwell, L. B., Barry, K. L., Adams, W., & Stauffacher, E. A. (1999). Brief physician advice for alcohol problems in older adults: A randomized community-based trial. *Journal of Family Practice, 48*(5), 378–384.

Fletcher, A. E., Price, G. M., Ng, E. S., Stirling, S. L., Bulpitt, C. J., Breeze, E., et al. (2004). Population-based multidimensional assessment of older people in UK general practice: A cluster-randomised factorial trial. *Lancet, 364*(9446), 1667–1677.

Fonkych, K., O'Leary, J. F., Melnick, G. A., & Keeler, E. B. (2008). Medicare HMO impact on utilization at the end of life. *The American Journal of Managed Care, 14*(8), 505–512.

Forette, F., Seux, M. L., Staessen, J. A., Thijs, L., Babarskiene, M. R., Babeanu, S., et al. (2002). The prevention of dementia with antihypertensive treatment: New evidence from the systolic hypertension in Europe (Syst-Eur) study. *Archives of Internal Medicine, 162*(18), 2046–2052.

Fortes, M. (1961). Pietas and ancestor worship. *Journal of the Royal Anthropological Society, 91*, 166–191.

Fortinsky, R. H., Kulldorff, M., Kleppinger, A., & Kenyon-Pesce, L. (2009). Dementia care consultation for family caregivers: Collaborative model linking an Alzheimer's association chapter with primary care physicians. *Aging and Mental Health, 13*(2), 162–170.

Foster, G., Taylor, S. J., Eldridge, S. E., Ramsay, J., Griffiths, C. J. (2007). Self-management education programmes by lay leaders for people with chronic conditions. *Cochrane Database of Systematic Reviews, 4*, CD005108.

Foster, L., Brown, R., Phillips, B., Schore, J., & Carlson, B. L. (2003). Improving the quality of Medicaid personal assistance through consumer direction. *Health Affairs* (web exclusive), w3-162–w3-175.

Franzini, L., Ribble, J. C., & Keddie, A. M. (2001). Understanding the Hispanic paradox. *Ethnicity & Disease, 11*(3), 496–518.

Freeborne, N., Lynn, J., & Desbiens, N. A. (2000). Insights about dying from the SUP-PORT project. The Study to Understand Prognoses and Preferences for Outcomes and Risks of Treatments. *Journal of the American Geriatrics Society, 48*(5 Suppl), S199–S205.

Freedman, V. A. (2000). Implications of asking "ambiguous" difficulty questions: An analysis of the second wave of the asset and health dynamics of the oldest old study. *The Journals of Gerontology. Series B, Psychological Sciences and Social Sciences, 55*, S288–S297.

Freedman, V. A. (2009). Adopting the ICF language for studying late-life disability: A field of dreams? Journal of Gerontology: Medical Sciences 64A, 1172-1174.

Freedman, V. A., & Agree, E. (2008). *Home modifications: Use, cost, and interactions with functioning among near-elderly and older adults.* Report to the Department of Health and Human Services Office of the Assistant Secretary for Planning and Evaluation. Retrieved September 20, 2009, from http://aspe.hhs.gov/daltcp/reports/2008/homemodes.htm

Freedman, V. A., Agree, E., & Cornman, J. (2005). *Development of an assistive technology and home environment assessment instrument for national survey: Final Report. Part 1. Recommended modules and instrument development process.* Report prepared for the Department of Health and Human Service's Office of the Assistant Secretary for Planning and Evaluation.

Freedman, V. A., Agree, E. M., Martin, L. G., & Cornman, J. C. (2006a). Trends in the use of assistive technology and personal care for late-life disability, 1992–2001. *Gerontologist, 46*(1), 124–127.

Freedman, V. A., Crimmins, E., Schoeni, R. F., Spillman, B. C., Aykan, H., Kramarow, E., et al. (2004). Resolving inconsistencies in trends in old-age disability: Report from a technical working group. *Demography, 41,* 417–441.

Freedman, V. A., Grafova, I. B., Schoeni, R. F., & Rogowski, J. (2007a, November 16–20). *Neighborhood associations with chronic disease prevalence and onset in later life.* Paper presented at the annual meeting of the Gerontological Society of America, San Francisco, CA.

Freedman, V. A., Grafova, I. B., Schoeni, R. F., & Rogowski, J. (2008). Neighborhoods and disability in later life. *Social Science & Medicine, 66*(11), 2253–2267.

Freedman, V. A., Hakan, A., & Martin, L. G. (2001). Aggregate changes in severe cognitive impairment among older Americans: 1993 and 1998. *The Journals of Gerontology, Psychological Sciences and Social Sciences, 56B*(2), S100.

Freedman, V. A., Hakan, A., & Martin, L. G. (2002a). Another look at aggregate changes in severe cognitive impairment: Further investigation into the cumulative effects of three survey design issues. *The Journals of Gerontology, Psychological Sciences and Social Sciences, 57B*(2), S126–S131.

Freedman, V. A., Hodgson, N., Lynn, J., Spillman, B., Waidmann, T., Wilkinson, A., et al. (2006b). Promoting declines in the prevalence of late-life disability: Comparisons of three potentially high-impact interventions. *Milbank Memorial Quarterly, 84*(3), 493–520.

Freedman, V. A., & Martin, L. G. (1998). Understanding trends in functional limitations among older Americans. *American Journal of Public Health, 88*(10), 1457–1462.

Freedman, V. A., & Martin, L. G. (1999). The role of education in explaining and forecasting trends in functional limitations among older Americans. *Demography, 36,* 461–473.

Freedman, V. A., Martin, L. G., & Schoeni, R. F. (2002b). Recent trends in disability and functioning among older adults in the United States: A systematic review. *Journal of the American Medical Association, 288*(24), 3137–3146.

Freedman, V. A., Schoeni, R. F., Martin, L. G., & Cornman, J. C. (2007b). Chronic conditions and the decline in late-life disability. *Demography, 44,* 459–477.

Freedman, V. A., & Soldo, B. J. (1994). *Forecasting disability: Workshop summary.* Washington, DC: Committee on National Statistics of the Commission on Behavioral and Social Sciences and Education.

Freiman, M., & Brown, E. (1996). *Research findings no. 6: Special care units in nursing homes—Selected characteristics.* Medical Expenditures Panel Study. Agency for Healthcare Research and Quality, 2001. Retrieved March 15, 2004, from http://www.meps.ahrq.gov/Papers/RF6_99-0017/RF6.htm

Fried, L. P., Bandeen-Roche, K., Chaves, P. H., & Johnson, B. A. (2000). Preclinical mobility disability predicts incident mobility disability in older women. *The Journals of Gerontology. Series A, Biological Sciences and Medical Sciences, 55*(1), M43–M52.

Fried, L. P., Bandeen-Roche, K., Kasper, J. D., & Guralnik, J. M. (1999). Association of comorbidity with disability in older women: The Women's Health and Aging Study. *Journal of Clinical Epidemiology, 52*(1), 27–37.

Fried, L. P., Bandeen-Roche, K., Williamson, J. D., Prasada-Rao, P., Chee, E., Tepper, S., et al. (1996). Functional decline in older adults: Expanding methods of ascertainment. *The Journals of Gerontology. Series A, Biological Sciences and Medical Sciences, 51*(5), M206–M214.

Fried, L. P., Carlson, M. C., Freedman, M., Frick, K. D., Glass, T. A., Hill, J., et al. (2004a). A social model for health promotion for an aging population: Initial evidence on the Experience Corps model. *Journal of Urban Health: Bulletin of the New York Academy of Medicine, 81,* 64–78.

Fried, L. P., Ferrucci, L., Darer, J., Williamson, J. D., & Anderson, G. (2004b). Untangling the concepts of disability, frailty, and comorbidity: Implications for improved targeting and care. *The Journals of Gerontology. Series A, Biological Sciences and Medical Sciences, 59,* 255–263.

Fried, L. P., Tangen, C. T., Walston, J., Newman, A. B., Hirsch, C., Gottdiener, J., et al. (2001). Frailty in older adults: Evidence for a phenotype. *The Journals of Gerontology. Series A, Biological Sciences and Medical Sciences, 56,* M146–M156.

Friedland, R. P., Fritsch, T., Smyth, K. A., Koss, E., Lerner, A. J., Chen, A. H., et al. (2001). Patients with Alzheimer's disease have reduced activities in midlife compared with healthy control-group members. *Proceedings of the National Academy of Sciences of the United States of America, 98,* 3440–3445.

Fries, J. F. (1980). Aging, natural death and the compression of morbidity. *New England Journal of Medicine, 303,* 130–135.

Fries, J. F. (1983). The compression of morbidity. *The Milbank Memorial Fund Quarterly. Health and Society, 61,* 397–419.

Fries, J. F. (2002). Reducing disability in older age. *Journal of the American Medical Association, 288*(24), 3164–3165.

Fries, J. F., & Crapo, L. M. (1981). *Vitality and aging.* San Francisco: W.H. Freeman and Company.

Fry, C. L. (1980). Cultural dimensions of aging. A multidimensional scaling analysis. In C. L. Fry (Ed.), *Aging in culture and society: Comparative viewpoints and strategies* (pp. 42–64). Brooklyn: JF Bergin.

Gallo, J. J., Rabins, P. V., Lyketsos, C. G., Tien, A. Y., Anthony, J. C. (1997). Depression without sadness: Functional outcomes of nondysphoric depression in later life. *Journal of the American Geriatrics Society, 45*(5), 570–578.

GAO. (1998). Alzheimer's disease: Estimates of prevalence in the U.S. Retrieved from http://www.gao.gov/archive/1998/he98016.pdf

Gaugler, J. E., Yu, F., Krichbaum, K., & Wyman, J. F. (2009). Predictors of nursing home admission for persons with dementia. *Medical Care, 47*(2), 191–198.

Gijsen, R., Hoeymans, N., Schellevis, F. G., Ruwaard, D., Satariano, W. A., van den Bos, et al. (2001). Causes and consequences of comorbidity: A review. *Journal of Clinical Epidemiology, 54,* 661–674.

Gill, T. M., Baker, D. I., Gottschalk, M., Peduzzi, P. N., Allore, H., & Byers, A. (2002). A program to prevent functional decline in physically frail, elderly persons who live at home. *New England Journal of Medicine, 347*(14), 1068–1074.

Gill, T. M., & Feinstein, A. R. (1994). A critical appraisal of the quality of quality-of-life measurements. *Journal of the American Medical Association, 272*(8), 619–626.

Gill, T. M., & Kurland, B. (2003). The burden and patterns of disability in activities of daily living among community-living older persons. *The Journals of Gerontology. Series A, Biological Sciences and Medical Sciences, 58*(1), 70–75.

Gill, T. M., Robison, J. T., & Tinetti, M. E. (1998). Difficulty and dependence: Two components of the disability continuum among community-living older persons. *Archives Internal Medicine, 128*, 96–101.

Gillick, M. R. (1994). *Choosing medical care in old age: What kind, how much, when to stop.* Cambridge: Harvard University Press.

Glass, A. P., Roberto, K. A., Brossoie, N., Teaster, P. B., & Butler, D. Q. (2008–2009). *Health Care Financing Review, 30*(2), 53–66.

Gold, M. (2008). *Medicare advantage in 2008.* Prepared for The Henry J. Kaiser Family Foundation. Retrieved August 15, 2008, from http://www.kff.org/medicare/upload/7775.pdf

Goldman, D. P., Shang, B., Bhattacharya, J., Garger, A. M., Hurd, M., Joyce, G. F., et al. (2005). Consequences of health trends and medical innovation for the future elderly. *Health Affairs, 24* (Suppl 2), W5R5–W5R17.

Goodman, S. N. (2002). The mammography dilemma: A crisis for evidence-based medicine? *Annals of Internal Medicine, 137*(5 Part 1), 363–365.

Gotzsche, P. C., & Olsen, O. (2000). Is screening for breast cancer with mammography justifiable? *Lancet, 355*, 129–134.

Grady, D., Yaffe, K., Kristof, M., Lin, F., Richards, C., & Barrett-Connor, E. (2002). Effect of postmenopausal hormone therapy on cognitive function: The Heart and Estrogen/progestin Replacement Study. *American Journal of Medicine, 113*(7), 543–548.

Gravelle, H., Dusheiko, M., Sheaff, R., Sargent, P., Boaden, R., Pickard, S., et al. (2007). Impact of case management (Evercare) on frail elderly patients: Controlled before and after analysis of quantitative outcome data. *British Medical Journal, 334*(7583), 31.

Green, C. R., Mohs, R. C., Schmeidler, J., Aryan, M., & Davis, K. L. (1993). Functional decline in Alzheimer's disease: A longitudinal study. *Journal of the American Geriatrics Society, 41*, 654–661.

Gregg, E. W., Yaffe, K., Cauley, J. A., Rolka, D. B., Blackwell, T. L., Narayan, K. M., et al. (2000). Is diabetes associated with cognitive impairment and cognitive decline among older women? Study of Osteoporotic Fractures Research Group. *Archives of Internal Medicine, 160*(2), 174–180.

Gruenberg, E. M. (1977). The failures of success. *The Milbank Memorial Fund Quarterly. Health and Society, 55*(1), 3–24.

Gruneir, A., Lapane, K. L., Miller, S. C., & Mor, V. (2008). Is dementia special care really special? A new look at an old question. *Journal of the American Geriatrics Society, 56*(2), 199–205.

Guralnik, J. M., & Ferrucci, L. (2009). The challenge of understanding the disablement process in older persons: Commentary responding to Jette, A.M. Toward a common language of disablement. *Journal of Gerontology: Medical Sciences.* (Advance Access published on July 23, 2009; doi: doi:10.1093/gerona/glp094)

Guralnik, J. M., Ferrucci, L., Penninx, B. W., Kasper, J. D., Leveille, S. G., Bandeen-Roche, K., et al. (1999). New and worsening conditions and change in physical and cognitive performance during weekly evaluations over 6 months: The Women's Health and Aging Study. *The Journals of Gerontology Series A, Biological and Medical Sciences, 54*(8), M410–M422.

Guralnik, J. M., Ferrucci, F., Pieper, C. F., Leveille, S. B., Markides, K. S., Ostir, G. V., et al. (2000). Lower extremity function and subsequent disability: Consistency across studies. *The Journals of Gerontology Series A, Biological and Medical Science, 55A,* M221–M231.

Guralnik, J. M., Ferrucci, L., Simonsick, E. M., Salive, M. E., & Wallace, R. B. (1995a). Lower-extremity function in persons over the age of 70 years as a predictor of subsequent disability. *New England Journal of Medicine, 332*(9), 556–561.

Guralnik, J. M., Fried, L. P., Simonsick, E. M., Kasper, J. D., & Lafferty, M. E. (Eds.) (1995b). *The Women's Health and Aging Study.* NIH 95-4009. Bethesda, MD: National Institutes of Health.

Guralnik, J. M., Simonsick, E. M., Ferrucci, L., Glynn, R. J., Berkman, L. F., Blazer, D. G., et al. (1994). A short physical performance battery assessing lower extremity function: Association with self-reported disability and prediction of mortality and nursing home admission. *Journal of Gerontology, 49*(2), M85–M94.

Gurland, B. J., Wilder, D. E., Chen, J., Lantigua, R., Mayeux, R., & Van Nostrand, J. (1995). A flexible system of detection for Alzheimer's disease and related dementias. *Aging (Milano), 7*(3), 165–172.

Hadley, E. (1992). Cause of death among the oldest old. In R. M. Suzman, D. P. Willis, & K. G. Manton (Eds.), *The oldest old* (pp. 183–198). New York: Oxford University Press.

Hanlon, J. T., Schmader, K. E., Ruby, C. M., & Weinberger, M. (2001). Suboptimal prescribing in older inpatients and outpatients. *Journal of the American Geriatrics Society, 49,* 200–209.

Hardy, S. E., & Gill, T. M. (2004). Recovery from disability among community-dwelling older persons. *Journal of the American Medical Association, 291,* 1596–1602.

Hayward, M. D., & Gorman, B. K. (2004). The long arm of childhood: The influence of early-life social conditions on men's mortality. *Demography, 41*(1), 87–107.

Hebert, L. E., Scherr, P. A., Bienias, J. L., Bennett, D. A., & Evans, D. A. (2003). Alzheimer disease in the U.S. population: Prevalence estimates using the 2000 census. *Archives of Neurology, 60*(8), 1119–1122.

Heiss, F., McFadden, D., & Winter, J. (2006). Who failed to enroll in Medicare Part D, and why? Early results. *Health Affairs (Project Hope), 25,* w344–54.

Helmes, E., Csapo, K. G., & Short, J.-A. (1987). Standardization and validation of the Multidimensional observation scale for elderly subjects (MOSES). *Journal of Gerontology, 42,* 395–405.

Helzner, E. P., Luchsinger, J. A., Scarmeas, N., Cosentino, S., Brickman, A. M., & Glymour, M. M., et al. (2009). Contribution of vascular risk factors to the progression in Alzheimer disease. *Archives of Neurology, 66*(3), 343–348.

Helzner, E. P., Scarmeas, N., Cosentino, S., Portet, F., & Stern, Y. (2007). Leisure activity and cognitive decline in incident Alzheimer disease. *Archives of Neurology, 64*(12), 1749–1754.

Helzner, E. P., Scarmeas, N., Cosentino, S., Tang, M. X., Schupf, N., & Stern, Y. (2008). Survival in Alzheimer disease: A multiethnic, population-based study of incident cases. *Neurology, 71*(19), 1489–1495.

Henderson, V. W. (2009). Estrogens, episodic memory, and Alzheimer's disease: A critical update. *Seminars in Reproductive Medicine, 27*(3), 283–293.

Hennessey, C. H., Moriarty, D. G., Scherr, P. A., & Brackbill, R. (1994). Measuring health-related quality of life for public health surveillance. *Public Health Reports, 109*(5), 665–672.

Herndon, L. A., Schmeissner, P. J., Dudaronek, J. M., Brown, P. A., Listner, K. M., Sakano, Y., et al. (2002). Stochastic and genetic factors influence tissue-specific decline in ageing *C. elegans. Nature, 419*, 808–814.

Hetzel, B. S., & Leeder, S. R. (2001). Half a century of healthcare in Australia. *The Medical Journal of Australia, 174*(1), 33–36.

Hetzel, D. M. (2001). Death, disease and diversity in Australia, 1951 to 2000. *The Medical Journal of Australia, 174*(1), 21–24.

Hetzel, L., & Smith, A. (2001). *Census 2000 brief, the 65 years and over population: 2000.* Washington DC: U.S. Census Bureau.

Heuts, P. H., de Bie, R., Drietelaar, M., Aretz, K., Hopman-Rock, M., Bastiaenen, C. H., et al. (2005). Self-management in osteoarthritis of hip or knee: A randomized clinical trial in a primary healthcare setting. *Journal of Rheumatology, 32*, 543–549.

Hirtz, D., Thurman, D. J., Gwinn-Hardy, K., Mohamed, M., Chaudhuri, A. R., & Zalutsky, R. (2007). How common are the "common" neurologic disorders? *Neurology, 68*(5), 326–337.

Hoadley, J. (2008). *Medicare Part D: Simplifying the program and improving the value of information for beneficiaries.* Commonwealth Fund Issue Brief. Available at http://www.commonwealthfund.org.

Hoffman, C., Rice, D., & Sung, H. Y. (1996). Persons with chronic conditions. Their prevalence and costs. *Journal of the American Medical Association, 276*(18), 1473–1479.

Hogan, C., Junney, J., Gabel, J., & Lynn, J. (2001). Medicare beneficiaries' costs of care in the last year of life. *Health Affairs, 20*(4), 188–195.

Hogervorst, E., Yaffe, K., Richards, M., & Huppert, F. (2002). Hormone replacement therapy to maintain cognitive function in women with dementia. *Cochrane Database of Systematic Reviews, 3*, CD003799

Hokenstad, A., Ramirez, M., Haslanger, K., & Finneran, K. (1997). *Medicaid home care services in New York City: Demographics, health conditions, and impairment levels of New York City's Medicaid home care population.* New York, United Hospital Fund.

Hokenstad, A., & Shineman, M. (2009). *An overview of Medicaid long-term care programs in New York.* New York: Medicaid Institute, United Hospital Fund.

Holmes, D., Teresi, J. A., & Ory, M. G. (2000). Overview of the volume. In D. Holmes, J. A. Teresi, & M. G. Ory (Eds.), *Special care units* (pp. 7–18). Paris: Serdi Publishers; New York: Springer Press.

Holtzer, R., Verghese, J., Wang, C., Hall, C. B., & Lipton, R. B. (2008). Within-person across-neuropsychological test variability and incident dementia. *Journal of the American Medical Association 300*(7), 823–830.

Hooyman, N., Gonyea, J., & Montgomery, R. (1985). The impact of in-home services termination on family caregivers. *Gerontologist, 25*(2), 141–145.

Horiuchi, S. (2003). Age patterns of mortality. In P. Demeny and G. McNicoll (Eds.), *The encyclopedia of population.* Farmington Hills, MI: Macmillan Reference.

Hornbrook, M. C., Stevens, V. J., Wingfield, D. J., Hollis, J. F., Greenlick, M. R, & Ory, M. G. (1994). Preventing falls among community-dwelling older persons: Results from a randomized trial. *The Gerontologist, 34*, 16–23.

Hsu, J., Price, M., Huang, J., Brand, R., Fung, V., Hui, R., et al. (2006). Unintended consequences of caps on Medicare drug benefits. *New England Journal of Medicine, 354*(22), 2349–2359.

Hughes, C. P., Berg, L., Danziger, W. L., Cohen, L. A., & Martin, R. L. (1982). A new clinical scale for the staging of dementia. *British Journal of Psychology, 140,* 566–572.

Hughes, S. L., Seymour, R. B., Campbell, R., Pollak, N., Huber, G., & Sharma, L. (2004). Impact of the fit and strong intervention on older adults with osteoarthritis. *Gerontologist, 44*(2), 217–228.

Human Mortality Database. University of California, Berkeley (USA), and Max Planck Institute for Demographic Research (Germany). Available at www.mortality.org and www.humanmortality.de

Humphrey, L. L., Chan, B. K. S., Detlefsen, S., & Helfand, M. (2002a). Screening for breast cancer. *Systematic Evidence Review No. 15* (Prepared by the Oregon Health & Science University. Practice Center under Contract No. 290-97-0018.) Rockville, MD: Agency for Healthcare Research and Quality.

Humphrey, L. L., Helfand, M., & Chan, B. K. S. (2002b). Breast cancer screening: A summary of the evidence for the U.S. Preventive Services Task Force. *Annals of Internal Medicine, 137,* 347–360.

Hurley, A. C., Volicer, B. J., Hanrahan, P. A., Houde, S., & Volicer, L. (1992). Assessment of discomfort in advanced Alzheimer patients. *Research in Nursing and Health, 15,* 369–377.

Iezzoni, L. I., & Freedman, V. A. (2008). Turning the disability tide: The importance of definitions. *Journal of the American Medical Association, 299*(3), 332–334.

Inouye, S. K., Bogardus, S. T., Jr., Charpentier, P. A., Leo-Summers, L., Acampora, D., Holford T. R., et al. (1999). A multicomponent intervention to prevent delirium in hospitalized older patients. *New England Journal of Medicine, 340*(9), 669–676.

Institute of Medicine. (1998). *Approaching death: Improving care at the end of life.* M. J. Field & C. K. Cassel (Eds.). Washington, DC: National Academy Press.

Institute of Medicine. (2002). *Care without coverage: Too little, too late.* Washington, DC: National Academy Press.

Institute of Medicine. (2007). *The future of disability in America.* Washington, DC: National Academies Press.

Institute of Medicine. (2008). *Retooling for an aging America: Building the health care workforce.* Washington, DC: National Academies Press.

Jackson, R., & Howe, N. (2007). *The graying of the great powers.* Washington, DC: Center for Strategic and International Studies.

Jackson, V. (2002). Screening mammography: Controversies and headlines. *Radiology, 225,* 323–326.

Jaeschke, R., Singer, J., & Guyatt, G. H. (1989). Measurement of health status. Ascertaining the minimal clinically important difference. *Controlled Clinical Trials, 10*(4), 407–415.

Janevic, M. R., Janz, N. K., Dodge, J. A., Wang, Y., Lin, X., & Clark, N. M. (2004). Longitudinal effects of social support on the health and functioning of older women with heart disease. *International Journal of Aging & Human Development, 59*(2), 153–175.

Jarvik, G. P., Wijsman, E. M., Kukull, W. A., Schellenberg, G. D., Yu, C., & Larson, E. B. (1995). Interaction of apolipoprotein E genotype, total cholesterol level, and sex in prediction of Alzheimer disease in a case-control study. *Neurology, 45,* 1092–1096.

Jette, A. M. (2009). Toward a common language of disablement. Journal of Gerontology: Medical Sciences, 64A, 1165-1168.

Jette, A. M., Assmann, S. F., Rooks, D., Harris, B. A., & Crawford, S. (1998). Inter-relationships among disablement concepts. *The Journals of Gerontology. Series A, Biological Sciences and Medical Sciences, 53*(5), M395–M404.

Jette, A.M., Haley, S. M., & Kooyoomjian, J. T. (2003). Are the ICF activity and participation dimensions distinct? *Journal of Rehabilitation Medicine, 35*(3), 145–149.

Jette, A. M., Lachman, M., Giorgetti, M. M., Assmann, S. F., Harris, B. A., Levenson, C., et al. (1999). Exercise—it's never too late: The strong-for-life program. *American Journal of Public Health, 89*(1), 66–72.

Jette, A. M., Tao, W., & Haley, S. M. (2007). Blending activity and participation sub-domains of the ICF. *Disability and Rehabilitation, 29*(22), 1742–1750.

Johnson, R. W., Toohey, D., & Wiener, J. W. (2007). *Meeting the long-term care needs of the baby boomers: How changing families will affect paid helpers and institutions.* Washington, DC: Urban Institute. Retrieved September 29, 2009, from http://www.urban.org/UploadedPDF/311451_Meeting_Care.pdf

Jorm, A. F., Christensen, H., Korten, A. E., Jacomb, P. A., & Henderson, A. S. (2000). Informant ratings of cognitive decline in old age: Validation against change on cognitive tests over 7 to 8 years. *Psychological Medicine, 30*, 981–985.

Kaiser Family Foundation. (2006a). *Prescription drug coverage among Medicare beneficiaries.* Retrieved May 15, 2009, from http://www.kff.org/medicare/upload/7453.pdf

Kaiser Family Foundation. (2006b). *Dual eligibles.* Retrieved May 15, 2009, from http://www.kff.org/medicaid/upload/Dual-Eligibles-Medicaid-s-Role-for-Low-Income-Medicare-Beneficiaries-Feb-2006.pdf

Kaiser Family Foundation. (2008). *Employer health benefits 2008 summary of findings—Report.* Retrieved May 15, 2009, from http://ehbs.kff.org/images/abstract/7791.pdf.

Kane, R. A. (1995). Expanding the home care concept: blurring distinctions among home care, institutional care, and other long-term-care services. *The Milbank Quarterly, 73*(2), 161–186.

Kane, R. L., & Kane, R. A. (2000). Assessment in long-term care. *Annual Review of Public Health, 1*, 659–686.

Kaplan, E., Goodglass, H., & Weintraub, S. (1983). *Boston naming test.* Philadelphia: Lea & Febiger.

Kaplan, R. M., & Anderson, J. P. (1996). The general health policy model: An integrated approach. In B. Spilker (Ed.), *Quality of life and pharmacoeconomics in clinical trials* (pp. 203–225). Philadelphia: Lippincott-Raven.

Karagiozis, H., Gray, S., Sacco, J., Shapiro, M., & Kawas, C. (1998). The Direct Assessment of Functional Abilities (DAFA): A comparison to an indirect measure of instrumental activities of daily living. *Gerontologist, 38*(1), 113–121.

Karlawish, J., Kim, S. Y., Knopman, D., van Dyck, C. H., James, B. D., & Marson, D. (2008). The views of Alzheimer disease patients and their study partners on proxy consent for clinical trial enrollment. *The American Journal of Geriatric Psychiatry. 16*(3), 240–247.

Katz, S., Branch, L. G., Branson, M. H., Papsidero, J. A., Beck, J. C., & Greer, D. S. (1983). Active life expectancy. *New England Journal of Medicine, 309*, 1218–1224.

Katz, S., Ford, A. B., Moscowitz, A. W., et al. (1963). Studies of illness in the aged: The index of ADL: A standardized measure of biological and psychosocial function. *Journal of the American Medical Association, 185*, 914–919.

Kaufman, S. (2005). *And a time to die: How American hospitals shape the end of life.* New York: Scribner.

Kelly-Hayes, M., Jette, A. M., Wolf, P. A., D'Agostino, R. B., & Odell, P. M. (1992). Functional limitations and disability among elders in the Framingham Study. *American Journal of Public Health, 82*(6), 841–845.

Kemper, P., Komisar, H. L., & Alecxih, L. (2005–2006). Long-term care over an uncertain future: What can current retirees expect? *Inquiry, 42*(4), 335–350.

Kemper, P., & Murtaugh, C. M. (1991). Lifetime use of nursing home care. *New England Journal of Medicine, 324*(9), 595–600.

Keysor, J. (2006). How does the environment influence disability? Examining the evidence. In M. Field, A. Jette, & L. Martin (Eds.), *Workshop on disability in America: A new look—Summary and background papers* (pp. 88–100). Washington, DC: National Academies Press.

Keysor, J., Jette, A., & Haley, S. M. (2005). Development of the home and community environment (HACE) instrument. *Journal of Rehabilitation Medicine, 37*(1), 37–44.

Kim, H., & Lee, J. (2006). The impact of comorbidity on wealth changes in later life. *The Journals of Gerontology. Series B, Psychological Sciences and Social Sciences, 61*(6), S307–S314.

Kim, S. Y., Kim, H. M., Langa, K. M., Karlawish, J. H., Knopman, D. S., & Appelbaum, P. S. (2009). Surrogate consent for dementia research: A national survey of older Americans. *Neurology, 72*(2), 149–155.

King, A. C., Baumann, K., O'Sullivan, P., Wilcox, S., & Castro, C. (2002). Effects of moderate-intensity exercise on physiological, behavioral, and emotional responses to family caregiving: A randomized controlled trial. *The Journals of Gerontology. Series A, Biological Sciences and Medical Sciences, 57*(1), M26–M36.

Kinsella, K., & He, W. (2009). *An aging world: 2008.* Washington, DC: Government Printing Office.

Kinsella, K., & Velkoff, V. A. (2001). *An aging World: 2001.* Washington, DC: Government Printing Office.

Kitchener, M., Carrillo, H., & Harrington, C. (2003). Medicaid community-based programs: A longitudinal analysis of state variation in expenditures and utilization. *Inquiry, 40*(4), 375–389.

Kleinmeier, R. W. (1962). Intellectual change in the scenium. In *Proceedings of the Social Statistics Section, American Statistical Association* (pp. 290–295). Washington, DC: American Statistical Association.

Klinenberg, E. (2004). *Heat wave. A social autopsy of disaster in Chicago.* Chicago: University of Chicago Press.

Kluger, A., Gianutos, J. G., Golumb, J., Ferris, S. H., George, A. E., Franssen, E., et al. (1997). Patterns of motor impairment in normal aging, mild cognitive decline, and early Alzheimer's disease. *The Journals of Gerontology. Series B, Psychological Sciences and Social Sciences, 52*, P28–P39.

Klunk, W. E., Engler, H., Nordberg, A., Wang, Y., Blomqvist, G., Holt, D. P., et al. (2004). Imaging brain amyloid in Alzheimer's disease with Pittsburgh Compound-B. *Annals of Neurology, 55*(3), 306–319.

Knopman, D. S., Berg, J. D., Thomas, R., Grundman, M., Thal, L. J., & Sano, M. (1999). Nursing home placement is related to dementia progression: Experience from a clinical trial. Alzheimer's Disease Cooperative Trial. *Neurology, 52*, 714–718.

Knopman, D. S., Rocca, W. A., Cha, R. H., Edland, S. D., & Kokmen, E. (2003). Survival study of vascular dementia in Rochester, Minnesota. *Archives of Neurology, 60*(1), 85–90.

Komisar, H. L., & Thompson, L. S. (2007). *National spending for long-term care. Fact Sheet.* Washington, DC: Georgetown University Long-Term Care Financing Project.

Kovar, M. G. (1986). *Aging in the eighties, preliminary data for the Supplement on Aging to the National Health Interview Survey, US, Jan–Jun, 1984.* Advance Data from Vital and Health Statistics, No. 115 DHHS 86-1250. Hyattsville, MD: National Center for Health Statistics/Public Health Service. Retrieved March 15, 2004, from http://www.cdc.gov/nchs/data/ad/ad115acc.pdf

Kovar, M. G., & Lawton, M. P. (1994). Functional disability: Activities and instrumental activities of daily living. *Annual Review of Geriatrics and Gerontology* (Vol. 14.). New York: Springer Press.

Krach, C. A., & Velkoff, V. A. (1999). *Centenarians in the United States* (U.S. Bureau of the Census, Current Population Reports, Series P23-199RV). Washington, DC: U.S. Government Printing Office.

Kramer, M. (1980). The rising pandemic of mental disorders and associated chronic diseases and disabilities. *Acta Psychiatrica Scandinavia, Symposium Supplement, 285,* 62-85.

Kuh, D., Bassey, J., Hardy, R., Sayer, A. A., Wadsworth, M., & Cooper, C. (2002). Birth weight, childhood size, and muscle strength in adult life: Evidence from a birth cohort study. *American Journal of Epidemiology, 156,* 627–633.

Kung, H.-C., Hoyert, D. L., Xu, J., & Murray, S. L. (2008, April 24). Deaths: Final data for 2005. *National Vital Statistics Reports, 56*(10). Retrieved September 15, 2009, from http://www.cdc.gov/nchs/data/nvsr/nvsr56/nvsr56_10.pdf

Kutner, N. G., & Bliwise, D. L. (2000). Observed agitation and the phenomenon of "sundowning" among SCU residents. In D. Holmes, J. A. Teresi, & M. G. Ory (Eds.), *Special care units* (pp. 151–162). Paris: Serdi Publishers; New York: Springer Press.

Lachs, M. S., & Pillemer, K. (2004). Elder abuse. *Lancet, 364*(9441), 1263–1272.

Lachs, M. S., Williams, C. S, O'Brien, S., & Pillemer, K. A. (2002). Adult protective service use and nursing home placement. *The Gerontologist, 42*(6), 734–739.

Lachs, M. S., Williams, C. S., O'Brien, S., Pillemer, K. A., & Charlson, M. E. (1998). The mortality of elder mistreatment. *Journal of the American Medical Association, 280*(5), 428–432.

LaCroix, A. Z., Leveille, S. G., Hecht, J. A., Grothaus, L. C., & Wagner, E. H. (1996). Does walking decrease the risk of cardiovascular disease hospitalizations and death in older adults? *Journal of the American Geriatrics Society, 44*(2), 113–120.

Lakdawalla, D. N., Bhattacharya, J., & Goldman, D. P. (2004). Are the young becoming more disabled? *Health Affairs (Project Hope), 23*(1), 168–176.

Lamb, S. (2009). Elder residences and outsourced sons: Remaking aging in cosmopolitan India. In J. Sokolovsky (Ed.), *The cultural context of aging* (pp. 418–440). Westport, CT: Praeger Publishers.

Landefeld, C. S., Palmer, R. M., Kresevic, D. M., Fortinsky, R. H., & Kowal, J. (1995). A randomized trial of care in a hospital medical unit especially designed to improve functional outcomes of acutely ill older patients. *New England Journal of Medicine, 332,* 1338–1344.

Lang, J. E., Benson, W. F., & Anderson, L. A. (2005). Aging and public health: Partnerships that can affect cardiovascular health programs. *American Journal of Preventive Medicine, 29*(5 Suppl 1), 158–163.

Langa, K. M., Larson, E. B., Karlawish, J. H., Cutler, D. M., Kabeto, M. U., Kim, S. Y., et al. (2008). Trends in the prevalence and mortality of cognitive impairment in the United States: Is there evidence of a compression of cognitive morbidity? *Alzheimers & Dementia, 4*(2), 134–144.

Langa, K. M., Plassman, B. L., Wallace, R. B., Herzog, A. R., Heeringa, S. G., Ofstedal, M. B., et al. (2005). The Aging, Demographics, and Memory Study: Study design and methods. *Neuroepidemiology, 25*(4), 181–191.

Larson, E. B., Shadlen, M. F., Wang, L., McCormick, W. C., Bowen, J. D., Teri, L., et al. (2004). Survival after initial diagnosis of Alzheimer disease. *Annals of Internal Medicine, 140*(7), 501–509.

Larson, R., Zuzanek, J., & Mannell, R. (1985). Being alone versus being with people: Disengagement in the daily experience of older adults. *Journal of Gerontology, 40*(3), 375–381.

Launer, L. J., Anderson, K., Dewey, M. E., Lentenneur, L., Ott, A., Amaducci, L. A., Brayne, C., et al. (1999). Rates and risk factors for dementia and Alzheimer's disease: Results from EURODEM pooled analyses. *Neurology, 52,* 78–84.

Lawton, M. P. (1991). A multidimensional view of quality of life in frail elders. In J. E. Birren (Ed.), *The concept and measurement of quality of life in the frail elderly.* San Diego: Academic Press.

Lawton, M. P., & Brody, E. M. (1969). Assessment of older people: Self-maintaining and instrumental activities of daily living. *Gerontologist, 9*(3), 179–186.

Lawton, M. P., Brody, E., & Pruchno, R. (1991). *Respite for caregivers of Alzheimer patients: Research and practice.* New York: Springer.

Lawton, M. P., Moss, M., & Glicksman, A. (1993). The quality of the last year of life of older persons. *Milbank Quarterly, 68,* 1–28.

Lawton, M. P., Parmelee, P. A., Katz, I. R., & Nesselroade, J. (1996). Affective states in normal and depressed older people. *The Journals of Gerontology. Series B, Psychological Sciences and Social Sciences, 51*(6), P309–P316.

Lawton, M. P., Van Haitsma, K., Perkinson, M., & Ruckdeschel, K. (2001). Observed affect and quality of life in dementia. In S. M. Albert & R. G. Logsdon (Eds.), *Assessing quality of life in Alzheimer's disease* (pp. 3–16). New York: Springer Publishing.

Lazirides, E. N., Rudberg, M. A., Furner, S. E., & Cassel, C. K. (1994). Do activities of daily living have a hierarchical structure? An analysis using the Longitudinal Study of Aging. *Journal of Gerontology, 49*(2), M47–M51.

Leber, P. (1991). *Global assessment measures. Letter to companies involved in antidementia research.* Washington, DC: Food and Drug Administration.

LeBlanc, A. J., Tonner, M. C., & Harrington, C. (2001). State Medicaid programs offering personal care services. *Health Care Financing Review, 22*(4), 155–173.

Lee, S. J., Lindquist, K., Segal, M. R., & Covinsky, K. E. (2006). Development and validation of a prognostic index for 4-year mortality in older adults. *Journal of the American Medical Association, 295*(7), 801–808.

Leibson, C., Owens, T., O'Brien, P., Waring, S., Tangalos, E., Hanson V., et al. (1999). Use of physician and acute care services by persons with and without Alzheimer's

disease: A population-based comparison. *Journal of the American Geriatrics Society,*
47, 864–869.

Lemieux, J., Chovan, T., & Heath, K. (2008). Medigap coverage and Medicare spending:
A second look. *Health Affairs (Millwood), 27*(2), 469–477.

Leplege, A., & Hunt, S. (1997). The problem of quality of life in medicine. *Journal of the*
American Medical Association, 278(1), 47–50.

Leveille, S. G., Phelan, E. A., Davis, C., LoGerfo, M., & LoGerfo, J. P. (2004). Preventing disability through community-based health coaching. *Journal of the American*
Geriatrics Society, 52(2), 328–329.

Leveille, S. G., Wagner, E. H., Davis, C., Grothaus, L., Wallace, J., LoGerfo, M., et al.
(1998). Preventing disability and managing chronic illness in frail older adults: A randomized trial of a community-based partnership with primary care. *Journal of the*
American Geriatrics Society, 46(10), 1191–1198.

Levine, C., Albert, S. M., Hokenstad, A., Halper, D., Hart, A. Y., & Gould, D. A. (2006).
"This case is closed": The transition in family caregiving when home health care services end. *Milbank Quarterly, 84*(2), 305–331.

Levy, G., Tang, M. X., Louis, E. D., Cote, L. J., Alfaro, B., Mejia, H., et al. (2002). The association of incident dementia with mortality in PD. *Neurology, 59*(11), 1708–1713.

Levy, R. (1994). Aging-associated cognitive decline. *International Psychogeriatrics, 6,*
63–68.

Levy-Storms, L., Schnelle, J. F., & Simmons, S. F. (2007). What do family members notice
following an intervention to improve mobility and incontinence care for nursing home
residents? An analysis of open-ended comments. *The Gerontologist, 47*(1), 14–20.

Liao, Y., McGee, D. L., Cao, G., & Cooper, R. S. (2000). Quality of life in the last year
of life of older adults: 1986 vs. 1993. *Journal of the American Medical Association,*
283(4), 512–518.

Lieberman, A. (2002). *Dementia in Parkinson's disease.* National Parkinson's Disease
Foundation. Retrieved April 15, 2004, from http://www.parkinson.org/pddement.htm

Lin, E. H., Katon, W., Von Korff, M., Tang, L., Williams, J. W., Jr., Kroenke, K., et al.
(2003). Effect of improving depression care on pain and functional outcomes among
older adults with arthritis: A randomized controlled trial. *Journal of the American*
Medical Association, 290(18), 2428–2429.

Lindeman, D. A., Arnsberger, P., & Owens, D. (2000). Staffing and specialized dementia
care units: Impact of resident outcomes. In D. Holmes, J. A. Teresi, & M. G. Ory
(Eds.), *Special care units* (pp. 217–228). Paris: Serdi Publishers; New York: Springer
Press.

Loewenstein, D. A., Ardila, A., Rosselli, M., Hayden, S., Duara, R., Berkowitz, N.,
et al. (1992). Comparative analysis of functional status among Spanish- and English-
speaking patients with dementia. *Journal of Gerontology, 47,* P389–P394.

Logsdon, R. G., Gibbons, L. E., McCurry, S. M., & Teri, L. (2001). Quality of life in
Alzheimer's disease: Patient and caregiver reports. In S. M. Albert & R. G. Logs-
don (Eds.), *Assessing quality of life in Alzheimer's disease* (pp. 17–30). New York:
Springer Publishing.

Loong, T.-W. (2003). Understanding sensitivity and specificity with the right side of the
brain. *British Medical Journal, 327,* 716–719.

Lopez, O. L., Kuller, L. H., Fitzpatrick, A., Ives, D., Becker, J. T., & Beauchamp, N.
(2003). Evaluation of dementia in the cardiovascular health cognition study. *Neuro-*
epidemiology, 22(1), 1–12.

Lorig, K., Holman, H., Sobel, D., Laurent, D., Gonzalez, V., & Minor, M. (2000). *Living a healthy life with chronic conditions* (2nd ed.). Boulder, CO: Bull.

Lorig, K. R., Ritter, P. L., Dost, A., Plant, K., Laurent, D. D., & McNeil, I. (2008). The Expert Patients Programme online, a 1-year study of an Internet-based self-management programme for people with long-term conditions. *Chronic Illness, 4*(4), 247–256.

Lorig, K., Ritter, P., Stewart, A. L., Sobel, D., Brown, B. W., Bandura, A., et al. (2001). Chronic disease self-management program: Two-year health status and health care utilization outcomes. *Medical Care, 39*(11), 1217–1223.

Lorig, K. R., Sobel, D. S., Stewart, A. L., Brown, B. W., Jr., Bandura, A., Ritter, P., et al. (1999). Evidence suggesting that a chronic disease self-management program can improve health status while reducing hospitalization: A randomized trial. *Medical Care, 37*(1), 5–14.

Lubitz, J., Cai, L., Kramarow, E., & Lentzner, H. (2003). Health, life expectancy, and health care spending among the elderly. *New England Journal of Medicine, 349*(11), 1048–1055.

Lubitz, J. D., & Riley, G. R. (1993). Trends in Medicare payments in the last year of life. *New England Journal of Medicine, 328*(15), 1092–1096.

Luchsinger, J. A., & Gustafson, D. R. (2009). Adiposity, type 2 diabetes, and Alzheimer's disease. *Journal of Alzheimers Disease, 16*(4), 693–704.

Luchsinger, J. A., Tang, M. X., Stern, Y., Shea, S., & Mayeux, R. (2001). Diabetes mellitus and risk of Alzheimer's disease and dementia with stroke in a multiethnic cohort. *American Journal of Epidemiology, 154*(7), 635–641.

Luepker, R. V., Rastam, L., Hannan, P. J., Murray, D. M., Gray, C., Baker, W. L., et al. (1996). Community education for cardiovascular disease prevention. Morbidity and mortality results from the Minnesota Heart Health Program. *American Journal of Epidemiology, 144*(4), 351–362.

Lunney, J. R., Lynn, J., & Hogan, C. (2002). Profiles of older Medicare decedents. *Journal of the American Geriatrics Society, 50,* 1108–1112.

Lydick, E., & Epstein, R. S. (1993). Interpretation of quality of life changes. *Quality of Life Research, 2,* 221–226.

Lynn, J. (2001). Serving patients who may die soon and their families: The role of hospice and other services. *Journal of the American Medical Association, 285,* 925–932.

Lynn, J., & Adamson, D. M. (2003). *Living well at the end of life. Adapting health care to serious. chronic illness in old age.* Santa Monica, CA: RAND Health.

Lynn, J., Teno, J. M., Phillips, R. S., Wu, A. W., Desbiens, N., Harrold, J., et al. (1997). Perceptions by family members of the dying experience of older and seriously ill patients. SUPPORT Investigators. Study to understand prognoses and preferences for outcomes and risks of treatments. *Annals of Internal Medicine, 126*(2), 97–106.

Mack, K., & Thompson, L. (2001). *Data profiles, family caregivers of older persons: Adult children.* Washington, DC: Georgetown University, The Center on an Aging Society.

Maestre, G., Ottman, R., Stern, Y., Gurland, B., Chun, M., Tang, M. X., Shelanski, M., et al. (1995). Apolipoprotein E and Alzheimer's disease: Ethnic variation in genotypic risks. *Annals of Neurology, 37*(2), 254–259.

Magaziner, J., Hawkes, W., Hebel, J. R., Zimmerman, S. I., Fox, K. M., Dolan, M., et al. (2000). Recovery from hip fracture in eight areas of function. *Journals of Gerontology: Biological and Medical Sciences, 55,* M498–507.

Magaziner, J., Simonsick, E. M., Kashner, T. M., & Hebel, J. R. (1988). Patient-proxy response comparability on measures of patient health and functional status. *Journal of Clinical Epidemiology, 41*(11), 1065–1074.

Manly, J. J., Bell-McGinty, S., Tang, M. X., Schupf, N., Stern, Y., & Mayeux, R. (2005). Implementing diagnostic criteria and estimating frequency of mild cognitive impairment in an urban community. *Archives of Neurology, 62*(11), 1739–1746.

Manly, J. J., Jacobs, D. M., Touradji, D., Small, S. A., & Stern, Y. (2002). Reading level attenuates differences in neuropsychological performance between African-American and White elders. *Journal of the International Neuropsychological Society, 8*(3), 341–348.

Manly, J. J., Tang, M. X., Schupf, N., Stern, Y., Vonsattel, J. P., & Mayeux, R. (2008). Frequency and course of mild cognitive impairment in a multiethnic community. *Annals of Neurology, 63*(4), 494–506.

Manton, K. G. (1989). Epidemiological, demographic, and social correlates of disability among the elderly. *Milbank Quarterly, 67*(Suppl 2 Pt 1), 13–58.

Manton, K. G. (1992). Mortality and life expectancy changes among the oldest old. In R. M. Suzman, D. P. Willis, & K. G. Manton (Eds.), *The oldest old* (pp. 157–182). New York: Oxford University Press.

Manton, K. G., Corder, L. S., & Stallard, E. (1993). Estimates of change in chronic disability and institutional incidence and prevalence rates in the U.S. elderly population from the 1982, 1984, and 1989 National Long Term Care Survey. *Journals of Gerontology 1993, 48*(4), S153–S166.

Manton, K. G., Corder, L., & Stallard, E. (1997). Chronic disability trends in elderly United States populations: 1982–1994. *Proceedings of the National Academy of Sciences of the United States of America, 94*(6), 2593–2598.

Manton, K. G., & Gu, X. (2001). Changes in the prevalence of chronic disability in the United States Black and nonblack population above age 65 from 1982 to 1999. *Proceedings of the National Academy of Sciences of the United States of America, 98*(11), 6354–6359.

Manton, K. G., Gu, X., & Lamb, V. L. (2006). Change in chronic disability from 1982 to 2004/2005 as measured by long-term changes in function and health in the U.S. elderly population. *Proceedings of the National Academy of Sciences of the United States of America, 103*(48), 18374–18379.

Manton, K. G., Stallard, E., & Corder, L. (1995). Changes in morbidity and chronic disability in the U.S. elderly population: Evidence from the 1982, 1984, and 1989 National Long Term Care Surveys. *The Journals of Gerontology. Series B, Psychological Sciences and Social Sciences, 50*(4), S194–S204.

Manton, K. G., Suzman, R., & Willis, D. (Eds.) (1992). *The oldest old.* New York: Oxford University Press.

Manton, K. G., & Vaupel, J. W. (1995). Survival after the age of 80 in the United States, Sweden, France, England, and Japan. *New England Journal of Medicine, 333*, 1232–1235.

Marengoni, A., Rizzuto, D., Wang, H. X., Winblad, B., & Fratiglioni, L. (2009). Patterns of chronic multimorbidity in the elderly population. *Journal of the American Geriatrics Society, 57*(2), 225–230.

Markides, K. S., & Eschbach, K. (2005). Aging, migration, and mortality: Current status of research on the Hispanic paradox. *The Journals of Gerontology. Series B, Psychological Sciences and Social Sciences, 60*(Spec No 2), 68-75.

Markides, K. S., Rudkin, L., Angel, R. J., & Espino, D. V. (1997). Health status of Hispanic elderly in the United States. In L. G. Martin & B. Soldo (Eds.), *Racial and ethnic differences in the health of older Americans* (pp. 285–300). Washington, DC: National Academy Press.

Martin, L. G., Freedman, V. A., Schoeni, R. F., & Andreski, P. M. (2009). Health and functioning among baby boomers approaching 60. *The Journals of Gerontology. Series B, Psychological Sciences and Social Sciences, 64*(3), 369–377.

Mattis, S. (1976). Mental status examination for organic mental syndrome in the elderly patient. In L. Bellek & T. B. Karasu (Eds.), *Geriatric psychiatry.* New York: Grune & Stratton.

Mausner, J. S., & Kramer, S. (1985). *Epidemiology: An introductory text.* Philadelphia: W.B. Saunders.

Mayeux, R., Small, S. A., Tang, M., Tycko, B., & Stern, Y. (2001). Memory performance in healthy elderly without Alzheimer's disease: Effects of time and apolipoprotein-E. *Neurobiology of Aging, 22*(4), 683–689.

McCann, J. J., Bienas, J. L., & Evans, D. A. (2000). Change in performance tests of activities of daily living among residents of dementia special care and traditional nursing home units. In D. Holmes, J. A. Teresi, & M. G. Ory (Eds.), *Special care units* (pp. 141–150). Paris: Serdi Publishers; New York: Springer Press.

McClure, R., Turner, C., Peel, N., Spinks, A., Eakin, E., & Hughes, K. (2005). Population-based interventions for the prevention of fall-related injuries in older people. *Cochrane Database of Systematic Reviews,* Issue 2. Art. No.: CD004441.

McCluskey, A. (2000). Paid attendant carers hold important and unexpected roles which contribute to the lives of people with brain injury. *Brain Injury, 14*, 943–957.

McCullough, D. (2008). *My mother, your mother: Embracing "slow medicine," the compassionate approach to caring for your aging loved ones.* New York: HarperCollins.

McKhann, G., Drachman, D., Folstein, M., Katzman, R., Price, D., & Stadlan, E. M. (1984). Clinical diagnosis of Alzheimer's disease: Report of the NINCDS-ADRDA Work Group under the auspices of Department of Health and Human Services Task Force on Alzheimer's Disease. *Neurology, 34*(7), 939–944.

Medicare Payment Advisory Commission (MedPac). (2004). Hospice in Medicare: Recent trends and review of the issues. Washington, D.C. In *Report to the Congress: New approaches in Medicare* (Chap. 6). Available at http://www.medpac.gov/publications%5Ccongressional_reports%5CJune04_ch6.pdf

Medicare Payment Advisory Commission (MedPac). (2009). *Health care spending and the Medicare Program.* Washington, D.C. Retrieved from http://www.medpac.gov/documents/Jun09DataBookEntireReport.pdf

Meier, D. (1999). Impact of palliative interventions and mortality rate in hospitalized patients with advanced dementia. In A. van der Heiude (Ed.), Clinical and epidemiological aspects of end of life decision-making. *Akad. Van Wetensch Verhandl. Natuur, Reeks 2, 102,* 217–227.

Miller, S.C., Gozalo, P., & Mor, V. (2000). Outcomes and utilization for hospice and non-hospice nursing facility decedents. Washington, DC: U.S. Department of Health and Human Services (HHS), Office of Disability, Aging and Long-Term Care Policy. Retrieved September 25, 2009, from http://aspe.hhs.gov/daltcp/Reports/oututil.htm

Miller, T. (2001). Increasing longevity and Medicare expenditures. *Demography, 38,* 215–226.

Miniño, A. M., Heron, M., Smith, B. L. & Kochanek, K. D. (2007). *Deaths: Final data for 2004.* National Center for Health Statistics. Retrieved September 15, 2009, from http://www.cdc.gov/nchs/data/hestat/finaldeaths04/finaldeaths04.htm

Mittelman, M. S., Ferris, S. H., Shulman, E., Steinberg, G., & Levin, B. (1996). A family intervention to delay nursing home placement of patients with Alzheimer's disease. *Journal of the American Medical Association, 276*(21), 1725–1731.

Mohs, R. C., Doody, R. S., Morris, J. C., Leni, J. R., Rogers, S. L., Perdomo, C. A., et al. (2001). A 1-year, placebo controlled preservation of functional survival study of donepezil in AD patients. *Neurology, 57,* 481–488.

Moon, M. (2006). Organization and financing of health care. In *Handbook of aging and the social sciences* (6th ed., pp. 381–395). Burlington, MA: Academic Press.

Mor, V., Zinn, J., Angelelli, J., Teno, J. M., & Miller, S. C. (2004). Driven to tiers: Socioeconomic and racial disparities in the quality of nursing home care. *Millbank Quarterly, 82*(2), 227–256.

Morris, J. C., Storandt, M., Miller, J. P., McKeel, D. W., Price, J. L., Rubin, E. H., et al. (2001). Mild cognitive impairment represents early-stage Alzheimer's disease. *Archives of Neurology, 58,* 397–405.

Morris, J. N., & Emerson-Lombardo, N. (1994). A national perspective on SCU service richness: Findings from the AARP survey. *Alzheimer Disease and Associated Disorders, 8*(suppl), S87–S96.

Morrison, R. S., & Siu, A. L. (2000). Survival in end-stage dementia following acute illness. *Journal of the American Medical Association, 284*(1), 47–52.

Morrison, R. S., Chichin, E., Carter, J., Burack, O., Lantz, M., & Meier, D. E. (2005). The effect of a social work intervention to enhance advance care planning documentation in the nursing home. *Journal of the American Geriatrics Society, 53,* 290–294.

Moss, M., & Lawton, M. P. (1982). Time budgets of older people: A window on four lifestyles. *Journal of Gerontology, 37,* 115–123.

Mossey, J., & Moss, M. (2002). *Subthreshold depression in elders living at home: A public health problem.* Washington, DC: American Public Health Association.

Muharin, R. K., DeBettignies, B. H., & Pirozzolo, F. J. (1991). Structured assessment of independent living skills: Preliminary analysis of functional abilities in dementia. *The Journals of Gerontology. Series B, Psychological Sciences and Social Sciences, 46,* P58–P66.

Mulsant, B. H., Alexopoulos, G. S., Reynolds, C. F., 3rd, Katz, I. R., Abrams, R., Oslin, D., et al. (2001). Pharmacological treatment of depression in older primary care patients: The PROSPECT algorithm. *International Journal of Geriatric Psychiatry, 16*(6), 585–592.

Murray, C. J., & Lopez, A. D. (1996). Evidence-based health policy—lessons from the Global Burden of Disease Study. *Science, 274*(5288), 740–743.

Myers, R. H., Schaefer, E. J., Wilson, P. W. F., et al. (1996). Apolipoprotein E allele 4 is associated with dementia in a population based study: The Framingham Study. *Neurology, 46,* 673–677.

National Caregiver Alliance and AARP. (2004). *Caregiving in the U.S.* Retrieved September 29, 2009, from http://www.caregiving.org/data/04finalreport.pdf

National Caregiver Alliance and MetLife Mature Market Institute. (in press). *Why should we be concerned about our working caregivers?*

National Center for Health Statistics. (2002). *National Health Interview Survey, 2000. Early release of selected estimates based on data from the January–June, NHIS.*

Retrieved June 15, 2004, from http://www.cdc.gov/nchs/about/major/nhis/released 200212.htm

National Center for Health Statistics. (2006). *Deaths by place of death, age, race, and sex: United States, 1999–2004.* June 6, 2007, p. 1 Worktable 309.

National Center for Health Statistics. (2008). *Health, United States, 2007, with chartbook on trends in health of Americans.* Hyattsville, MD.: Government Printing Office.

National Center for Health Statistics. (2009). *Health, United States, 2008.* Hyattsville, MD: US Government Printing Office. Retrieved May 15, 2009, from http://www.cdc.gov/nchs/hus.htm

National Council on Aging. (2001). *Myths and Realities of Aging, 2000.* New York: Harris Interactive.

National Council on Aging. (2006a). *Using the evidence base to promote healthy aging.* Issue Brief 1. Washington, DC: Center for Healthy Aging.

National Council on Aging. (2006b). *Evidence-based programs for the elderly initiative.* Issue Brief 3. Washington, DC: Center for Healthy Aging.

Nelson, D. E., Shayne, B., Powell-Griner, E., Klein, R., Wells, H. E., Hogelin, G., et al. (2002b). State trends in health risk factors and receipt of clinical preventive services among US adults during the 1990s. *Journal of the American Medical Association, 287,* 2659–2667.

Nelson, H. D., Humphrey, L. L., Nygren, P., Teutsch, S. M., & Allan, J. D. (2002a). Postmenopausal hormone replacement therapy: Scientific review. *Journal of the American Medical Association, 288*(7), 872–881.

Nerenberg, L. (2007). *Elder abuse prevention: Emerging trends and promising strategies.* New York: Springer Publishing Company.

Newcomer, R., Clay, T., Luxenberg, J. S., & Miller, R. H. (1999). Misclassification and selection bias when identifying Alzheimer's disease solely from Medicare claims records. *Journal of the American Geriatrics Society, 47,* 215–219.

Newman, A. B., Gottdiener, J. S., McBurnie, M. A., Hirsch, H. H., Kop, W. J., Tracy, R., et al. (2001). Cardiovascular Health Study Research Group. Associations of subclinical disease with frailty. *The Journals of Gerontology. Series A, Biological Sciences and Medical Sciences, 56A,* M158–M166.

Newman, J. P., Engel, R. J., & Jensen, J. E. (1991). Age differences in depressive symptom experiences. *Psychology of Aging, 46,* 224–235.

Nichol, K. L., Nordin, J., Mullooly, J., Lask, R., Fillbrandt, K., & Iwane, M. (2003). Influenza vaccination and reduction in hospitalizations for cardiac disease and stroke among the elderly. *New England Journal of Medicine, 348*(14), 1322–1332.

Nichol, K. L., Nordin, J. D., Nelson, D. B., Mullooly, J. P., & Hak, E. (2007). Effectiveness of influenza vaccine in the community-dwelling elderly. *New England Journal of Medicine, 357*(14), 1373–1381.

Olsen, O., & Gotzsche, P. C. (2001). Cochrane review on screening for breast cancer with mammography. *Lancet, 35,* 1340–1342.

Olshansky, S. J., & Ault, A. B. (1986). The fourth stage of the epidemiologic transition: The age of delayed degenerative diseases. *Milbank Quarterly, 64*(3), 355–391.

Olshansky, S. J., Carnes, B. A., & Butler, R. N. (2001). If humans were built to last. *Scientific American, 284*(3), 50–55.

Olshansky, S. J., Carnes, B. A., & Cassel, C. (1990). In search of Methuselah: Estimating the upper limits to human longevity. *Science, 250*(4981), 634–640.

Onder, G., Penninx, B. W., Lapuerta, P., Fried, L. P., Ostir, G. V., Guralnik, J. M., et al. (2002). Change in physical performance over time in older women: The Women's Health and Aging Study. *The Journals of Gerontology. Series A, Biological Sciences and Medical Sciences, 57*(5), M289–M293.

Ormond, B. A., Black, K. J., Tilly, J., & Thomas, S. (2004). *Supportive services programs in naturally occurring retirement communities.* Washington, DC: Urban Institute.

Orpana, H. M., Ross, N., Feeny, D., McFarland, B., Bernier, J., & Kaplan, M. (2009). The natural history of health-related quality of life: A 10-year cohort study. *Health Report, 20*(1), 29–35.

Pacala, J. T., Boult, C., Reed, R. L., & Aliberti, E. (1997). Predictive validity of the Pra instrument among older recipients of managed care. *Journal of the American Geriatrics Society, 45,* 614–617.

Pahor, M., Blair, S. N., Espeland, M., Fielding, R., Gill, T. M., Guralnik, J. M., et al. LIFE Study Investigators. (2006). Effects of a physical activity intervention on measures of physical performance: Results of the lifestyle interventions and independence for Elders Pilot (LIFE-P) Study. *The Journals of Gerontology. Series A, Biological Sciences and Medical Sciences, 61,* 1157–1165.

Palloni, A., & Arias, E. (2004). Paradox lost: Explaining the Hispanic adult mortality advantage. *Demography, 41*(3), 385–415.

Palloni, A., & Morenoff, J. D. (2001). Interpreting the paradoxical in the Hispanic paradox: Demographic and epidemiologic approaches. *Annals of the New York Academy of Science, 954,* 140–174.

Palmore, E. B. (1999). *Ageism* (2nd ed.). New York: Springer Press.

Panza, F., D'Introno, A., Colacicco, A. M., Capurso, C., Del Parigi, A., Caselli, R. J., et al. (2009, in press). Temporal relationship between depressive symptoms and cognitive impairment: The Italian Longitudinal Study on Aging. *Journal of Alzheimers Disease.*

Patrick, D. L., Danis, M. L., Southerland, L. I., & Hong, G. (1988). Quality of life following intensive care. *Journal of General Internal Medicine, 3,* 218–223.

Patrick, D. L., & Erikson, P. (1993). *Health status and health policy.* Oxford: Oxford University Press.

Patrick, D. L., Sittampalam, Y., Somerville, S. M., Carter, W. B., & Bergner, M. (1986). A cross-cultural comparison of health status values. *American Journal of Public Health, 75*(12), 1402–1407.

Pearlin, L. I., & Schooler, C. (1978). The structure of coping. *Journal of Health Social Behavior, 19*(1), 2–21.

Penninx, B. W., Guralnik, J. M., Ferrucci, L., Simonsick, E. M., Deeg, D. J., & Wallace, R. B. (1998). Depressive symptoms and physical decline in community-dwelling older persons. *Journal of the American Medical Association, 279*(21), 1720–1726.

Peterson, R. C. (2000). Mild cognitive impairment: Transition between aging and Alzheimer's disease. *Neurologia, 15,* 93–101.

Peterson, R. C., Smith, G. E., Waring, S. C., Ivnik, R. J., Kokmen, E., & Tangelos, E. G. (1997). Aging, memory, and mild cognitive impairment. *International Psychogeriatrics, 9,* 65–69.

Peterson, R. C., Stevens, J. C., Ganguli, M., Tangelos, E. G., Cummings, J. L., & DeKosky, S. T. (2001). Practice parameter: Early detection of dementia: Mild cognitive impairment (an evidence-based review). *Neurology, 56,* 1133–1142.

Pfeffer, R. I., Kurosaki, C. H., Chance, J. M., & Filos, S. (1982). Measurement of functional activities in older adults in the community. *Journal of Gerontology, 37*, 323–329.

Phelan, E. A., Williams, B., Leveille, S., Snyder, S., Wagner, E. H., & LoGerfo, J. P. (2002). Outcomes of a community-based dissemination of the health enhancement program. *Journal of the American Geriatrics Society, 50*(9), 1519–1524.

Phillips, C. D., Sloan, P. D., Hawes, C., Koch, G., Han, J., Spry, K., Dunteman, G., et al. (1997). Effects of residence in Alzheimer disease special care units on functional outcomes. *Journal of the American Medical Association, 276*, 1341–1343.

Pickle, L. W., Mungiole, M., Jones, G. K., & White, A. A. (1996). *Atlas of United States mortality.* Hyattsville, MD: National Center for Health Statistics.

Pillemer, K., & Finkelhor, D. (1998). The prevalence of elder abuse: A random sample survey. *Gerontologist, 28*(1), 51–57.

Plassman, B. L., Langa, K. M., Fisher, G. G., Heeringa, S. G., Weir, D. R., Ofstedal, M. B., et al. (2007). Prevalence of dementia in the United States: The aging, demographics, and memory study. *Neuroepidemiology, 29*(1–2), 125–132.

Plassman, B. L., Langa, K. M., Fisher, G. G., Heeringa, S. G., Weir, D. R., Ofstedal, M. B., et al. (2008). Prevalence of cognitive impairment without dementia in the United States. *Annals of Internal Medicine, 148*(6), 427–434.

Population Reference Bureau. (2004). Transitions in world population. *Population Bulletin, 59*(1). Washington, DC: Population Reference Bureau.

Posner, H. B., Tang, M. X., Luchsinger, J., Lantigua, R., Stern, Y., & Mayeux, R. (2002). The relationship of hypertension in the elderly to AD, vascular dementia, and cognitive function. *Neurology, 58*(8), 1175–1181.

Poulshock, S. W., & Deimling, G. T. (1984). Families caring for elders in residence: Issues in the measurement of burden. *Journal of Gerontology, 39*(2), 230–239.

President's Council on Bioethics. (2005). *Taking care: Ethical caregiving in our aging society.* Washington, DC: Author.

Preston, S. H., Himes, C., & Eggers, M. (1989). Demographic conditions responsible for population aging. *Demography, 26*(4), 691–704.

Preston, S. H., & Martin, L. G. (1994). *Demography of aging.* Washington, DC: National Academy Press.

Public Papers of the Presidents of the United States: Lyndon B. Johnson, 1965. Volume II, entry 394, pp. 811-815. Washington, D. C.: Government Printing Office, 1966. Retrieved October 28, 2009 from: http://www.lbjlib.utexas.edu/johnson/archives.hom/speeches.hom/650730.asp

Quijano, L., Stanley, M., Petersen, N., Casado, B., Steinberg, E., Cully, J., et al. (2007). Healthy IDEAS: A depression intervention delivered by community-based case managers serving older adults. *Journal of Applied Gerontology, 26*(2), 139–156.

Rabins, P., Kasper, J., Kleinman, L., Black, B., & Patrick, D. L. (2001). Concepts and methods in the development of the ADQOL: An instrument for assessing health-related quality of life in persons with Alzheimer's disease. In S. M. Albert & R. G. Logsdon (Eds.), *Assessing quality of life in Alzheimer's disease* (pp. 51–68). New York: Springer Publishing Company.

Rabkin, J. G., Albert, S. M., Del Bene, M. L., O'Sullivan, I., Tider, T., Rowland, L. P., et al. (2005). Prevalence of depressive disorders and change over time in late-stage ALS. *Neurology, 65*(1), 62–67.

Rabkin, J.G., Wagner, G. J., & Del Bene, M. (2000). Resilience and distress among amyotrophic lateral sclerosis patients and caregivers. *Psychosom Med, 62,* 271–279.

Raebel, M. A., Delate, T., Ellis, J. L., & Bayliss, E. A. (2008). Effects of reaching the drug benefit threshold on Medicare members' healthcare utilization during the first year of Medicare Part D. *Medical Care, 46*(10), 1116–1122.

Rantanen, T., Guralnik, J. M., Ferrucci, L., Leveille, S., & Fried, L. P. (1999a). Coimpairments: Strength and balance as predictors of severe walking disability. *The Journals of Gerontology. Series A, Biological Sciences and Medical Sciences, 54*(4), M172–M176.

Rantanen, T., Guralnik, J. M., Foley, D., Masaki, K., Leveille, S., Curb, J. D., et al. (1999b). Midlife hand grip strength as a predictor of old age disability. *Journal of the American Medical Association, 281*, 558–560.

Ravitsky, V., Fiester, A., & Caplan, A. (2009). *The Penn Center guide to bioethics.* New York: Springer Publishing Company.

Reed, A. E., Mikels, J. A., & Simon, K. I. (2008). Older adults prefer less choice than young adults. *Psychology of Aging, 23*(3), 671–675.

Reinhard, S. C. (2004). The work of caregiving: What do ADLs and IADLs tell us? In C. Levine (Ed.), *Family caregivers on the job: Moving beyond ADLs and IADLs.* New York: United Hospital Fund of New York.

Reinhard, S. C., & Horwitz, A. (1995). Caregiver burden: Differentiating the content and consequences of family caregiving. *Journal of Marriage and the Family, 57*, 741–750.

Reuben, D. B., Borok, G. M., Wolde-Tsadik, G., Ershoff, D. H., Fishman, L K., Ambrosini, V. L., et al. (1995). A randomized trial of comprehensive geriatric assessment in the care of hospitalized patients. *New England Journal of Medicine, 332*, 1345–1350.

Reynolds, C. F., 3rd. (2008). Preventing depression in old age: It's time. *American Journal of Geriatric Psychiatry, 16*(6), 433–434.

Rich, M W., Beckkam, V., Wittenberg, C., Leven, C. V., Freedland, K. E., & Carney, R. M. (1995). A multidisciplinary intervention to prevent the readmission of elderly patients with congestive heart failure. *New England Journal of Medicine, 333*, 1190–1195.

Richards, M., Touchon, J., Ledesert, B., & Ritchie, K. (1999). Cognitive decline in ageing: Are AAMI and AACD distinct entities? *International Journal of Geriatric Psychiatry, 14*, 534–540.

Ritchie, K., Artero, S., & Touchon, J. (2001). Classification criteria for mild cognitive impairment: A population-based validation study. *Neurology, 56*, 37–42.

Roberts, R. E., Kaplan, G. A., Shema, S. J., & Strawbridge, W. J. (1997). Prevalence and correlates of depression in an aging cohort: The Alameda County Study. *The Journals of Gerontology. Series B, Psychological Sciences and Social Sciences, 52*(5), S252–S258.

Robine, J. M., & Michel, J. P. (2004). Looking forward to a general theory on population aging. *The Journals of Gerontology. Series A, Biological Sciences and Medical Sciences, 59*(6), M590–M597.

Robine, J. M., Romieu, I., Cambois, E., van de Water, H. P. A., & Boshuizen, H. C. (1995). *Contribution of the network on health expectancy and the disability process.* World Health Report (WHR95). Geneva, Switzerland: World Health Organization.

Rockwood, K., Andrew, M., & Mitnitski, A. (2007). A comparison of two approaches to measuring frailty in elderly people. *The Journals of Gerontology. Series A, Biological Sciences and Medical Sciences, 62*(7), 738–743.

Rodgers, W., & Miller, B. (1997). A comparative analysis of ADL questions in surveys of older people. *The Journals of Gerontology. Series B, Psychological Sciences and Social Sciences, 52*(Spec No), 21–36.

Rosen, W. (1981). *The Rosen Drawing Test.* Bronx, NY: Veteran's Administration Medical Center.

Rosenberg, H. G. (2009). Complaint discourse, aging, and caregiving among the Ju/'hoansi of Botswana. In J. Sokolovsky (Ed.), *The cultural context of aging* (pp. 30–52). Westport, CT: Praeger Publishers.

Roses, A. D., Strittmatter, W. J., Pericak-Vance, M. A., Corder, E. H., Saunders, A M., & Schmechel, D. E. (1994). Clinical application of apolipoprotein E genotyping to Alzheimer's disease. *Lancet, 343*(8912), 1564–1565.

Ross, G. W., Abbot, R. D., Petrovitch, H., Masaki, K. H., Murdaugh, C., Trockman, C., et al. (1997). Frequency and characteristics of silent dementia among elderly Japanese-American men. The Honolulu-Asia Aging Study. *Journal of the American Medical Association, 277,* 800–805.

Roth, D. L., Stevens, A. B., Burgio, L. D., & Burgio, K. L. (2002). Timed-event sequential analysis of agitation in nursing home residents during personal care interactions with nursing assistants. *The Journals of Gerontology. Series B, Psychological Sciences and Social Sciences, 57*(5), P461–P468.

Rothenberg, R. B., & Koplan, J. P. (1990). Chronic disease in the 1990s. *Annual Review of Public Health, 11,* 267–296.

Roubenoff, R., & Castaneda, C. (2001). Sarcopenia—Understanding the dynamics of aging muscle. *Journal of the American Medical Association, 286*(10), 1230–1231.

Rowe, J. W., & Kahn, R. L. (1987). Human aging: Usual and successful. *Science, 237,* 143–149.

Rozzini, R., Frisoni, G. B., Sabatini, T., & Trabucchi, M. (2002). The association of depression and mortality in elderly persons. *The Journals of Gerontology. Series A, Biological Sciences and Medical Sciences, 57*(2), M144–M145.

Rubenstein, L. Z. (1990). The importance of including the home environment in assessment of frail older persons. *Journal of the American Geriatrics Society, 47*(1), 111–112.

Rubenstein, L. Z., Stuck, A. E., Siu, A. L., & Wieland, G. D. (1991). Impacts of geriatric evaluation and management programs on defined outcomes: Overview of evidence. *Journal of the American Geriatrics Society, 38S,* 8S–16S.

Russell, D. W., Cutrona, C. E., de la Mora, A., & Wallace, R. B. (1997). Loneliness and nursing home admission among rural older adults. *Psychology & Aging, 12*(4), 574–589.

Russell, L. B. (2009). Preventing chronic disease: An important investment, but don't count on cost savings. *Health Affairs (Project Hope), 28*(1), 42–45.

Ryan, E. B., Bourhis, R. Y., & Knops, U. (1991). Evaluative perceptions of patronizing speech addressed to elders. *Psychology of Aging, 6*(3), 442–450.

Satariano, W. (2006). *Epidemiology of aging: An ecological approach.* Sudbury, MA: Jones and Bartlett.

Saunders, A. M., Strittmatter, W. J., Schmechel, D., George-Hyslop, P. H., Pericak-Vance, M. A., Joo, S. H., et al. (1993). Association of apolipoprotein E allele epsilon-4 with late-onset familial and sporadic Alzheimer's disease. *Neurology, 43,* 1467–1472.

Scarmeas, N., Albert, S. M., Manly, J. J., & Stern, Y. (2006). Education and rates of cognitive decline in incident Alzheimer's disease. *Journal of Neurology, Neurosurgery, and Psychiatry, 77*(3), 308–316.

Scarmeas, N., Luchsinger, J. A., Mayeux, R., & Stern, Y. (2007). Mediterranean diet and Alzheimer disease mortality. *Neurology, 69*(11), 1084–1093.

Scarmeas, N., Zarahn, E., Anderson, K. E., Habeck, C. G., Hilton, J., Flynn, J., et al. (2003). Association of life activities with cerebral blood flow in Alzheimer disease: Implications for the cognitive reserve hypothesis. *Archives of Neurology, 60*(3), 359–365.

Scheffler, R. M., Brown, T. T., Syme, L., Kawachi, I., Tolstykh, I., & Iribarren, C. (2008). Community-level social capital and recurrence of acute coronary syndrome. *Social Science & Medicine, 66*(7), 1603–1613.

Schmidt, T. A., Hickman, S. E., & Tolle, S. W. (2004a). Honoring treatment preferences near the end of life: The Oregon physician orders for life-sustaining treatment (POLST) program. *Advances in Experimental Medicine and Biology, 550*, 255–262.

Schmidt, T A., Hickman, S. E., Tolle, S. W., & Brooks, H. S. (2004b). The Physician Orders for Life-Sustaining Treatment program: Oregon emergency medical technicians' practical experiences and attitudes. *Journal of the American Geriatrics Society, 52*(9), 1430–1434.

Schneider, L. S., & Olin, J. T. (1996). Clinical global impressions in Alzheimer's clinical trials. *International Psychogeriatrics, 8*(2), 277–288; discussion 288–290.

Schneider, L. S., Tariot, P. N., Dagerman, K. S., Davis, S. M., Hsiao, J. K., Ismail, M. S., et al. (2006). Effectiveness of atypical antipsychotic drugs in patients with Alzheimer's disease. *New England Journal of Medicine, 355*(15), 1525–1538.

Schnelle, J. F., Bertrand, R., Hurd, D., White, A., Squires, D., Feuerberg, M., et al. (2009). Resident choice and the survey process: The need for standardized observation and transparency. *The Gerontologist, 49*(4), 517–524.

Schoeni, R. F., Freedman, V. A., & Martin, L. G. (2008). Why is late-life disability declining? *Milbank Quarterly, 86*(1), 47–89.

Schoeni, R. F., Freedman, V. A., & Wallace, R. B. (2001). Persistent, consistent, widespread, and robust? Another look at recent trends in old-age disability. *Journal of Gerontology, 56B*(4), S206.

Schoeni, R., Martin, L. M., Andreski, P., & Freedman, V. A. (2005). Persistent and growing socioeconomic disparities in disability among the elderly: 1982–2002. *American Journal of Public Health, 95*(11), 2065–2070.

Schootman, M., Andresen, E. M., Wolinsky, F. D., Malmstrom, T. K., Miller, J. P., & Miller, D. K. (2006). Neighborhood conditions and risk of incident lower-body functional limitations among middle-aged African Americans. *American Journal of Epidemiology, 163*(5), 450–458.

Schulz, R., & Beach, S. R. (1999). Caregiving as a risk factor for mortality: The Caregiver Health Effects Study. *Journal of the American Medical Association, 282*(23), 2215–2219.

Schulz, R., Beach, S. R., Ives, D. G., Martire, L. M., Ariyo, A. A., & Kop, W. J. (2000). Association between depression and mortality in older adults: The Cardiovascular Health Study. *Archives of Internal Medicine, 160*(12), 1761–1768.

Schulz, R., & Martire, L. (in press). Caregiving and employment. In S. Czaja (Ed.).

Scitovsky, A. (1994). The high costs of dying revisited. *Milbank Quarterly. 72.* 561–591.

Seeman, T. E., Merkin, S. S., Crimmins, E. M., Karlamangla, A. S. (in press). Are disability trends worsening among recent cohorts of older Americans?: NHANES 1999–2004 versus 1988–1994. *American Journal of Public Health.*

Sehl, M. E., & Yates, F. E. (2001). Kinetics of human aging: I. Rates of senescence between ages 30 and 70 years in healthy people. *The Journals of Gerontology. Series A, Biological Sciences and Medical Sciences, 56A*, B198–B208.

Shumaker, S. A., Legault, C., Rapp, S. R., Thal, L., Wallace, R. B., Ockene, J. K., et al.; WHIMS Investigators. (2003). Estrogen plus progestin and the incidence of dementia and mild cognitive impairment in postmenopausal women: The Women's Health Initiative Memory Study: A randomized controlled trial. *Journal of the American Medical Association, 289*(20), 2651–2662.

Shumway-Cook, A., Patla, A., Stewart, A., Ferrucci, L., Ciol, M. A., & Guralnik, J. M. (2003). Environmental components of mobility disability in community-living older persons. *Journal of the American Geriatrics Society, 51*(3), 393–398.

Silliman, R. A. (2000). Caregiving issues in the geriatric medical encounter. *Clinics in Geriatric Medicine, 16*(1), 51–60.

Silliman, R. A., Bhatti, S., Khan, A., Dukes, K. A., & Sullivan, L. M. (1996). The care of older persons with diabetes mellitus: Families and primary care physicians. *Journal of the American Geriatrics Society, 44*(11), 1314–1321.

Simmons, S. F., Keeler, E., Zhuo, X., Hickey, K. A., Sato, H. W., & Schnelle, J. F. (2008). Prevention of unintentional weight loss in nursing home residents: A controlled trial of feeding assistance. *Journal of the American Geriatrics Society, 56*(8), 1466–1473.

Simonsick, E. M., Kasper, J. D., & Phillips, C. L. (1998). Physical disability and social interaction: Factors associated with low social contact and home confinement in disabled older women (The Women's Health and Aging Study). *The Journals of Gerontology. Series B, Psychological Sciences and Social Sciences, 53*(4), S209–S217.

Sloane, P. D., Mitchell, C. M., Calkins, M., & Zimmerman, S. I. (2000). Light and noise levels in Alzheimer's disease special care units. In D. Holmes, J. A. Teresi, M. G. Ory (Eds.), *Special care units*. Paris: Serdi Publishers; New York: Springer Press.

Sloane, P. D., Mitchell, C. M., Weisman, G., Zimmerman, S., Foley, K. M., Lynn, M., et al. (2002). The Therapeutic Environment Screening Survey for Nursing Homes (TESS-NH): An observational instrument for assessing the physical environment of institutional settings for persons with dementia. *The Journals of Gerontology. Series B, Psychological Sciences and Social Sciences, 57*(2), S69–S78.

Small, S. A., Tsai, W. Y., DeLaPaz, R., Mayeux, R., & Stern, Y. (2002). Imaging hippocampal function across the human life span: Is memory decline normal or not? *Annals of Neurology, 51*(3), 290–295.

Snowdon, D. A., Kemper, S. J., Mortimer, J. A., Greiner, L. H., Wekstein, D. R., & Markesberry, W. R. (1996). Linguistic ability in early life and cognitive function and Alzheimer's disease in late life. Findings from the Nun Study. *Journal of the American Medical Association, 275*(7), 528–532.

Soldo, B., Mitchell, O., Tfaily, R., & McCabe, J. (2007). Cross-cohort differences in health on the verge of retirement. In B. Madrian, O. Mitchell, & B. Soldo (Eds.), *Redefining retirement: How will boomers fare?* (pp. 138–158). New York, NY: Oxford University Press.

Sonn, U., Frandin, K., & Grimby, G. (1995). Instrumental activities of daily living related to impairments and functional limitation in 70 year olds. *Scandinavian Journal of Rehabilitation Medicine, 27,* 119–128.

Spain, D., & Bianchi, S.M. (1996) *Balancing Act.* New York: Russell Sage Foundation.

Special Committee on Aging, United States Senate. (1991). *Lifelong learning for an aging society—An information paper.* Serial No. 102. Washington, DC: U.S. Government Printing Office.

Spilker, B., & Revicki, D. A. (1999). Taxonomy of quality of life. In B. Spilker (Ed.), *Quality of life and pharmacoeconomics in clinical trials*. Philadelphia: Lippincott-Raven.

Spillman, B. C. (2004). Changes in elderly disability rates and the implications for health care utilization and cost. *Milbank Quarterly, 82*(1), 157–194.

Spitzer, R. L., Kroenke, K., & Williams, J. B. (1999). Validation and utility of a self-report version of PRIME-MD: The PHQ primary care study. Primary Care Evaluation of Mental Disorders. Patient Health Questionnaire. *Journal of the American Medical Association, 282*(18), 1737–1744.

Stern, Y., Albert, S. M., Sano, M., Richards, M., Miller, L., Folstein, M., et al. (1994). Assessing dependency in Alzheimer's disease. *The Journals of Gerontology. Series A, Biological Sciences and Medical Sciences, 49*, M216–M221.

Stevens, J. A., & Sogolo, E. D. (2008). *Preventing falls: What works.* A CDC Compendium of Effective Community-based Interventions from Around the World. Atlanta, GA: National Center for Injury Prevention and Control.

Stewart, A. L., Greenfield, S., Hays, R. D., Wells, K., Rogers, W. H., Berry, S. D., et al. (1989). Functional status and well-being of patients with chronic conditions. Results from the Medical Outcomes Study. *Journal of the American Medical Association, 262*(7), 907–913.

Stewart, S., Pearson, S., & Horowitz, J. D. (1998). Effects of a home-based intervention among patients with congestive heart failure discharged from acute hospital care. *Archives of Internal Medicine, 158*(10), 1067–1072.

Strawbridge, W. J., Wallhagan, M. I., & Cohen, R. D. (2002). Successful aging and well-being: Self-rated compared with Rowe and Kahn. *The Gerontologist, 42*(6), 727–733.

Stroeken, K. (2002). From shrub to log: The ancestral dimension of elderhood among the Sukuma in Tanzania. In S. Makoni & K. Stroeken (Eds.), *Ageing in Africa: Sociolinguistic and anthropological approaches*. Burlington, VT: Ashgate.

Stuck, A. E. (2001). Management of polypharmacy in community-dwelling older persons. *Very Old Patient Centered Medicine: Assessment and management of geriatric syndromes.* Retrieved May 15, 2009, from http://www.healthandage.com/html/min/eama/eama4/publi/

Stuck, A E., Aronow, H. U., Steiner, A., Alessi, C. A., Bula, C. J., Gold, M. N., et al. (1995). A trial of annual in-home comprehensive geriatric assessments for elderly people living in the community. *New England Journal of Medicine, 333*, 1184–1189.

Stuck, A. E., Beers, M. H., Steine, A., Aronow, H. U., Rubenstein, L. Z., & Beck, J. C. (1994). Inappropriate medication use in community-resident older persons. *Archives of Internal Medicine, 154*, 2195–2200.

Stuck, A. E., Egger, M., Hammer, A., Minder, C. E., & Beck, J. C. (2002). Home visits to prevent nursing home admission and functional decline in elderly people: Systematic review and meta-regression analysis. *Journal of the American Medical Association, 287*(8), 1022–1028.

Stuck, A. E., Siu, A. L., Wieland, G. D., & Rubenstein, L. Z. (1993). Comprehensive geriatric assessment: A meta-analysis of controlled trials. *Lancet, 342*, 1032–1036.

Stuck, A. E., Walthert, J. M., Nikolaus, T., Bula, C. J., Hohmann, C., & Beck, J. C. (1999). Risk factors for functional status decline in community-living elderly people: A systematic literature review. *Social Science and Medicine, 48*, 445–469.

Sturm, R., Ringel, J. S., & Andreyeva, T. (2004). Increasing obesity rates and disability trends. *Health Affairs (Project Hope), 23*(2), 199–205.

Sullivan, D. F. (1966). Conceptual problem in developing an index of health. *Vital and Health Statistics, 2*(16), 1–18.

Sullivan, D. F. (1971). A single index of mortality and morbidity. *HSMHA Health Reports, 86*(4), 347–354.

Surgeon General. (1999). *Surgeon General's report on mental health.* Retrieved from http://www.surgeongeneral.gov/library/mentalhealth/home.html

Susser, M. (1997). Steps toward discovering causes: Divergence and convergence of epidemiology and clinical medicine. *Epidemiology & Prevention, 21*(3), 160–168.

Suzman, R. M., Willis, D. P., & Manton, K. G. (1992). *The oldest old.* New York: Oxford University Press.

Tabert, M. H., Albert, S. M., Borukhova-Milov, L., Camacho, Y., Pelton, G., Liu, X., et al. (2002). Functional deficits in patients with mild cognitive impairment: Prediction of AD. *Neurology, 58*(5), 758–764.

Talbot, C., Lendon, C., Craddock, N., Shears, S., Morris, J. C., & Goate, A. (1994). Protection against Alzheimer's disease with apoe e2. *Lancet, 343,* 1432–1433.

Tang, M.-X., Cross, P., Andrews, H., Jacobs, D., Small, S., Bell, K., et al. (2001). Incidence of AD in African-Americans, Caribbean Hispanics, and Caucasians in northern Manhattan. *Neurology, 56,* 49–56.

Tang, M.-X, Jacobs, D., Stern, Y., Marder, K., Schofield, P., Gurland, B., et al. (1996). Effect of oestrogen during menopause on risk and age at onset of Alzheimer's disease. *Lancet, 348*(9025), 429–432.

Tang, M.-X., Stern, Y., Marder, K., Bell, K., Gurland, B., Lantigua, R., et al. (1998) The APOE-epsilon4 allele and the risk of Alzheimer disease among African Americans, Whites, and Hispanics. *Journal of the American Medical Association, 279*(10), 751–755.

Tattersall, R. (2002). The expert patient: A new approach to chronic disease management for the twenty-first century. *Clinical Medicine, 2*(3), 227–229.

Teresi, J. A., Holmes, D., Ramirez, M., & Kong, J. (1998). Staffing patterns, staff support, and training in special care and nonspecial care units. *Journal of Mental Health and Aging, 4*(4), 443–458.

Testa, M. A., & Simonson, D. C. (1996). Assessment of Quality-of-Life Outcomes. *New England Journal of Medicine, 334*(13), 835–840.

Tierney, M. C., Szalai, J. P., Snow, W. G., Fisher, R. H., Nores, A., Nadon, G., et al. (1996). Prediction of probable Alzheimer's disease in memory-impaired patients: A prospective longitudinal study. *Neurology, 46,* 661–665.

Tinetti, M. E., Baker, D. I., McAvay, G., Claus, E. B., Garrett, P., Gottschalk, M., et al. (1994). A multifactorial intervention to reduce the risk of falling among elderly people living in the community. *New England Journal of Medicine, 331,* 821–827.

Tinetti, M. E., McAvay, G., & Claus, E. (1996). Does multiple risk factor reduction explain the reduction in fall rate in the Yale FICSIT trial? *American Journal of Epidemiology, 144,* 389–399.

Tinetti, M. E., Speechley, M., & Ginter, S. F. (1988). Risk factors for falls among elderly persons living in the community. *New England Journal of Medicine, 319,* 1701–1707.

Tinetti, M. E., & Williams, C. S. (1998). The effect of falls and fall injuries on functioning in community-dwelling older persons. *The Journals of Gerontology. Series A, Biological Sciences and Medical Sciences, 53*(2), 112–119.

Torrance, G. W. (1987). Utility approach to measuring health-related quality of life. *Journal of Chronic Diseases, 40*(6), 593–603.

Torrance, G. W., Erickson, P., Patrick, D., & Feldman, J. J. (1995). *Technical Notes. Years of Healthy Life 1995* (April (PHS) 95-1237). Atlanta, GA: Centers for Disease Control and Prevention.

Torstan, L. (2005). *Gerotranscendence: A developmental theory of positive aging.* New York: Springer Publishing Company.

Touchon, J., & Ritchie, K. (1999). Prodromal cognitive disorder in Alzheimer's disease. *International Journal of Geriatric Psychiatry, 14,* 556–563.

Trinh, N.-H., Hoblyn, J., Mohanty, S., & Yaffe, K. (2003). Efficacy of cholinesterase inhibitors in the treatment of neuropsychiatric symptoms and functional impairment in Alzheimer's disease. *Journal of the American Medical Association, 289,* 210–216.

Tseng, C.-W., Brook, R. H., Keeler, E., Steers, W. N., & Mangione, C. M. (2004). Cost-lowering strategies used by Medicare beneficiaries who exceed drug benefit caps and have a gap in drug coverage. *Journal of the American Medical Association, 292,* 952–960.

University Center on Social and Urban Research. (2005). *State of Aging in Allegheny County.* University of Pittsburgh.

Unutzer, J., Katon, W., Callahan, C. M., Williams, J. W., Jr., Hunkeler, E., Harpole, L., et al. (2002a). Collaborative care management of late-life depression in the primary care setting: A randomized controlled trial. *Journal of the American Medical Association, 288*(22), 2836–2845.

Unutzer, J., Patrick, D. L., Marmon, T., Simon, G. E., & Katon, W. J. (2002b). Depressive symptoms and mortality in a prospective study of 2,558 older adults. *American Journal of Geriatric Psychiatry, 10*(5), 521–530.

U.S. Census Bureau. (2004a). Population projections. Interim projections consistent with Census 2000. Table 2a. Projected Population of the United States, by Age and Sex: 2000 to 2050. Retrieved March 23, 2008, from http://www.census.gov/ipc/www/usinterimproj/natprojtab02a.xls

U.S. Census Bureau. (2004b). Population projections. Interim projections consistent with Census 2000. Population pyramids and demographic summary indicators for U.S. Regions and Divisions. Retrieved March 23, 2008, from http://www.census.gov/population/projections/52PyrmdUS1.pdf and http://www.census.gov/population/projections/52PyrmdUS3.pdf

U.S. Census Bureau, International Data Base. (2008). Retrieved March 23, 2008, from http://www.census.gov/ipc/www/idbnew.html

U.S. General Accounting Office (GAO). (1998). *Alzheimer's disease: Estimates of prevalence in the U.S.* Retrieved April, 15, 2004, from http://www.gao.gov/archive/1998/he98016.pdf

U.S. Preventive Services Task Force. (2002). *Screening for breast cancer: Recommendations and rationale.* Rockville, MD: Agency for Healthcare Research and Quality. Retrieved May 15, 2009, from http://www.ahrq.gov/clinic/3rduspstf/breastcancer/brcanrr.htm

U.S. Preventive Services Task Force. (1996, 2002, 2008, 2009). *Pocket guide to clinical preventive services.* Retrieved November 16, 2009 from http://www.ahrq.gov/clinic/pocketgd09/

Van den Block, L., Deschepper, R., Drieskens, K., Bauwens, S., Bilsen, J., Bossuyt, N., et al. (2007). Hospitalisations at the end of life: Using a sentinel surveillance network to study hospital use and associated patient, disease and healthcare factors. *BMC Health Services Research, 7,* 69.

van der Steen, J. T., Ooms, M. E., van der Wal, G., & Ribbe, M. W. (2002). Pneumonia: The demented patient's best friend? Discomfort after starting or withholding antibiotic treatment. *Journal of the American Geriatrics Society, 50*(10), 1681–1688.

van Duijn, C. M., de Knijff, P., Wehnert, A., De Voecht, J., Bronzova, J. B., Havekes, L. M., et al. (1995). The apolipoprotein E epsilon-2 allele is associated with an increased risk of early-onset Alzheimer's disease and a reduced survival. *Annals of Neurology, 37,* 605–610.

Van Haitsma, K., Lawton, M. P., & Kleban, M. H. (2000). Does segregation help or hinder? Examining the role of homogeneity in behavioral and emotional aspects of quality of life in persons with cognitive impairment in the nursing home. In D. Holmes, J. A. Teresi, M. G. Ory (Eds.), *Special care units* (pp. 163–178). Paris: Serdi Publishers; New York: Springer Press.

Vaupel, J. W. (1997). The remarkable improvements in survival at older ages. *Philosophical Transactions of the Royal Society of London. Series B, Biological Sciences, 352*(1363), 1799–1804.

Verbrugge, L. M., & Jette, A. M. (1994). The disablement process. *Social Science & Medicine, 38*(1), 1–14.

Verbrugge, L. M., & Patrick, D. L. (1995). Seven chronic conditions: Their impact on US adults' activity levels and use of medical services. *American Journal of Public Health, 85,* 173–182.

Verbrugge, L. M., & Sevak, P. (2002). Use, type, and efficacy of assistance for disability. *The Journals of Gerontology. Series B, Psychological Sciences and Social Sciences, 57*(6), S366–S379.

Visser, M., Kritchevsky, S. B., Goodpaster, B. H., Newman, A. B., Nevitt, M., Stamm, E., et al. (2002a). Leg muscle mass and composition in relation to lower extremity performance in men and women aged 70 to 79: The Health, Aging, and Body Composition Study. *Journal of the American Geriatrics Society, 50,* 897–904.

Visser, M., Pahor, M., Taafe, D. R., Goodpaster, B. H., Simonsick, E. M., Newman, A. B., et al. (2002b). Relationship of interleukin-6 and tumor necrosis factor-(alpha) with muscle mass and muscle strength in elderly men and women: The Health ABC Study. *Journal of Gerontology, 57A,* M326–M332.

Wallace, J. I., Buchner, D. M., Grothaus, L., Leveille, S., Tyll, L., LaCroix, A. Z., et al. (1998). Implementation and effectiveness of a community-based health promotion program for older adults. *The Journals of Gerontology. Series A, Biological Sciences and Medical Sciences, 53*(4), M301–M306.

Wallace, R. B. (1997). Variability in disease manifestations in older adults: Implications for public and community health programs. In T. Hickey, M. A. Spears, & T. R. Prahaska (Eds.), *Public health and aging* (pp. 75–86). Baltimore: Johns Hopkins.

Wallace, S.P. (2005). The public health perspective on aging. *Generations, 24*(2), 5–10.

Wallace, S. P., & Gutierrez, V. F. (2005). Equity of access to health care for older adults in four major Latin American cities. *Revista Panamericana de Salud Pública, 17*(5–6), 394–409.

Walter-Ginzburg, A., Blumstein, T., & Guralnik, J. M. (2004). The Israeli kibbutz as a venue for reduced disability in old age: Lessons from the Cross-sectional and Longitudinal Aging Study (CALAS). *Social Science & Medicine, 59*(2), 389–403.

Ware, J. E., & Stewart, A. L. (1992). *Measuring function and well-being.* Cambridge, MA: Harvard University Press.

Wechsler, D. (1981). *Wechsler adult intelligence scale-revised.* New York: The Psychological Corporation.

Weinberger, M., Murray, M. D., Marrero, D. G., Brewer, N., Lykens, M., Harris, L. E., et al. (2002). Effectiveness of pharmacist care for patients with reactive airways disease: A randomized controlled trial. *Journal of the American Medical Association, 288*(13), 1594–1602.

Weinberger, M., Oddone, E. Z., & Henderson, W. G. (1996). Does increased access to primary care reduce hospital readmissions? Veterans Affairs Cooperative Study Group on Primary Care and Hospital Readmission. *New England Journal of Medicine, 334*(22), 1441–1447.

Weiner, J. M., Hanley, R. J., Clark, R., & Van Nostrand, J. F. (1990). Measuring the activities of daily living: Comparisons across national surveys. *Journal of Gerontology, 45*(6), S229–S237.

Weir, D. (2007). Are Baby Boomers living well longer? In B. Madrian, O. Mitchell, & B. Soldo (Eds.), *Redefining retirement: How will boomers fare?* (pp. 95–111). New York, NY: Oxford University Press.

Weiss, C. O., Hoenig, H. M., & Fried, L. P. (2007). Compensatory strategies used by older adults facing mobility disability. *Archives of Physical Medicine and Rehabilitation, 88,* 1217–1220.

Weissert, W., Chernow, M., & Hirth, R. (2003). Titrating versus targeting home care services to frail elderly clients; An application of agency theory and cost-benefit analysis to home care policy. *Journal of Aging and Health, 15*(1), 99–123.

Wells, K. B., Stewart, A., Hays, R. D., Burnam, M. A., Rogers, W., Daniels, M., Berry, S., et al. (1989). The functioning and well-being of depressed patients. Results from the Medical Outcomes Study. *Journal of the American Medical Association, 262*(7), 914–919.

Wennberg, J. E., Fisher, E. S., Skinner, J. S., & Bronner, K. K. (2007). Extending the P4P agenda, part 2: How Medicare can reduce waste and improve the care of the chronically ill. *Health Affairs (Project Hope), 26*(6), 1575–1585.

West, C. G, Reed, D. M., & Gildengorin, G. L. (1998). Can money buy happiness? Depressive symptoms in an affluent older population. *Journal of the American Geriatrics Society, 46*(1), 49–57.

Whalley, L. J., & Deary, I. J. (2001). Longitudinal cohort study of childhood IQ and survival up to age 76. *British Medical Journal, 322,* 1–5.

Whalley, L. J., Starr, J. M., Athawes, R., Hunter, D., Pattie, A., & Deary, I. J. (2000). Childhood mental ability and dementia. *Neurology, 55,* 1455–1459.

Whiteneck, G. G., Harrison-Felix, C. L., Mellick, D. C., Brooks, C. A., Charlifue, S. B., & Gerhart, K. A. (2004). Quantifying environmental factors: A measure of physical, attitudinal, service, productivity, and policy barriers. *Archives of Physical Medicine and Rehabilitation, 85*(8), 1324–1335.

Wight, R. G., Aneshensel, C. S., Miller-Martinez, D., Botticello, A. L., Cummings, J. R., Karlamangla, A. S., et al. (2006). Urban neighborhood context, educational attainment, and cognitive function among older adults. *American Journal of Epidemiology, 163*(12), 1071–1978.

Willcox, S. M., Himmselstein, D. U., & Woolhandler, S. (1994). Inappropriate drug prescribing in the community-dwelling elderly. *Journal of the American Medical Association, 272*, 292–296.

Willis, S. L., Tennstedt, S. L., Marsiske, M., Ball, K., Elias, J., Koepke, K. M., et al. (2006). Long-term effects of cognitive training on everyday functional outcomes in older adults. *Journal of the American Medical Association, 296*(23), 2805–2814.

Wilson, P. W. F., Myers, R. H., Larson, M. G., Ordovas, J. M., Wolf, P. A., & Schaefer, E. J. (1994). Apolipoprotein E alleles, dyslipidemia, and coronary heart disease. *Journal of the American Medical Association, 272*, 1666–1671.

Wilson, R. S., Beckett, L. A., Bienias, J. L., Evans, D. A., & Bennett, D. A. (2003). Terminal decline in cognitive function. *Neurology, 60*(11), 1782–1787.

Wilson, R. S., Bennett, D. A., Bienias, J. L., Aggarwal, N. T., Mendes de Leon, C. F., Morris, M. C., et al. (2002). Cognitive activity and incident AD in a population-based sample of older persons. *Neurology, 59*(12), 1910–1914.

Wilson, R. S., Hebert, L. E., Scherr, P. A., Barnes, L. L., Mendes de Leon, C. F., & Evans, D. A. (2009). Educational attainment and cognitive decline in old age. *Neurology, 72*(5), 460–465.

Wilson, R. S., Li, Y., Aggarwal, N. T., Barnes, L. L., McCann, J. J., Gilley, D. W., et al. (2004). Education and the course of cognitive decline in Alzheimer disease. *Neurology, 63*(7), 1198–1202.

Wolff, J., Starfield, B., & Anderson, G. (2002). Prevalence, expenditures, and complications of multiple chronic conditions in the elderly. *Archives of Internal Medicine, 162*, 2269–2276.

Wolfson, C., Wolfson, D. B., Asgharian, M., M'Lan, C. E., Ostbye, T., Rockwood, K., et al. (2001). Clinical Progression of Dementia Study Group. A reevaluation of the duration of survival after the onset of dementia. *New England Journal of Medicine, 344*(15), 1111–1116.

Wolinsky, F. D., Unverzagt, F. W., Smith, D. M., Jones, R., Stoddard, A., & Tennstedt, S. L. (2006). The ACTIVE cognitive training trial and health-related quality of life: Protection that lasts for 5 years. *The Journals of Gerontology. Series A, Biological Sciences and Medical Sciences, 61*(12), 1324–1329.

Wolinsky, F. D., Vander Weg, M. W., Martin, R., et al. (2009). The effect of speed-of-processing training on depressive symptoms in ACTIVE. *The Journals of Gerontology. Series A, Biological Sciences and Medical Sciences, 64*(4), 468–472.

World Bank. (1995). *The disability-adjusted life year (DALY) definition, measurement, and potential use.* Human Capital Development and Operations Policy, HCO Working Papers. Retrieved March 2004, from www.worldbank.org/html

World Health Organization. (1981). *International classification of impairment, disability and handicap.* Geneva, Switzerland: Author.

World Health Organization. (2001). *International classification of functioning, disability and health.* Geneva, Switzerland: Author. Retrieved September 26, 2009, from http://www.who.int/classifications/icf/en/

World Health Organization. (2002). *Towards a common language for functioning, disability, and health: ICF.* Geneva, Switzerland: Author. Retrieved September 26, 2009, from http://www.who.int/classifications/icf/training/icfbeginnersguide.pdf

Wu, W., Brickman, A., Luchsinger, J., Ferrazzano, P., Pichiule, P., Yoshita, M., et al. (2008). The brain in the age of old: The hippocampal formation is targeted differentially by diseases of late life. *Annals of Neurology, 64*(6), 698–706.

Wunderlich, G. S., & Kohler P. O., (Eds.). (2001). *Improving the quality of long-term care.* Committee on Improving Quality in Long-Term Care, Institute of Medicine. Washington, DC: National Academy Press.

Yaffe, K., Blackwell, T., Gore, R., Sands, L., Reus, V., & Browner, W. S. (1999a). Depressive symptoms and cognitive decline in nondemented elderly women: A prospective study. *Archives of General Psychiatry, 56*(5), 425–430.

Yaffe, K., Browner, W., Cauley, J., Launer, L., & Harris, T. (1999b). Association between bone mineral density and cognitive decline in older women. *Journal of the American Geriatrics Society, 47*(10), 1176–1182.

Yesavage, J. A., Brink, T. L., Rose, T. L, Lum, O., Huang, V., Adey, M. B., et al. (1983). Development and validation of a geriatric depression screening scale: A preliminary report. *Journal of Psychiatric Research, 17,* 37–49.

Zilkens, R. R., Spilsbury, K., Bruce, D. G., & Semmens, J. B. (in press). Clinical epidemiology and in-patient hospital use in the last year of life (1990–2005) of 29,884 Western Australians with dementia. *Journal of Alzheimers Disease.*

Zimmerman, S., Sloane, P. D., Williams, C. S., Reed, P. S., Preisser, J. S., Eckert, J. K., et al. (2005). Dementia care and quality of life in assisted living and nursing homes. *Gerontologist, 45*(1), 133–146.

Zwahr, M. D., Park, D. C., & Shifren, K. (1999). Judgments about estrogen replacement therapy: The role of age, cognitive abilities, and beliefs. *Psychology of Aging, 14*(2), 179–191.

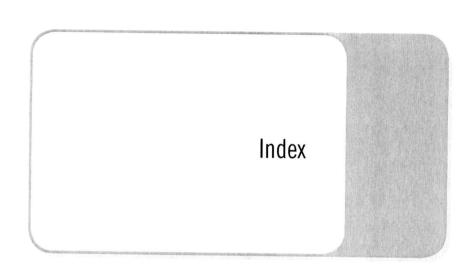

Index